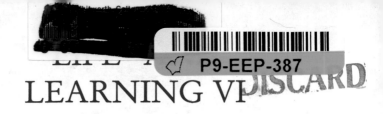

LEARNING VI

PROCEEDINGS OF THE SIXTH
UNIVERSITY FACULTY FOR LIFE
CONFERENCE

JUNE 1996
AT GEORGETOWN UNIVERSITY

edited by
Joseph W. Koterski, S.J.

Washington, D.C.
University Faculty for Life

Published by University Faculty for Life
120 New North Building
Georgetown University
Washington, D.C., 20057

Printed in the United States of America

ISBN 1-886387-04-4

Preface

The present volume contains papers presented at the sixth annual conference of the University Faculty for Life, held on the Georgetown University campus in Washington, D.C., in June 1996.

Our sincere gratitude is due to Georgetown University and especially to the host of our meeting, Fr. Thomas King, S.J., who has served as President of UFL since its foundation in 1989. We would also like to thank all the benefactors who have supported this organization and made possible its annual meetings and the publication of its newsletter and of its volumes of proceedings.

In the first two sections of this volume we are pleased to present papers on some of the life-issues that are at present among the most intensely debated. The studies by Richard Doerflinger and by Dwight Duncan and Peter Lubin examine the recent court decisions on physician-assisted suicide. Among the other current topics treated are infanticide (Bottum), world population and recent UN conferences (Simon, Carey, Wilson), and health-care reform (Conn).

Philosophical and theological perspectives on the life-questions have been a regular feature of presentations at UFL meetings. This year we are pleased to include essays on the problems of cooperation within an abortive culture (Conley), embodiment (Crosby), intention (Garcia), and the politics of a culture of life (Miller), as well as three papers on sexual ethics (Fehring, Nicholas, and O'Connell).

One of the most interesting features of each year's UFL meeting has been the presence of so many different academic disciplines. This year's proceedings also includes papers with a basis in law (Strahan), literature (Koloze), and history (Cassidy, Stanislaus, Brennan, Hunt).

Joseph W. Koterski, S.J.
Fordham University

Acknowledgements

"The Use and Abuse of History in *Compassion in Dying*" is reprinted by the permission of *Harvard Journal of Law and Public Policy*, where it appeared in volume 20 (fall 1996) 175-214.

J. L. A. Garcia, "Intentions in Medical Ethics" is reprinted with the author's permission from *Human Lives*, ed. D. Oderberg & J. Laing, Macmillan, 1996.

"More People, Greater Wealth, More Resources, Healthier Environment" by Julian Simon is reprinted from *Economic Affairs* (April 1994) 22-29 by permission of the author.

Life and Learning VI

Table of Contents

LIFE AND LEARNING VI

THE EUTHANASIA DEBATE TODAY

Richard M. Doerflinger

"EU-THANASIA," FROM GREEK WORDS meaning a good or easy death, has taken on a very different meaning today: the killing of a patient by his or her doctor.

Some people draw a distinction between euthanasia (active killing by physicians) and physician-assisted suicide (prescribing or providing lethal drugs for the patient to self-administer). But the intent, that of causing the patient's premature death, is the same; the means, a lethal drug-overdose, is the same; and as Derek Humphry, founder of the Hemlock Society, has acknowledged, allowing assisted suicide inevitably forces us to consider allowing active euthanasia. Humphry says that suicide by oral overdose goes badly about 25% of the time, so a doctor should be standing by in every case "to administer the *coup de grace* if necessary."[1] Even recent court rulings favoring assisted suicide have found no real distinction between the two practices. So for all practical purposes, we can treat assisted suicide and active euthanasia together.

How are we faring in our struggle against legalized euthanasia? Until very recently, not too badly. Consider the following:

■ The voters of Washington (in 1991) and California (in 1992) defeated referenda designed to legalize euthanasia.

■ In November 1994, Oregon voters narrowly approved a measure to legalize assisted suicide, 51 to 49 percent; but it was enjoined by a federal court and has never gone into effect.

■ More importantly, despite predictions to the contrary, efforts to expand the Oregon agenda to other states have been a dismal failure. In 1995 and the first half of 1996 bills like Oregon's were introduced in at least 15 states but all were defeated. Some state legislatures allowed these bills to die without a hearing. Even states carefully chosen by euthanasia groups as ideal battlegrounds defeated such bills by lopsided margins: 6-to-1 in a committee of the New Mexico

3

legislature (even though the state medical society refused to oppose the bill); 256-to-90 in the New Hampshire House of Representatives.

▪ In fact the only new laws being enacted on this issue are laws that absolutely *ban* assisted suicide.   Iowa became the 34ᵗʰ state with a specific ban on assisted suicide on March 1, 1996; at this writing Rhode Island seems poised to become the 35ᵗʰ, differently worded bills having been overwhelmingly approved in both House and Senate.

▪ Finally, until a few weeks ago, *no* jurisdiction in the country had a court ruling recognizing any "right" to assisted suicide.   Indeed, three courts had recently ruled that there is no such right: a three-judge panel of the Ninth Circuit Court of Appeals (upholding Washington State's law against assisted suicide); a U. S. District Court in New York (upholding that state's similar ban); and the State Supreme Court of Michigan.   And a federal judge had ruled that Oregon's new law selectively *allowing* assisted suicide for the terminally ill violated constitutional guarantees of equal protection under law.

THE APPELLATE RULINGS

Into this rather promising situation, two federal appellate court decisions this spring fell like hand grenades tossed into a hospital ward.   Having failed almost universally to win the support of the American people and their elected representatives, euthanasia supporters stepped up their efforts in the federal courts and won two resounding victories.   On March 6, an 11-judge panel of the Ninth Circuit Court of Appeals voted 8-to-3 to knock down Washington's ban on assisted suicide as it applies to terminally ill adults, arguing that the Due Process clause of the 14ᵗʰ Amendment guarantees the "right" of such patients to receive "life-ending medication" to hasten their deaths.   (An odd choice of words: If lethal poison is "medica-tion," the disease it "cures" must be life itself.)   On April 2, the Second Circuit Court of Appeals denied the existence of such a fundamental right, but still knocked down New York's law against assisted suicide.   Here the argument was that there is no "rational basis" for banning the prescribing of lethal drugs to terminally ill patients when the State already recognizes their right to hasten death by refusing unwanted medical treatment.

These two rulings are worth reviewing because, far from striking a blow in favor of assisted suicide, their logic shows very clearly why our society should *never* start down this path.

THE 9TH CIRCUIT RULING IN *COMPASSION IN DYING V. WASHINGTON*

The lethal inevitability of euthanasia's "slippery slope" is most glaringly evident in the Ninth Circuit decision. Knocking down traditional distinctions between withdrawal of medical treatment and killing, the court defines a new constitutional right to assisted suicide for all "terminally ill, competent adults who wish to hasten their own deaths."[2] At first there seem to be three limits on this right: it applies only to assisting a suicide, so the patient himself has to administer the drugs; it must be by a competent adult's own voluntary decision; and it applies only to the terminally ill. The court then proceeds to take each of these limits away, one by one.

First, the Court admits that "it may be difficult to make a principled distinction" between assisting a patient's suicide and simply injecting that patient with lethal drugs. "We would be less than candid," says the court, "if we did not acknowledge that for present purposes we view the critical line in right-to-die cases as the one between the voluntary and involuntary termination of an individual's life.... *We consider it less important who administers the medication than who determines whether the terminally ill person's life shall end.*"[3] So ends any firm barrier against lethal injections by physicians; instead we are to rely on the voluntariness of the patient's own decision. That is the next limit to disappear.

Second, the court notes approvingly that life-sustaining treatment is withdrawn from incompetent patients by surrogate decision makers all the time. These surrogates may be family members, proxies appointed by the patient, or even guardians appointed by the State. The court transfers all this delegated decision making over to the euthanasia context: "Finally, we should make it clear that a decision of a duly appointed surrogate decision maker *is for all legal purposes the decision of the patient himself.*"[4] So the "voluntary decision" safeguard is gone as well: "Substituted judgment" and other doctrines will be used to decide that incompetent patients should be killed, and those decisions will be treated as though they came from the patients themselves. The court notes that some surrogates may make decisions based on unworthy motives, or even for economic reasons—but it says this also happens in decisions to withdraw treatment, so it should not slow us down in approving this new "right." In any case, the court says, the risk of abuse here is greatly reduced because these patients are terminally ill and "will die shortly in any event."[5] So the final barrier to widespread killing is the restriction to patients who are truly terminally ill.

Third, this final limitation drops away when the court defines what it means by "terminally ill." It notes that there are many different definitions in over 40 state laws, and that some of these laws define the term "without reference to a fixed time period." For example, some laws define it to include people in a coma or "persistent vegetative state" even if they could survive for many years with continued feeding and nursing care. Of special interest to the court is the Uniform Rights of the Terminally Ill Act, which defines a condition as "terminal" if it will lead to death in a relatively short time "*without* administering life-sustaining treatment." Anyone who needs medical assistance to continue living—a diabetic who needs insulin, or a physically disabled person who needs a ventilator to assist breathing—could be seen as "terminal" under such definitions. The court decides that "*all* of the persons described in the various statutes would appear to fall within an appropriate definition of the term."[6]

So much for any meaningful restriction to cases of "terminal" illness. Combined with the other expansions of the "right" outlined above, this new definition of "terminal" lays the groundwork for giving lethal injections to patients who are helpless and incompetent (therefore "terminal" in this new sense) who never asked for death, based on the wishes of proxies or state-appointed guardians.

THE 2ND CIRCUIT RULING IN *QUILL V. VACCO*

The Second Circuit Court of Appeals does not draw out these same consequences so openly. Yet its analysis clearly sets the groundwork for the same expansions of the right to kill. It does so by constructing an "equal protection" argument: Terminally ill patients who are on life support now have a right to hasten their deaths by refusing that support; but terminally ill patients who are not sick enough to need such artificial support cannot presently enjoy that same right, because there is nothing for them to refuse so they can die. Therefore the State must allow them to exercise their right to hasten death by receiving lethal drugs from their doctors.[7]

There are many flaws in this analysis, to say the least. Among other things it seems to imply that your right to receive lethal drugs is stronger the *healthier* you are—for only the completely strong and healthy person can be sure that he will need lethal drugs (and not a mere refusal of outside support) in order to exercise the coveted "right to hasten death."

But the central confusion in this ruling is the denial of any "rational" difference between refusing unwanted or burdensome treatment and committing suicide. To be sure, there are borderline cases where a patient or family may refuse some easily provided form of care precisely in order to hasten death; but such motives are generally hidden from the eyes of the law. Most often, life-extending treatment is refused because it will have little benefit in curing or ameliorating the disease, or because it would impose unnecessary suffering and other burdens on a patient who is already weak and vulnerable. As Dr. Leon Kass said at a congressional hearing on assisted suicide on April 29, 1996, these decisions are generally not about seeking death but about "how we choose to *live*, even while we are dying."

In fact, from a doctor's legal viewpoint the two situations are opposites. The patient's refusal of treatment gives a doctor no new legal power or authority, but places a firm *limit* on that power and authority: he *may not* provide or continue such treatment without the patient's consent, or he will be performing a battery. By contrast, giving legal validity to a request for lethal drugs gives the physician a new power to take life that has never existed since the advent of the Hippocratic oath.

Until this spring, almost every state or federal judge to address the issue had found that refusal of medical treatment was qualitatively different from suicide or euthanasia. Courts have consistently ruled that a seriously ill patient's decision to refuse treatment does not cause death, but allows the patient to die of natural causes; death is really caused by his or her underlying illness.

Most courts establishing the legal right to refuse treatment have insisted so firmly on the distinction between refusing treatment and committing suicide, that if they are no longer allowed to draw that distinction they might well reconsider whether the right to refuse treatment exists either.   But the Second Circuit judges assume that the opposite course is correct: Having rejected the grounds on which most courts have defended the right to refuse treatment, the judges nonetheless assume that it exists and then piggyback onto it a right to receive assistance in suicide.

If the two rights really are the same under the Constitution, what follows? Well, what follows is the same set of consequences that we have already seen in the Ninth Circuit decision. The right to refuse treatment, after all, belongs to everyone and not just to the terminally ill; so the right to assisted suicide can hardly be restricted to the terminally ill in any narrow sense of the term.   (Unlike the Ninth Circuit, the Second Circuit judges do not try to define terminal illness but proclaim that everyone knows what it is; "everyone" presumably includes the legislators who wrote those 41 different laws cited by the Ninth Circuit.) The right to refuse treatment is often exercised on behalf of incompetent patients by family members, appointed proxies, and even state-appointed guardians.   And once the obvious and traditional distinction between allowing nature to take its course and actively intervening to provide lethal means for suicide is destroyed, does anyone really think the court will find a new and convincing basis for the far more precarious distinction between assisted suicide and active euthanasia? In short, while the Second Circuit decision is not so explicit in drawing out the consequences of its legal reasoning, it takes us to the same place as the Ninth Circuit decision.

THE SLIPPERY SLOPE

Clearly the "slippery slope" of euthanasia already has its illustrations in our history.   No society—I repeat, no society—that has officially endorsed voluntary suicide or euthanasia has ever failed to move on to killing people without their consent. Greek and Roman society are sometimes cited as honoring an idea of "noble" suicide—yet this practice also became a means of execution by the State, as in Socrates' forced "suicide" by hemlock.   Nazi Germany's experiment with euthanasia of the retarded and mentally ill was never based on the voluntary request of the victim, though it began with a request from the parents of a handicapped child and was often publicly defended in terms of the victims' "right to die." And according to the Dutch government's own 1991 study, the Netherlands' experiment in "voluntary" euthanasia produces more killing of patients without their request every year than with their request.

Physicians in the Netherlands have moved fairly quickly from ending the lives of the terminally ill to doing so to the physically disabled and to people who have no physical illness but are elderly or depressed.   Now we know that doctors give lethal injections to handicapped newborn infants at least 10 times a year—infants with disabilities like Down's Syndrome or spina bifida, who certainly never asked to be killed.

In one recent case reported by American psychiatrist Herbert Hendin, a Dutch physician gave a lethal injection to a Catholic nun who was in considerable pain while dying.   She never asked for euthanasia, but he felt that was because her religion wouldn't let her—so he simply gave it to her without asking.

These cases are frightening enough.   But by "constitutionalizing" the issue, our American courts have managed to do in days what it took the Dutch twenty years to do.   In our legal system the slippery slope is more like a leap from the edge of a cliff.   But perhaps this is a good thing if it demonstrates to Americans all at once where this agenda leads.   In our country there will be no gradual raising of the temperature, so that we are heated up to boiling without knowing exactly when to cry out.   We should be crying out right now—especially to the Supreme Court, which is about to take up the Second and Ninth Circuit cases.   (In this context, of course, we will have to cry out very articulately and with all the appropriate footnotes.)

EQUAL DIGNITY UNDER LAW

What should we say to the Court, at the level of principled legal argument? I think we would do well to study U. S. District Judge Michael Hogan's ruling in *Lee v.   Oregon*, which found Oregon's law *allowing* assisted suicide for the terminally ill to be unconstitutional.

Hogan's ruling is a mirror image of the Second Circuit decision now on its way to the Supreme Court. He argues that laws allowing assisted suicide for certain classes of citizens violate constitutional guarantees of equal protection under law, by depriving a class of citizens of the protections against killing that all other citizens continue to enjoy.

Surely there is no rational basis for treating terminally ill people and other people in completely opposite ways when they are tempted to commit suicide. Suicidal people are found in every demographic group—especially among the young, the very old and members of certain high-stress professions. From the viewpoint of suicidal persons in any such group, their pain and suffering is more real and more intolerable than any physical pain that could be relieved by morphine and other painkillers. Persistent suicidal desires among the terminally ill are not significantly more common, no more "free," and no less caused by treatable depression than such desires felt by people in these other groups. Yet an entire legal and political movement has dedicated itself to facilitating suicide for the seriously ill, even while the law continues to forbid such "assistance" for everyone else.

Why would the State continue to view assisting the suicide of anyone else as a homicide, but view assisting the suicide of certain seriously ill or disabled people as a decent and lawful act? The only possible answer is: Because the State has made its own supposedly "objective" judgment that these patients, unlike any other citizens, have lives not worth protecting. When these particular people think they have lives not worth living, government can think of no reason to disagree.

Imagine the scenario: two people come forward wanting to commit suicide. Both have made a suicidal decision that they see as free and rational; both say they find nothing but pain and suffering in continuing with life. But one is able-bodied, while the other has an illness or disability that two physicians say is "terminal." On this basis, a law like the one recently approved in Oregon says to the first person that his life is too valuable to throw away—that we will provide counseling and psychological assistance to relieve these suicidal feelings, and legally forbid anyone to provide "aid" in suicide. To the second person the State will say: "Go right ahead. In fact we've anticipated your request, by proclaiming in advance that we have no interest in preventing the suicide of someone with your condition. Officially the government doesn't care whether you live or die."

This is not a recipe for greater freedom. It gives to government a new power that no human being should have: the power to decide which citizens' lives will be protected by law, and which will not. As one columnist put it very succinctly during the debate on the California euthanasia referendum, this is "Death With a Note from Big Brother."[8]

Clearly, judges and others who support such legal developments do not think they are practicing invidious discrimination against people with serious illnesses and disabilities. They believe they are giving these people a new "right" to end their lives painlessly. Yet they say they are not interested in granting this right to able-bodied people like themselves. If a law gave such selective "freedom" for assisted suicide to other defined classes of people—solely to women, or to members of a particular ethnic or religious group—howls of protest would rise up from civil rights organizations, and rightly so. The fact that many people do not see such invidious discrimination in the assisted-suicide agenda is an indication of how deep some of our prejudices about frail or seriously ill people really are. Physically healthy people simply assume that in some objective sense these patients are indeed "better off dead," that their suicides are rational and legitimate when other people's suicides are not.

In fact this prejudice is directly contrary to the views of those with the most experience of serious illness or old age. Whatever opinion polls may show at any moment—and many of the polls have greatly exaggerated public support for assisted suicide by asking vague questions filled with euphemisms—every major poll shows that senior citizens are far more opposed to assisted suicide than younger voters.[9] Low-income voters, black and Hispanic citizens, and others who are relatively powerless in our society are also more opposed to it than others—perhaps because they can well imagine assisted suicide becoming the "treatment of choice" for people like them when public health clinics are strapped for resources. Physicians who have treated many terminally ill patients also oppose assisted suicide more strongly than those without such experience.[10]

In my view, Judge Hogan was absolutely correct when he found that a law allowing assisted suicide for the terminally ill "withholds from terminally ill citizens the same protections from suicide the majority enjoys." After finding that the Ore-gon law provided "little assurance that only competent termi-nally ill persons will voluntarily die," he added: "The majority has not accepted this situation for themselves, and there is no rational basis for imposing it on the terminally ill."[11]

"SAFEGUARDS" AND THE BOTTOM LINE

Some people think the exploitation of vulnerable patients under a regime of legalized assisted suicide can be prevented by incorporating various "safeguards" into the law. In fact, to some extent the Ninth Circuit's new ruling renders that question moot, by indicating that some widely supported "safeguards" may well be found unconstitutional once the courts view assisted suicide as a fundamental right. For example, the Court says any waiting periods to think over the euthanasia decision must be "short."[12] Further, it says that "constitutional concerns" would be raised by any requirement that family members be consulted and agree with the decision.[13] By noting that minor children have the same "right to die" as adults do, the Court invites all the battles about euthanasia for minors and parental consent that we have already fought for many years in the abortion context.[14]

In any event, calls for safeguards miss the point. Any law that singles out a class of citizens for disparate treatment under the law of homicide perpetrates the same basic injustice. Once that unjust decision has been made, efforts to "fix" the law by tightening its loopholes only have the effect of defining ever more clearly the isolated class of patients to be singled out for exclusion from the law's protection. Such an unfair law cannot be "fixed." Government will still be making a pre-emptive judgment that citizens of a certain description—the vast majority of whom have never expressed any desire to die—are good candidates for a premature death by lethal drugs.

It defies belief to claim that insurance companies, health maintenance organizations and state governments struggling to save money will not also act on such judgments. Even before it legalized assisted suicide, Oregon instituted a Medicaid rationing plan under which terminally ill patients who are poor will simply not be able to receive various life-supporting treatments for their conditions. Once the assisted suicide measure passed, the state Medicaid director announced that assisted suicide *will* be covered for *every* patient—it will be very high on the priority list, under the title "comfort care." (One wonders whether the state treasury really receives the greatest "comfort" from this policy.) So the State will take away all the *other* treatments patients might have wanted to *support* life, and give them assisted suicide free of charge. This idea of essentially offering patients an economic *incentive* to assisted suicide by giving it public funds has been endorsed by that bastion of individual freedom in our society, the American Civil Liberties Union.

WHAT TO DO?

What is being done to oppose this, and what can we do?
We can tell others what this issue really entails—through articles, opinion pieces, letters to the editor, call-in shows and private conversation. We can write to our state and federal legislators, urging them to oppose legalization of assisted suicide and to pass new laws against it where necessary. We can promote compassionate care of the dying by supporting, and volunteering at, local hospices and respite care programs. And we can pray that our society will come to a full recognition of the dignity of each and every human life.

In Washington, D.C., some groups are working together to advance a federal policy on this problem. Both President Clinton and Senate Majority Leader Dole recently announced their opposition to assisted suicide. A bill will soon be introduced in Congress to prevent all funding and support for assisted suicide in federal health programs. Recently 40 members of Congress wrote to the U. S. Solicitor General, urging the Clinton Administration to file a brief urging the Supreme Court to review and reverse the Second Circuit decision. And the U. S. Catholic Conference has joined with Lutheran, Southern Baptist and Evangelical Christian groups to file its own brief urging the Supreme Court to take these cases.

In short, the current situation has many alarming features, and there is much work to be done. But if I have to offer one assessment of where we stand in the national debate on assisted suicide, it is this:

We're not dead yet.

NOTES

1. Derek Humphry, Letter to the Editors, *The New York Times* (12/3/94) 22.

2. *Compassion in Dying v. Washington*, No. 94-35534, slip op. at 3117 (9th Cir. March 6, 1996).

3. *Ibid.* at 3201-2.

4. *Ibid.* at 3201 n. 120.

5. *Ibid.* at 3189.

6. *Ibid.* at 3200.

7. *Quill v. Vacco*, No. 95-7028, slip op. at 29-31 (2d Cir. April 2, 1996).

8. D. Saunders, in *The San Francisco Chronicle* (8/31/92) A18.

9. Even polls by the Hemlock Society show that "the younger the person, the more likely he or she is to favor this legislation" allowing assisted suicide (Hemlock *TimeLines* [Jan.-Feb. 1994] 9). A recent national survey by the *Washington Post* showed 50% support for making physician-assisted suicide legal (*Washington Post* [4/4/96] A18); but support dropped to 38% among those aged 65 or over. A July 1995 poll by The Tarrance Group found that "voters aged 18 to 34 years old support assisted suicide, 56% to 40%. But those aged 65 and over—whom some would see as the primary beneficiaries of a legal 'right to die'—oppose the practice 55% to 37%, with 48% strongly opposed" ("Poll: Americans Divided on Euthanasia" in *Life at Risk: A Chronicle of Euthanasia Trends in America* [June/July 1995] 1).

10. In a recent survey of Michigan physicians, legalization was favored by 73% of those who "never" treat terminally ill patients but by only 44% of those who treat them "very often" (J. Bachman *et al.*, "Attitudes of Michigan physicians and the public toward legalizing physician-assisted suicide and voluntary euthanasia" in *New England Journal of Medicine* (2/1/96) 306. The same correlation is found among Washington physicians: see J. Cohen *et al.*, "Attitudes toward assisted suicide and euthanasia among physicians in Washington State" in *New England Journal of Medicine* (7/14/94) 93.

11. *Lee v. Oregon*, 891 F. Supp. 1429, 1438 (D. Or. 1995).

12. *Compassion in Dying* at 3204.

13. *Ibid.* at 3192 n. 100.

14. *Ibid.* at 3164.

THE USE AND ABUSE OF HISTORY IN *COMPASSION IN DYING*

Dwight G. Duncan* and Peter Lubin**

> We must never forget that it is a *constitution* we are
> expanding.   - From a 21ˢᵗ century casebook
>   on constitutional law.
> All our final resolutions are made in a state of mind that is
> not going to last.   - Marcel Proust[1]

I. INTRODUCTION

Barely thirty years ago, in *Griswold v. Connecticut*,[2] the Supreme Court discovered that there were certain fundamental rights not expressly to be found in the Constitution, but rather to be teased out of the Bill of Rights by way of the Fourteenth Amendment's Due Process Clause. In that case, a Connecticut statute made it a crime to use any contraceptive device; the question the Court addressed was whether a married couple could be prosecuted for using such devices. The Court held that the Connecticut law was unconstitutional. In the opinion of Justice Douglas, certain explicit constitutional guarantees—the First, Third, Fourth, Fifth, and Ninth Amendments—gave rise to a new, general right of privacy. To use Justice Douglas's famous phrasing: "specific guarantees in the Bill of Rights have penumbras, formed by emanations from those guarantees that help give them life and substance."[3] Thus, the commonly understood "right of privacy" (which all polite people respected) became quite a different

---

* I would like to thank Associate Dean David Prentiss for his advice and encouragement and my research assistant David Kiernan.

** Both authors would like to acknowledge gratefully the assistance of their colleagues Philip E. Cleary, Matthew Pauley, and Frances Rudko; librarian Gordon Russell, who provided bibliographic references; and the library staff at Southern New England School of Law, especially Korin Munsterman, who provided instant electronic searches. Sally Fitzgerald also helped us with her comments.

constitutional right.

In the succeeding thirty years, the penumbras have lengthened. *Griswold* was followed by a series of cases that found new avatars of the "right of privacy," particularly in the abortion cases[4] and other related decisions on procreation and child rearing.[5]

II. THE USE OF HISTORY IN CONSTITUTIONAL DECISION-MAKING

The Supreme Court, mindful of the need to limit the creativity of its own members, has continued to insist on the importance of history in determining what implicit fundamental rights were to be recognized. Despite *Roe v. Wade* and its progeny, the Court insisted that there should not be automatic recognition of other, novel fundamental rights. In *Bowers v. Hardwick*,[6] for example, the Court refused to find a fundamental constitutional right to homosexual sodomy. In *Cruzan*,[7] the Court addressed the problem of withdrawal of medical treatment from a patient in a persistent vegetative state, but did not recognize a right to physician-assisted suicide or even a fundamental right to suicide *tout court*.

Indeed, *Cruzan* expressly recognized that "there can be no gainsaying" the interest of the state in the protection and preservation of human life, noting that "all civilized nations... demonstrate their commitment to life by treating homicide as a serious crime" and that "the majority of States in this country have laws imposing criminal penalties on one who assists another to commit suicide."[8] There was no suggestion in *Cruzan* that the constitutionality of such laws was in question. Justice Scalia's concurrence noted the strong legal tradition against assisted suicide, and explained:

[a]lthough the States abolished the penalties imposed by the common law [on suicide] (*i.e.*, forfeiture and ignominious burial), they did so to spare the innocent family and not to legitimize the act.... Thus, "there is no significant support for the claim that a right to suicide is so rooted in our tradition that it may be deemed fundamental or implicit in the concept of ordered liberty."[9]

Nonetheless, earlier this year, the Ninth Circuit became the first appellate court in American history to hold that physician-assisted suicide of terminally ill patients is protected by the Constitution under the Fourteenth Amendment's Due Process Clause.[10] In so ruling, it struck down a Washington state statute that criminalized the practice. The case, *Compassion in Dying v. Washington*, was decided *en banc*,[11] 8-3, with the majority opinion written by Judge Stephen J. Reinhardt.

In *Bowers*, the Supreme Court had described the considerations appropriate in determining which fundamental rights should be recognized even though they are "not readily identifiable in the Constitution's text."[12] Such rights, said the Court, are either those that are "'implicit in the concept of ordered liberty,' such that 'neither liberty nor justice would exist if [they] were sacrificed'" or those "liberties that are 'deeply rooted in this Nation's history and tradition.'"[13] These seemingly alternative formulations both depend on history. For what else could serve as a reliable guide to locate those rights "implicit in the concept of ordered liberty" except history, which identifies those rights "deeply rooted in the nation's history and traditions"? Justice Cardozo, the source of the first phrase, immediately glossed it as equivalent to a "principle of justice so rooted in the traditions and conscience of our people as to be ranked as fundamental."[14]

Significantly, when *Bowers* held that "neither of these formulations would extend a fundamental right to homosexuals to engage in acts of consensual sodomy,"[15] the argument was strictly historical:

Proscriptions against that conduct have ancient roots. Sodomy was a criminal offense at common law and was forbidden by the laws of the original 13 States when they ratified the Bill of Rights. In 1868, when the Fourteenth Amendment was ratified, all but 5 of the 37 States in the Union had criminal sodomy laws. In fact, until 1961, all 50 States outlawed sodomy, and today 24 States and the District of Columbia continue to provide criminal penalties for sodomy performed in private and between consenting adults. Against this background, to claim that a right to engage in such conduct is "deeply rooted in this nation's history and tradition" or "implicit in the concept of ordered liberty" is, at best, facetious.[16]

The Court properly identified the danger of reckless invention of new fundamental rights:

The Court is most vulnerable and comes nearest to illegitimacy when it deals with judge-made constitutional law having little or no cognizable roots in the language or design of the Constitution. That this is so was painfully demonstrated by the face-off between the Executive and the Court in the

1930's, which resulted in the repudiation of much of the substantive gloss that the Court had placed on the Due Process Clauses of the Fifth and Fourteenth Amendments. There should be, therefore, great resistance to expand the substantive reach of those Clauses, particularly if it requires redefining the category of rights deemed to be fundamental. Otherwise, the Judiciary necessarily takes to itself further authority to govern the country without express constitutional authority.[17]

In fashioning a constitutional right to physician-assisted suicide, then, Judge Reinhardt could hardly—given *Bowers*—have avoided dealing with history. The overruled three-judge panel had said that the "constitutional right to aid in killing oneself" was "unknown to the past."[18] *Quill v. Vacco*, the Second Circuit case striking down New York's assisted suicide prohibition under the equal protection clause, similarly recognized that the right to assisted suicide is in no sense deeply rooted in the nation's history and traditions.[19]

III. JUDGE REINHARDT'S USE OF HISTORY

Judge Reinhardt employs three strategies to minimize the significance of what ought to have been the heart of the inquiry—history.

First, his historical inquiry is surprisingly brief. It consists of just four pages, in a fifty-page opinion, which give us a *tour d'horizon* of the subject, from the ancient Greeks to the present day. Second, his inquiry is not into the proper subject: his heading is "Historical Attitudes Toward Suicide," despite the fact that there is an enormous difference between suicide and physician-assisted suicide. Third, his inquiry is dishonest because, perhaps uncertain of the historical record, which he describes as "checkered,"[20] he claims that where the historical evidence does not support a position, it scarcely matters: "we believe that the [three-judge] panel's historical account is misguided, but even *if it were indisputably correct, historical evidence alone is not a sufficient basis for rejecting a claimed liberty interest.*"[21]

Those not inured to modern constitutional adjudication, and to the bland self-assurance of some of its practitioners, may be surprised. Even though neither the language of the Constitution, nor the historical record, supports the recognition of the "fundamental right" in question but actually supports the opposite, Judge Reinhardt is unwilling to allow "historical evidence alone" to stop him.

Let us, nonetheless, examine Judge Reinhardt's *Compassion in Dying* inquiry as if history mattered—for we allow ourselves to believe that it does. He claims that his four-page historical study[22] leads to no clear result. How accurate is his review of "Historical Attitudes Toward Suicide"? He begins by noting that the majority opinion of the three-judge panel, written by Judge John Noonan (a noted legal historian), claimed that "[a] constitutional right to aid in killing oneself" was "unknown to the past."[23] But Judge Reinhardt is quick to note that his own inquiry is "not so narrow" nor "[the *en banc* court's] conclusion so facile."[24] As he puts it:

the subject we must initially examine is not nearly so limited. Properly analyzed, the first issue to be resolved is whether there is a liberty interest in determining the time and manner of one's death. We do not ask simply whether there is a liberty interest in receiving "aid in killing oneself" because such a narrow interest could not exist in the absence of a broader and more important underlying interest—the right to die. In short, it is the end and not the means that defines the liberty interest.[25]

To justify his approach, Judge Reinhardt makes an analogy to the approach used by the Supreme Court in the abortion cases.[26] In those cases, he says, the Court initially determined whether a general liberty interest existed (an interest in having an abortion), not whether there was an interest in implementing that general liberty interest by a particular means (with medical assistance).

IV. ANTIQUITY
A. *The Hippocratic Oath*
If, as Judge Reinhardt argues, a historical inquiry ought to focus on a general "right to die," we should consider all three possibilities—suicide, assisted suicide, and euthanasia—in a continuum from the more to the less accepted. But he avoids all historical discussion of both physician-assisted suicide and euthanasia. It might be argued that there simply is not enough evidence to bring to bear on physician-assisted suicide. But there is at least one important bit of evidence from the past—the Hippocratic Oath.

Curiously, Judge Reinhardt does not mention the Hippocratic Oath in his historical survey. Instead, the Oath is dealt with in another section of the opinion. Nevertheless, it is the historical evidence most relevant to the issue of physician-assisted suicide. The language of the Oath, composed in classical antiquity, flatly forbade doctors from administering lethal drugs to patients. Doctors were not permitted even to suggest such a course.[27] The marginalization of this important piece of historical evidence is perhaps foreshadowed by Judge Reinhardt's quotation from *Roe v. Wade* that "'only the Pythagorean school of philosophers frowned upon the related act of suicide.'"[28] But the Hippocratic Oath was administered throughout the Western world for more than two millennia. Whatever one now makes of its original formulation, a survey devoted to "Historical Attitudes Toward Suicide" surely ought not overlook the Oath, correctly described by Justice Blackmun in *Roe* as "the apex of the development of strict ethical concepts in medicine."[29] The Oath expressly forbids administering poisons to patients *even when requested*. A clearer rejection of physician-assisted suicide cannot be imagined. What is important is not only the Oath itself, but also its wide acceptance, in so many countries, over so long a period, as the solemn accompaniment to full-fledged admission to the profession of medicine.

Elsewhere in the opinion, Judge Reinhardt notes that the Hippocratic Oath, in his view, is no longer relevant, because, according to him, it also forbade abortion.[30] His logic is: abortion is now allowed despite the Hippocratic Oath; *ergo* physician-assisted suicide should also be allowed. But this does not follow.

It is true that the Hippocratic Oath has recently fallen into desuetude. But there is ample evidence that the Hippocratic Oath's prohibition of physician-assisted suicide remains compelling to medical practitioners today. The dissent of Judge Beezer quotes the current AMA Code of Ethics:

While not legally binding, the AMA Code of Ethics provides clear guidance on the current position of medical ethicists. Section 2.211 of the American Medical Association's *Code of Medical Ethics and Current Opinions of the Council on Ethical and Judicial Affairs* ("AMA Code of Ethics") prohibits physician participation in physician-assisted suicide. In virtually identical language to its condemnation of euthanasia, section 2.211 provides:

Physician-assisted suicide occurs when a physician facilitates a patient's death by providing the necessary means and/or information to enable the patient to perform the life-ending act (e.g., the physician provides sleeping pills and information about the lethal dose, while aware that the patient may commit suicide).

It is understandable, though tragic, that some patients in extreme duress—such as those suffering from a terminal, painful, debilitating illness—may come to decide that death is preferable to life. However, *allowing physicians to participate in assisted suicide would cause more harm than good. Physician-assisted suicide is fundamentally incompatible with the physician's role as healer, would be difficult or impossible to control, and would pose serious societal risks.*[31]

This part of the Hippocratic Oath thus remains, in its AMA guise, still vital.

B. Literary Suicides

How accurate and complete an account does Judge Reinhardt give? How does he summarize views on suicide in classical antiquity? And how do these views accord with his sources? He relies on a handful of secondary sources, and never on the original texts themselves. Indeed, fully half of the footnotes in his historical survey refer to a single article.[32]

Judge Reinhardt begins by confounding history and literature. He states that "[i]n Greek and Roman times, far from being universally prohibited, suicide was often considered commendable in literature, mythology, and practice."[33] Hence in an "historical" survey he allows himself to start with "the first of all literary suicides," Jocasta, who chose "'an honorable way out of an insufferable situation.'"[34] As for Homer, he "records self-murder without comment, as something natural and heroic" and the "legends bear him out."[35] One legend is offered, presumably by way of example: "Aegeus threw himself into the sea—which therefore bore his name—when he mistakenly thought his son Theseus had been slain by the Minotaur."[36] This is breezily done, of course—no doubts, no weighing of evidence. "The legends bear him [Homer] out."

Aside from the eponymous tale of How the Aegean Got Its Name, how many Greek legends can Judge Reinhardt adduce in support of the proposition that the Greeks regarded suicide tolerantly? Is he so sure that it is proper to derive such a conclusion from that—or any—legend? As for Jocasta, neither her suicide, nor that of any other character in literature, whether deplorable or admirable, can be adduced to prove anything other than what all sensible people already know—that sometimes, feeling desperate or hopeless, people kill themselves. Jocasta and Aegeus do not exhaust the list. But we cannot claim that Cleopatra affixing that reluctant asp to her breast, nor Emma Bovary poisoning herself *en province*, nor Anna Karenina throwing herself under a St. Petersburg train, can tell us whether or not Elizabethan England, France under the Second Empire, or Czarist Russia, respectively, regarded suicide as noble or ignoble, practiced only by the very great or only by the very foolish. Judge Reinhardt's bizarre initial paragraph, fortunately, represents his only foray into world literature; he has other worlds to conquer.

C. *The Uses Of Ancient History*
1. The Hebrews

One might have expected Judge Reinhardt to begin with the Hebrews. The contribution of ancient Israel to Western civilization includes monotheism and the moral code enshrined in the Ten Commandments. The Hebrew Bible, as well as the traditions of the Jews, have helped form Western attitudes toward suicide. The opinion devotes one footnote of two sentences to the Bible: one for the Old Testament, and one for the New ("the stories of four suicides are noted in the Old Testament—Samson, Saul, Abimlech(sic), and Achitophel—and none is treated as an act worthy of censure").[37] To all of ancient Israel's history and religion and moral teachings Judge Reinhardt devotes not even a paragraph, but merely one sentence in one footnote: "Hundreds of Jews killed themselves at Masada in order to avoid being captured by Roman legions."[38]

This well-known fact, of course, tells us nothing about the accepted attitude toward suicide in ancient Israel.[39] But if we turn back to the text Judge Reinhardt uses with such assiduity, we find quite a different story. In the Old Testament the article finds, and lists, not four but eight suicides, and notes that:

With the exception of Samson, none of the eight who died by suicide are presented as heroes.

Only Samson's suicide was arguably heroic.... Since Samson does not appear directly to will his own death, but only the death of the Philistines at the cost of his own life, his intention is arguably not even suicidal.[40]

The article cites several scholars on the subject as well. One observes that "suicide may have been a relatively rare phenomenon in Biblical times."[41] Another scholar notes that "'those who did commit suicide were considered deranged....'"[42] A third says that "'[w]hen the act did occur, the victim and his family were punished by denial of a regular burial and the customary rituals of mourning.'"[43] It took time, however, for Jewish writers to develop their ideas more explicitly:

As the influence of Hellenism spread, Jewish writers developed a more philosophic posture and became more explicit in their treatment of moral problems such as suicide. The earliest known formal prohibition of suicide among the Jews occurred in the first century A.D., when Josephus, after his army had been conquered by the Romans, forbade his soldiers to kill themselves on the grounds that suicide was a cowardly act, contrary to nature and the law of God, who committed man's soul to his body. Josephus' order contrasted with that of Eleazer Ben Jair, who successfully urged his Zealot followers to commit mass suicide at Masada in order to avoid capture by the Romans. After the xile, prohibitions of suicide were included in the Rabbinic and Talmudic writings, expressed in stories and in mourning and funeral sanctions.[44]

Judge Reinhardt ignores all this.

Regardless of whether there are four or eight instances of suicide in the Hebrew Bible,[45] Judge Reinhardt says that "none is treated as an act worthy of censure." But there is at least one instance in which assisted suicide or mercy killing is clearly censured. That is the case of Saul, first King of Israel:

Saul was badly wounded in battle by a Philistine arrow. Afraid of being tortured and humiliated by his captors, he pleaded with his armour-bearer to kill him (I Sam 31:1-4; I Chron 10:1-4). There are two versions of what happened next. According to the first, the man refused, so Saul committed suicide by falling on his own sword (I Sam 31:5-6; I Chron 10:4). In the other account a young Amelikite came upon the wounded Saul leaning on his spear, perhaps attempting suicide. Saul begged him, "Stand beside me and slay me, for anguish has seized me and yet my life lingers." So the youth obliged (2 Sam 1:6-10) in what today we would call an act of voluntary euthanasia, assisted suicide or mercy killing.[46]

If the second story is followed, when David heard the news from the Amelikite, he "took hold on his clothes, and rent them...mourned, and wept, and fasted...."[47] Then he bade one of his men go up and make an end of the Amelikite, and when the blow had fallen, said over his dead body, "'Thy blood be on thy head; for thy mouth hath testified against thee, saying, I have slain the Lord's anointed.'"[48] Although the Amelikite's act was what we would today call assisting a suicide ("Saul begged him"), David treated it as the equivalent of murder.[49] One commentator has noted that "the undoubted conclusion of this story is that despite being done with the best will in the world, this was none the less a wicked act, deserving the severest of punishments."[50]

One would expect nothing less of a tradition that gave the world the Ten Commandments, with the categorical "Thou shalt not kill."[51] According to the Anchor Bible, this commandment is "formulated in the most absolute manner, without specifying the object of the crime, in order to include any possible object, any human being (including suicide)."[52]

Judge Reinhardt might have consulted Baruch Brody's meticulous study of rabbinical commentary on suicide,[53] which notes that "Judaism has not traditionally stressed patient autonomy, and it has on the whole opposed suicide and euthanasia."[54] Brody concludes more specifically that the "active euthanasia of a dying patient, even one who is in great pain, is prohibited in Jewish law because it is an act of killing, even if the goal in question—the death of the patient—is viewed as desirable."[55]

Of course, in the New Testament Judas commits suicide. But he is not exactly a role model. Judge Reinhardt, the revisionist, demurs: "In the New Testament, the suicide of Judas Iscariot is not treated as a further sin, rather as an act of repentance."[56] This is ludicrous exegesis. As one scholar has said:

the Jewish attitude toward suicide as infringing on God's rights makes it extremely unlikely that Judas' hanging himself would have been considered a divinely acceptable expiation.... To those who say that for various reasons it is noble to destroy oneself, Josephus replies with indignation, "It is an act of impiety towards God who created us."[57]

2. The Greeks

Judge Reinhardt's treatment of the Greeks does not inspire greater confidence. First, he says that "[i]n Athens, as well as the Greek colonies of Marseilles and Ceos, magistrates kept a supply of hemlock for those who wished to end their lives. The magistrates even supplied those who wished to commit suicide with the means to do so."[58] This passage relies on Emile Durkheim's *Suicide.*[59] But immediately above the quoted passage, we read the following:

Suicide was only considered illegal if it was not authorized by the state. Thus at Athens a man who had killed himself was punished with "atimia" [dishonor] for having committed an injustice to the city; the honors of regular burial were denied him; also his hand was cut from his body and buried separately. It was the same at Thebes with variations in detail, and also at Cyprus. The rule was so severe at Sparta that Aristodemus was punished for the way he sought and found death at the battle of Plataea.[60]

Furthermore, when one consults sources other than the polemical Durkheim, the historical record regarding state-authorized suicide seems more ambiguous: "The lack of clearness in the information [about suicide practices] is a strong indication that the customs of Ceos and Massilia [Marseilles] were exaggerated to meet the taste of a public that enjoyed hearing of strange situations 'abroad.'"[61]

When Judge Reinhardt turns his attention from Greek practices to philosophy, he deals with the pre-Socratics in short order. Here his scholarly source is the Supreme Court. He states:

In *Roe*, while surveying the attitudes of the Greeks toward abortion, the Court stated that "only the Pythagorean school of philosophers frowned on the related act of suicide," ...it then noted that the Pythagorean school represented a distinctly minority view.[62]

Unwittingly, perhaps, we are given a glimpse into the solidity of historical scholarship of the *Roe* court as well. To state that among the Greeks, "only the Pythagorean school of philosophers frowned on the related act of suicide" is to ignore Plato and Aristotle, an odd omission in a survey of Greek philosophy.

It is natural that Judge Reinhardt's discussion of the Greeks then turns to Socrates, whom some consider the most famous suicide in history. But it should be remembered that Socrates was under a death sentence. He took the hemlock rather than flee Athens or be killed by the state. Not everyone would consider this a classic suicide; some might consider it simply enforcing the state's punishment. As with his mention of Masada, however, Judge Reinhardt seems to think that the very circumstances of Socrates's end imply the culture's admiration, or approval, of suicide. It is humanly understandable that we are, in some sense, "impressed" with the obstinate bravery and self-sacrifice of the warriors at Masada, or with Socrates's willingness to die rather than be exiled, but this does not permit one to conclude that either ancient Israel or classical Greece approved of suicide.

Judge Reinhardt tells us that "[w]hile Socrates counseled his disciples against committing suicide, he willingly drank the hemlock as he was condemned to do, and his example inspired others to end their lives."[63] One might conclude from this that suicide met with approval in ancient Greece; Judge Reinhardt does nothing to dispel this misapprehension. He tells us further that "Plato, Socrates's most distinguished student, believed suicide was often justifiable."[64] According to Judge Reinhardt, Plato

suggested that if life itself became immoderate, then suicide became a rational, justifiable act. Painful disease, or intolerable constraint were sufficient reasons to depart. And this when religious superstitions faded was philosophic justification enough.[65]

But Judge Reinhardt's primary source—a source he carefully refrains from using in this portion of the opinion—arrives at quite a different conclusion concerning Plato's views. An examination of the *Phaedo*, the *Laws*, and the ethical system developed in the *Republic* and the *Timaeus*, shows that Plato certainly did not approve of suicide. In the *Phaedo*, Plato's narrative of Socrates's last hours,

Socrates compares the human relationship to the gods with that of slave to master: as the slave is the possession of the master, all humans are the possession of the gods, and none have the right themselves to dispose of their lives. Moreover, to commit suicide would provoke the anger of the gods and would thus entail consequent punishment. Even though the choice of death seems preferable to life in some cases, suicide is not morally justified....

In the time of Socrates, suicide is deemed immoral, not simply because it violates the "property rights" of the gods, but because it undermines the attainment of ultimate happiness.[66]

The rest of Plato's works bear out this conclusion:

In the *Laws*, Plato addresses the problem of suicide in the context of the individual's relationship with the social order. His treatment of the matter there can best be understood in light of the ethics he developed in the *Republic* and the *Timaeus*. In those works, Plato stressed an organic interrelationship between the individual person, the state, and the universe; morality ultimately being a matter of the human soul's disposition in the cosmic order.... Plato's public policy on suicide stated in the *Laws* presumes this ethical and cosmic perspective:

> the graves of such as perish thus must, in the first place, be solitary; they must have no companions whatsoever in the tomb. Furthermore, they must be buried ignominiously in waste and nameless spots... and the tomb shall be marked by neither headstone nor name.[67]

Therefore, at least for Judge Reinhardt's own major source, Plato

is concerned with suicide as a deliberate and reasoned decision, rather than as the result of passion, compulsion, or madness. In the latter cases, culpability is lacking and the fault of malice against society is not assumed; hence the state, while not condoning such action, suspends its judgment. *But when suicide is a rational and deliberate choice, it is deemed to be a flagrant act of contempt for the state and an abandonment of duty to society and the divine order.*[68]

If Judge Reinhardt's discussion of Plato can be criticized, the discussion of Aristotle cannot—but only because Aristotle is not mentioned by Judge Reinhardt. Again, however, Judge Reinhardt's major source correctly describes Aristotle as one who unconditionally condemned suicide. In Book V of the *Nicomachean Ethics,* Aristotle addresses the matter of "why the state punishes a man who kills himself (not merely why the state *should* punish him, it must be stressed, but why it in fact *does*)."[69] Aristotle, like Plato, believed that the individual has a moral obligation to serve society:

The law does not allow a man to kill himself... when a man voluntarily—that is, knowing who the victim and what the instrument is—injures another (not by way of retaliation) contrary to the law, he is acting unjustly. But a man who cuts his throat in a fit of anger is voluntarily doing, contrary to right principle, what the law does not allow; therefore he is acting unjustly, but towards whom? Surely not himself, but the state; because he suffers voluntarily, and nobody is voluntarily treated unjustly. It is for this reason that the state imposes a penalty, and a kind of dishonor is attached to a man who has taken his own life, on the ground that he is guilty of an offence against the state.[70]

Elsewhere, in a catalogue of virtues and vices, Aristotle defines the courageous as "those who are fearless in the face of honorable death, such as death in battle or any life threatening circumstance."[71] However, he draws a distinction between courageously facing death and the kind of suicide that results from a desire to "'escape from poverty or love or anything else that is distressing.'"[72] Suicide, "as an act of cowardice, was deemed a rejection of one's personal duty, both to society and to oneself."[73]

No doubt Aristotle's emphasis on the collective, on the duty of the individual to society, is foreign to, even antipathetic to, modern ears. But if the history of Western attitudes toward suicide is to be a guide, then passing over Aristotle is passing strange.

3. Roman Law

In discussing Roman history, the Ninth Circuit's opinion refers to Roman law. It acknowledges that the "Romans did sometimes punish suicide" in the case of those accused of a crime, whose property would escheat to the state unless the suicide was caused by "impatience of pain or sickness."[74] This does indeed seem to open a window for what we would call physician-assisted suicide. However, the opinion ignores the effect of the Roman *Lex Cornelia on Murderers and Poisoners*, which provided that:

someone is liable who kills any man.... He also is liable who makes up [and] administers poison for the purpose of killing a man.... [S]omeone is punished who makes, sells, or possesses a drug for the purpose of homicide.[75]

It would seem that the person who supplies the lethal drug would fall within the proscription of Roman law, regardless of how the individual suicide would be viewed. Gaius recognized that drugs may be either "harmful or beneficial."[76] In other words, regardless of how it treated the individual person who committed or attempted suicide, when it came to assisting suicide, Roman law came down exactly where the Hippocratic Oath did.[77] A recent treatise on Roman criminal law concluded that while suicide itself was not generally considered a crime, "a mercy killing would have still counted as murder."[78]

Roman law also provided that "[g]uilty intention could be presumed from the deed, which need not be direct, for furnishing the cause of death was expressly provided for."[79] When the Ninth Circuit's ruling extends the right to assist in suicide to "those whose services are essential to help the terminally ill patient obtain and take that medication and who act under the supervision or direction of a physician," including "the pharmacist..., the health care worker..., the family member or loved one who opens the bottle, places the pills in the patient's hand, advises him how many pills to take..., or the persons who help the patient to his death bed,"[80] the court departs from the historical liability imposed on poisoners. Justinian's *Institutes*, commenting on the *Lex Cornelia*, say, "This statute also inflicts punishment of death on poisoners, who kill men by their hateful arts of poison and magic, or who publicly sell deadly drugs."[81]

4. The Middle Ages

In the Christian world, at the end of antiquity, St. Augustine was—as the dissent notes—a clear and unambiguous voice for the tradition against self-killing. He viewed suicide as a simple violation of one of the Ten Commandments, "Thou shalt not kill."[82] Judge Reinhardt explains Augustine's opposition by saying, "Prompted in large part by the utilitarian concern that the rage for suicide would deplete the ranks of Christians, St. Augustine argued that committing suicide was a 'detestable and damnable wickedness' and was able to help turn the tide of public opinion."[83] The Ninth Circuit opinion fails to refer to any of Augustine's writings to substantiate the claim that he was against suicide because it depleted the ranks of Christians. In the *locus classicus* on suicide by Augustine, Book One of his *City of God*, there is no such reason for opposition to suicide given—only the categorical one of "Thou shalt not kill."[84] Indeed, if Augustine had been such a utilitarian, then given that suicide was a practice of his Donatist opponents, presumably he would not have objected to *their* use of suicide. But he clearly did object, which makes still more implausible the suggestion that his opposition to suicide was prompted by utilitarian considerations. Augustine's treatment of Judas's suicide is instructive, and differs from Judge Reinhardt's version:

We rightly abominate the act of Judas, and the judgement of truth is that when he hanged himself he did not atone for the guilt of his detestable betrayal but rather increased it, since he despaired of God's mercy and in a fit of self-destructive remorse left himself no chance of a saving repentance. How much lgss right has anyone to indulge in self-slaughter when he can find in himself no fault to justify such a punishment! For when Judas killed himself, he killed a criminal, and yet he ended his life guilty not only of

Christ's death, but also of his own; one crime led to another.[85]

Judge Reinhardt quotes Marzen as observing that "confusion regarding the distinction between suicide and martyrdom existed up until the time of St. Augustine (354-430 A.D.)."[86] Augustine was very clear on what constituted martyrdom. It was not the fact of dying, but the reason for the dying. *Non enim facit martyrem poena, sed causa.* "It is not, after all, the punishment that makes the martyr, but the cause."[87] Thus, for Augustine, the critical factor was the object and intent of the martyr, not simply the fatal result. The ham-handed way in which the majority confuses martyrdom and suicide is similar to the way it mangles the principle of double effect.[88] The court's view is that if death results it is suicide or it is intentional, whereas the tradition drew a careful distinction between what was directly intended and what was merely foreseeable as an unintended side-effect.[89] The martyr accepted death in order to be true to his beliefs. If he could have been faithful without dying, he would have done so. Similarly, the behavior of a person who uses medication to relieve pain and dies sooner than he would otherwise is acceptable and allowable. If the sick person could relieve his pain without hastening death, he would do so. In contrast, the potential suicide seeks death as a way of relieving suffering, either as an end or as a means, not as an unintended side-effect.

A glaring example of the tendentious quality of Judge Reinhardt's historical scholarship is his statement that Thomas More "strongly supported the right of the terminally ill to commit suicide and also expressed approval of the practice of assisting those who wished to hasten their deaths" in his book *Utopia*.[90] But the pro-suicide talk comes from the character Hythlodaeus, whose name literally means "learned in nonsense."[91] The character named "Thomas More" takes issue with those views.[92]

Professor Gerard Wegemer of the University of Dallas, author of a recent biography of Saint Thomas More as well as a study of More's writings on statesmanship,[93] states that to claim Thomas More's *Utopia* supports the right of the terminally ill to commit suicide is akin to saying that Jonathan Swift's *Modest Proposal* supports the right to kill Irish babies in order to provide food and fine gloves for English aristocrats.[94] Both works are satires.

Furthermore, *Utopia* was an early work of More. At the end of his life, while imprisoned in the Tower of London awaiting his execution, he wrote *A Dialogue of Comfort against Tribulation*. In that work, he devotes a lengthy passage of remarkable subtlety and perception to the ways to cure a person tempted by suicide. More himself used all legal means to avoid martyrdom, but in the end, he was ready to suffer death rather than violate the moral teachings and canon law of his Church. It is extremely unlikely that his *Utopia* urged repudiation of the same doctrines he was willing to be martyred to defend.

To be charitable, perhaps these criticisms of the Ninth Circuit can be regarded as quibbles. For Judge Reinhardt does acknowledge the prohibitions on suicide contained in canon law. Strangely, he mentions two regional and early councils[95]—those of Toledo and Braga—but ignores with regard to the latter its appearance in the standard canonical collection from the High Middle Ages, Gratian's *Decretum* (circa 1140),[96]

which fixed and enshrined the unequivocal prohibition of suicide for Western civilization. The *Decretum*'s incorporation of the canon from the Council of Braga thus promulgated it throughout Christendom:

Those who bring death on themselves voluntarily, whether by iron, or by poison, or by casting themselves down headlong, or by hanging, or in any way, let there be no commemoration of them in the oblation [at Mass], nor will their cadavers be brought to burial with psalms.[97]

Despite this, Judge Reinhardt correctly summarized the view of the Middle Ages on suicide: "Once established, the Christian view that suicide was in all cases a sin and crime held sway for 1,000 years...."[98]

V. THE ENGLISH COMMON LAW
A. Bracton
Henry de Bracton was a major figure in the development of the English common law, the writer who brought Roman law and English law into some kind of synthesis. Along with Sir Edward Coke and William Blackstone, Bracton is one of the three major figures in the common law before the modern period. Judge Reinhardt's treatment of him is instructive. Here is how he represents Bracton's view:

Suicide was a crime under the English common law, at least in limited circumstances, probably as early as the thirteenth century. Bracton, incorporating Roman Law as set forth in Justinian's Digest, declared that if someone commits suicide to avoid conviction of a felony, his property escheats to his lords. Bracton said "[i]t ought to be otherwise if he kills himself through madness or unwillingness to endure suffering." Despite his general fidelity to Roman law, Bracton did introduce a key innovation: "[I]f a man slays himself in weariness of life or because he is unwilling to endure further bodily pain... he may have a successor, but his movable goods [personal property] are confiscated. He does not lose his inheritance [real property], only his movable goods." Bracton's innovation was incorporated into English common law, which has thus treated suicides resulting from the inability to "endure further bodily pain" with compassion and understanding ever since a common law scheme was firmly established.[99]

Judge Reinhardt considers Bracton's innovation on Roman law as a manifestation of greater compassion for the person who committed suicide due to an inability "to endure further bodily pain." The historical record establishes just the opposite, as Judge Reinhardt had earlier noted by describing Roman law as holding that "suicide of a private citizen was not punishable if it was caused by 'impatience of pain or sickness, or by another cause,' or by 'weariness of life... lunacy, or fear of dishonor.'"[100]

The innovation made by the English common law with respect to suicide was really two-fold: to punish *all* suicides of sane people, rather than only certain kinds of suicide (those accused of crime, soldiers, slaves); and to *add* the penalty of confiscation of personal property to those suicides that were motivated by "impatience of pain or weariness of life." If the suicide was not so motivated, the real property would be confiscated as well. Can either of these common-law modifications of Roman law be viewed as Judge Reinhardt characterizes them, as treating "suicides resulting from the inability to 'endure further bodily pain' with compassion and understanding..."?[101]

This example nicely illustrates the shaky foundations of the majority opinion's purported survey of "Historical Attitudes Toward Suicide" (a rubric borrowed, incidentally, from the Marzen article that, carefully filleted, serves as Judge Reinhardt's major source). Judge Reinhardt offers three footnotes to Marzen in this section. Had Judge Reinhardt bothered to check Marzen's sources, however, he would have understood that the key passage in Marzen on which he relies lets him down here.

Here is the excerpt from Marzen on which Judge Reinhardt relies:

> Under Justinian's *Digest*, the concern with suicide was primarily with ensuring that those who were accused of a crime for which the Emperor would confiscate their property (disinheriting their heirs), would not evade familial impoverishment by committing suicide before judgment was passed. To prevent cheating the Emperor of otherwise confiscatable property, the Roman law provided, "Persons who have been caught while committing a crime, and, through fear of impending accusation, kill themselves, have no heirs." The Roman condemnation was not of suicide itself.[102]

Marzen then turns to Bracton, who naturally, in his *De Legibus et Consuetudinibus Anglie* [*On the Laws and Customs of England*], incorporated parts of Roman law as set forth in Justinian's *Digest*.

Bracton clearly repeats the statement of the *Digest:*

> But the goods of those who destroy themselves when they are not accused of a crime or taken in the course of a criminal act are not appropriated by the fisc, for it is not the wickedness of the deed that is reprehensible but that the fear of guilt in the accused takes the place of a confession.[103]

Yet Marzen writes that Bracton "could hardly have meant all that this language implies." Marzen bases his conclusion on what he describes as:

> [Bracton's] *key innovation:* [I]f a man slays himself in weariness of life or because he is unwilling to endure further bodily pain... he may have a successor, but his movable goods are confiscated. He does not lose his inheritance, only his movable goods. In other words, real property was to go to the heirs, but personal property was to be confiscated. *The principle that suicide of a sane person, for whatever reason, was a punishable felony was thus introduced into English common law.*[104]

As Marzen describes it, Bracton's innovation made the common law more lenient than Roman law:

> It thus became the common law that a sane suicide's personal property (movable goods or chattels) was confiscated, whereas his land would not be forfeited, as it generally had been under Roman law.[105]

However, land was not "generally" forfeitable under Roman law, as both Judge Reinhardt and Marzen had earlier recognized.[106]

Indeed, in the quoted passage, Marzen misstates the case that he had made just one paragraph previously. Under Roman law, a sane suicide's property—*whether personal property or land*—*would not be forfeited*. A person who "put[] an end to his life through *taedium vitae* or unendurable pain of some kind"[107] did not forfeit any property. Only those "who have been arraigned or who have been caught red-handed, and have committed suicide from fear of the impending charge"[108] would forfeit their property. To prevent cheating the state, the Roman law said that this class of suicide, and no other, will have all its property taken. The ordinary suicides would not have their property escheat. Further, attempted suicides would be punished if the attempt was "without any cause"; acceptable cause included "'weariness of life, or because he was compelled to take this step through pain of some description.'"[109] In other words, under Justinian, someone who committed suicide, not because he had been accused of a crime, but for a cause which included "pain of some description" or "weariness of life," would not forfeit either personal property or land.

Judge Reinhardt tells us that "Bracton's innovation was incorporated into English common law, which has thus treated suicides resulting from the inability to 'endure further bodily pain' with compassion and understanding ever since a common law scheme was firmly established."[110] This characterization of what Bracton did in the area of suicides is at least curious; some, less charitably, might describe it as bizarre. Bracton's innovation in fact made the legal position of the ordinary suicide worse than under Roman law. Further, far from treating the suicide with "compassion," the treatment of suicide under the common law was to become steadily more severe, as one can see in Blackstone. Yet relying solely on Judge Reinhardt's use of history and on his tone, an unsuspecting reader might well conclude the opposite.

B. Blackstone

After Bracton, the opinion devotes a paragraph to Sir Edward Coke, who, the opinion correctly observes, held that killing oneself was an offense and that people who committed suicide should forfeit their movable property. Judge Reinhardt then employs various rhetorical devices to minimize what an unwary reader can be excused for missing—the fact that in the English common law, there was a firm prohibition against suicide by the sane. Here is how the trick is performed:

Thus, although, formally, suicide was long considered a crime under English common law, in practice it was a crime that was punished leniently, if at all, because juries frequently used their power to nullify the law.[111]

But, as Justice Scalia wrote in his concurring opinion in *Cruzan*, "the States abolished the penalties imposed by the common law... to spare the innocent family and not to legitimize the act."[112] This is very different from approving of suicide—much less, of course, physician-assisted suicide—or thinking of it as a right.

The very next paragraph of Judge Reinhardt's opinion deploys to even greater effect the patronizing vocabulary of belittlement:

The traditional English experience was also shaped by the taboos that have long colored our views of suicide and perhaps still do today. English common law reflected the ancient fear that the spirit of someone who ended his own life would return to haunt the living.[113]

Note the words that evoke a pre-rational world of credulous peasants: views are shaped by "taboos" that have "long colored our views of suicide." And those credulous peasants with their "ancient fear" of a "spirit" that would "haunt the living" have their counterpart in those benighted souls who continue to regard suicide with horror (which is to say, who differ with Judge Reinhardt on his view of physician-assisted suicide): these are the people for whom those ancient "taboos... perhaps still [color their views] today." And then Judge Reinhardt becomes positively Transylvanian:

Accordingly, the traditional practice was to bury the body at a cross-roads—either so the suicide could not find his way home or so that the frequency of travelers would keep his spirit from rising. As added insurance, a stake was driven through the body.[114]

One would think, from this kind of tone, that none of those who over so many centuries had produced so many coherent arguments against suicide had ever existed—or that they were to be treated, tainted with a guilt by verbal association, as slack-jawed rustics

practicing a bit of apotropaic mumbo-jumbo. It is bizarre that while
Judge Reinhardt cites Blackstone's *Commentaries*, he never bothered
to look into those *Commentaries*. For if he had, he would have found
that Blackstone, certainly the most influential legal figure in Anglo-
American law from the Revolution to the Civil War, expresses no
ambiguity or doubt about where the English common law then stood
on this matter:

SELF-MURDER, the pretended heroism, but real cowardice, of the Stoic
philosophers, who destroyed themselves to avoid those ills which they had
not the fortitude to endure, though the attempting it seems to be counte-
nanced by the civil law, yet was punished by the Athenian law by cutting off
the hand, which committed the desperate deed. And also the law of England
wisely and religiously considers, that no man hath a power to destroy life,
but by commission from God, the author of it: and, as the suicide is guilty
of a double offence; one spiritual, in invading the prerogative of the
Almighty, and rushing into his immediate presence uncalled for; the other
temporal, against the king, who hath an interest in the preservation of all his
subjects; *the law has therefore ranked this among the highest crimes*, making it
a peculiar species of felony, a felony committed on oneself. A *felo de se*
therefore is he that deliberately puts an end to his own existence, or commits
any unlawful malicious act, the consequence of which is his own death: as if,
attempting to kill another, he runs upon his antagonist's sword; or, shooting
at another, the gun bursts and kills himself. The party must be of years of
discretion, and in his senses, else it is no crime. But this excuse ought not to
be strained to that length, to which our coroners' juries are apt to carry it,
viz., that the very act of suicide is an evidence of insanity; as if every man
who acts contrary to reason, had no reason at all: for the same argument
would prove every other criminal *non compos*, as well as the self-murderer.
The law very rationally judges, that every melancholy or hypochondriac fit
does not deprive a man of the capacity of discerning right from wrong; which
is necessary, as was observed in a former chapter, to form a legal excuse. And
therefore, if a real lunatic kills himself in a lucid interval, he is a *felo de se* as
much as another man.

But now the question follows, what punishment can human laws inflict on
one who has withdrawn himself from their reach? They can only act upon
what he has left behind him, his reputation and fortune: on the former, by
an ignominious burial in the highway, with a stake driven through his body;
on the latter, by a forfeiture of all his goods and chattels to the king: hoping
that his care for either his own reputation, or the welfare of his family,
would be some motive to restrain him from so desperate and wicked an act.
And it is observable, that this forfeiture has relation to the time of the act

done in the felon's lifetime, which was the cause of his death. As if husband and wife be possessed jointly of a term of years in land, and the husband drowns himself; the land shall be forfeited to the king, and the wife shall not have it by survivorship. For by the act of casting himself into the water he forfeits the term; which gives a title to the king, prior to the wife's title by survivorship, which could not accrue till the instant of her husband's death. And, though it must be owned that the letter of the law herein borders a little upon severity, yet it is some alleviation that the power of mitigation is left in the breast of the sovereign, who upon this (as on all other occasions) is reminded by the oath of his office to execute judgment in mercy.[115]

This quotation is adduced, not to provide readers with a frisson of horror at the way suicides were once treated, but simply to show that the exemplary punishment meted out to suicides—a punishment that could be mitigated by feelings "in the breast of the sovereign" who may "execute judgment in mercy"—reflects the English (and at that time American) common law's special abhorrence for suicide. That abhorrence was not lessened by the fact that mercy tempered justice and that frequently the official punishment was not inflicted. Nor was that disapproval in any sense diminished by the (growing) feeling that punishing the already-dead suicide was both futile and cruel. And certainly the existence of any such feeling had nothing to do with the notion of a fundamental right to physician-assisted suicide.

Further, it cannot be argued that Blackstone's *Commentaries* are unrepresentative, being either reactionary (that is, a statement of the law as it had been in ancient times, but was no longer) or revolutionary (a statement of the law not as it was, but as Blackstone wished it to be in the future). The *Commentaries* were a single-handed massive compilation that became authoritative for all judges and lawyers of what the common law was at the time of its writing: a kind of omnium-gatherum Restatement of the Common Law at the moment when the American Republic was founded.[116]

VI. THE AMERICAN EXPERIENCE
A. *The Declaration of Independence and John Locke*
Although one might expect that in an historical survey Judge Reinhardt would devote special attention to the American Republic, this is not the case. The English philosopher whose work stands most behind the Framers was John Locke. As Bernard Bailyn has written, "[T]he great virtuosi of the American Enlightenment—Franklin,

Adams, Jefferson—cited the classic Enlightenment texts.... In pamphlet after pamphlet the American writers cited Locke on natural rights and on the social and governmental contract...."[117] Yet Judge Reinhardt ignores Locke as though he had never existed.

Let us not make the same mistake. Locke's *Second Treatise of Government* is most relevant here; scholars of the Revolution have generally agreed that it is this work which most influenced Thomas Jefferson's draft of the Declaration of Independence.[118] Jefferson had in mind Locke's trinity of "life, liberty, and estate"[119] when he wrote that "all men are endowed by their creator with certain inalienable rights; that among these are life, liberty, and the pursuit of happiness."[120]

To understand what Jefferson meant by "inalienable rights to life [and] liberty" we have to look to Locke's *Second Treatise*. In his chapter on "The State of Nature," Locke observes that:

though this be a *State of Liberty*, yet it is *not a State of Licence*, though Man in that State have an uncontroleable Liberty, to dispose of his Person or Possessions, *yet he has not Liberty to destroy himself,* or so much as any Creature in his Possession, but where some nobler use, than its bare Preservation calls for it.... Every one as he is *bound to preserve himself,* and not to quit his Station wilfully; so by the like reason when his own Preservation comes not in competition, ought he, as much as he can, *to preserve the rest of Mankind,* and may not unless it be to do Justice on an Offender, take away, or impair the life, or what tends to the Preservation of the Life, the Liberty, Health, Limb or Goods of another.[121]

Later in the *Second Treatise,* Locke returns to the theme that "a Man" does not have "the Power of his own Life":

This *Freedom* from Absolute, Arbitrary Power, is so necessary to, and closely joyned with a Man's Preservation, that he cannot part with it, but by what forfeits his Preservation and Life together. For a Man, not having the Power of his own Life, *cannot,* by Compact, or his own Consent, *enslave himself* to any one, nor put himself under the Absolute, Arbitrary Power of another, to take away his Life, when he pleases. No body can give more Power than he has himself; and he that cannot take away his own Life, cannot give another power over it.[122]

Locke sounds his anti-suicide theme firmly and repeatedly: "yet he has not Liberty to destroy himself..."; "[e]very one as he is *bound to preserve himself*...";[123] "[f]or no Body can transfer to another more power than he has in himself; and no Body has an absolute Arbitrary Power over himself, or over any other, to destroy his own Life, or take away the Life or Property of another."[124] One cannot voluntarily give up either the right to life or the right to liberty: "he that cannot take away his own Life, cannot give another power over it."[125]

Another way of expressing this, one more familiar to Americans, is that these rights are "inalienable"—for Jefferson's formulation is an expression of the demands of Lockean natural rights.

Yet none of this—not Locke, not Jefferson, not the Declaration of Independence, and certainly not the Constitution—merits even passing mention in Judge Reinhardt's remorseless historical review. Nor does President Lincoln, whose comment on the *Dred Scott* decision illustrates what happens when judges ignore the meaning of the Declaration of Independence:

In those days, our Declaration of Independence was held sacred by all, and thought to include all; but now... it is assailed, and sneered at, and construed, and hawked at, and torn, till, if its framers could rise from their graves, they could not at all recognize it....

Chief Justice Taney, in his opinion in the Dred Scott case, ...[did] obvious violence to the plain unmistakable language of the Declaration.... [T]he authors of that notable instrument... defined with tolerable distinctness, in what respects they did consider all men created equal—equal in "certain inalienable rights, among which are life, liberty, and the pursuit of happiness." This they said, and this meant....

And now I appeal to all... are you really willing that the Declaration shall be thus frittered away?—thus left no more at most, than an interesting memorial of the dead past? thus shorn of its vitality, and practical value...?[126]

The "inalienable right to life" in the Declaration comes from Locke, and so it is Locke who supplies us with the part of its meaning that we tend to forget: that a man "has not Liberty to destroy himself," still less "give another power over [his life]."[127]

B. *The States*
Turning briefly to American law, Judge Reinhardt tells us that

[b]y 1798 six of the 13 original colonies had abolished all penalties for suicide

either by statute or state constitution. There is no evidence that any court ever imposed a punishment for suicide or attempted suicide under common law in post-revolutionary America.[128]

The question is, what are we to make of this information? Marzen's comment here is judicious:

It has sometimes been supposed that the abolition of forfeiture and ignominious burial as punishment for suicide occurred because the colonists had come to believe that suicide was an individual autonomous choice without adverse impact on the rights of others and society and that therefore government should not interfere with it. But as Stroud Milsom has warned, "Perhaps more than in any other kind of history, the historian of law is enticed into carrying concepts and even social frameworks back into periods to which they do not belong." The anachronistic assumption that our forebearers held and applied a political philosophy derived from Mills [sic] is not borne out by the available evidence.

The principal piece of evidence concerning the rationale of the colonists for their abolition of forfeiture is in a 1796 treatise by Zephaniah Swift, later Chief Justice of Connecticut, that clearly establishes that rationale.

There can be no act more contemptible, than to attempt to punish an offender for a crime, by exercising a mean act of revenge upon lifeless clay, that is insensible of the punishment. There can be no greater cruelty, than the inflicting a punishment, as the forfeiture of goods, which must fall solely on the innocent offspring of the offender. This odious practice has been attempted to be justified upon the principle, that such forfeiture will tend to deter mankind from the commission of such crimes, from a regard to their families. But it is evident that where a person is so destitute of affection for his family, and regardless of the pleasures of life, as to wish to put an end to his existence, that he will not be deterred by a consideration of their future subsistence. Indeed, this crime is so abhorrent to the feelings of mankind, and that strong love of life which is implanted in the human heart, that it cannot be so frequently committed, as to become dangerous to society. There can of course be no necessity of any punishment. This principle has been adopted in this state, and no instances have happened of a forfeiture of estate, and none lately of an ignominious burial.

Swift makes clear that the traditional penalties were abolished *not* because suicide itself was viewed as a lesser evil or as a human right, but because the penalties punished the innocent family of the suicide, without in any way reaching the real perpetrator of the act.[129]

Although criminalizing suicide does tell us something about society's attitudes, it is far less certain that we can conclude anything about whether or not a society regards suicide as a right merely from its refusal to punish suicides. Judge Reinhardt does not hesitate over the significance of this evidence. It means, in his review, what he wants it to mean. Because the excerpt above is from *his* principal source, he must have read it; it is too bad that Judge Reinhardt did not take this example of historical judiciousness as a model.

The Ninth Circuit's opinion tells us that "[b]y the time the Fourteenth Amendment was adopted in 1868, suicide was generally not punishable, and in only nine of the 37 states is it clear that there were statutes prohibiting assisting suicide."[130] The footnote goes on, however, to provide information that ought better to have been in the text:

Nevertheless, extrapolating from incomplete historical evidence and drawing inferences from States' treatment of suicide and from later historical evidence, Marzen hypothesized that in 1868, "twenty-one of the thirty-seven states, and eighteen of the thirty ratifying states prohibited assisting suicide."[131]

When one goes back to Marzen, Judge Reinhardt's source for this footnote, one finds that his conclusion—sneeringly described merely as a "hypothesi[s] derived" by "extrapolating" from "incomplete" evidence, and "drawing inferences" from "later historical evidence"—is far more precise than Judge Reinhardt would have us believe. The following paragraph gives a flavor of Marzen's method:

When the fourteenth amendment was ratified in 1868, nine of the thirty-seven states had statutes that prohibited assisting suicide. Of these, all but one state's legislature voted to ratify; Mississippi did not vote. In addition, Massachusetts, which voted to ratify, had case law to the same effect, and since South Carolina (which voted to ratify) had a statute condemning suicide as a felony while retaining the common law of crimes, it may be presumed that that state also criminalized assisting suicide. Under the same principle of imputation employed with regard to the ninth amendment, ten additional states (Alabama, Connecticut, Georgia, Kentucky, Maryland, Michigan, North Carolina, Pennsylvania, Tennessee, and Virginia) can be held to have prohibited assisting suicide under the common law of crimes. Of these, all but two voted to ratify; the legislatures of Kentucky and Maryland voted against the fourteenth amendment.

Of four states that ratified the fourteenth amendment (Nevada, New Hampshire, Rhode Island and West Virginia), and one that voted against ratification (Delaware), it can be said with confidence that although these states recognized the common law of crimes, there is insufficient evidence, apart from that, to establish their positions on attempting suicide or assisting suicide. Vermont, which voted to ratify, and California, which did not vote, applied the common law, but it is unclear whether they included the common law of crimes.

Illinois, Indiana, Iowa, Louisiana, Maine, Nebraska, and Texas, which voted to ratify, and Ohio, which voted against ratification, had no prohibition on assisting suicide. The status of New Jersey is unclear. Of the ten existing territories, Washington prohibited assisting suicide by statute; Colorado, the District of Columbia, Idaho, and Wyoming recognized the common law of crimes but, again, there is insufficient evidence to establish their position on assisting suicide; Arizona and Utah applied the common law, but it is unclear whether they included the common law of crimes; New Mexico and North Dakota had no prohibition on assisting suicide; and the status of Montana is unclear.

In short, twenty-one of the thirty-seven states, and eighteen of the thirty ratifying states prohibited assisting suicide. Only eight of the states, and seven of the ratifying states, definitely did not.[132]

The reader can now judge for himself who is being sloppy by "extrapolating from incomplete historical evidence," who has "hypothesized," and who, on the other hand, has specified in meticulous fashion how he arrived at his conclusions. Should one really describe as "extrapolating from incomplete historical evidence" and "drawing inferences" the assumption that if a State treats suicide as a crime, then it can be presumed to have "also criminalized assisting suicide"? How plausible is the assumption that such a State would *not* do so?

In Judge Reinhardt's entire historical survey, only one legal case is actually discussed:

The New Jersey Supreme Court declared in 1901 that since suicide was not punishable it should not be considered a crime. "[A]ll will admit that in some cases it is ethically defensible," the court said, as when a woman kills herself to escape being raped or "when a man curtails weeks or months of agony of an incurable disease."[133]

Again, Judge Reinhardt misleads through his selective quotation.

Here is what appears immediately *above* the discussion in his cited source:

> Perhaps a better candidate for Engelhardt and Malloy's title of "Aberrant Jurisdiction" (though the jurisdiction quickly repudiated it), would be New Jersey. In a 1901 insurance case, *Campbell v. Supreme Conclave Improved Order Heptasophs*, nine of the seventeen members of the state's highest court joined an opinion by Justice Gilbert Collins stating that since suicide was not punished with forfeiture, it was not a crime.[134]

And here is what *follows* the discussion of the case in the source:

> It is, however, the only pre-1980 case we have found that articulates such a view. It is isolated not only in contrast to cases in other jurisdictions, but within New Jersey as well. Two years later, an inferior appellate court took the extraordinary step not only of criticizing the Justice Collins' opinion but also of rendering a holding directly contrary to its language, which it characterized as dictum.[135]

Burke Balch, one of the co-authors of the article,[136] noted recently:

> "Indeed, in 1922, New Jersey's highest court... wrote, 'So strong is this concern of the state [in the preservation of the life of each of its citizens] that it does not even permit a man to take his own life....'"[137]

And of course, even if those cases in which suicide was not punished were held to mean that it was not a crime, there is a great difference between declaring something not a crime and recognizing it as a constitutional right.

VII. CONCLUSION

The use of history in *Compassion in Dying* is disturbing on several counts. It is wildly inaccurate in part, as when Bracton's "innovation" to Roman law is portrayed as lessening, rather than increasing, the punishment for sane suicides who kill themselves in order to "avoid pain." It is peculiar in the manner in which it deals with topics of major importance. The practices and moral code of ancient Israel are limited to one sentence in one footnote. Aristotle is not mentioned. Plato is discussed, but only in a paragraph quoted, not from Plato himself, nor from any of the modern experts on Plato, but in a few sentences lifted whole from Durkheim's polemical book *Suicide*.

Blackstone, one of the essential figures in the common law, whose
Commentaries served as the law school for generations of Americans
from independence until the mid-nineteenth century, is mentioned
only as the source for one footnote. And Western history, from the
founding of the American Republic until the present, is summed up
in two breathless paragraphs. There is no mention, for example, of
the Nazi experience in euthanasia, which at times retained some
elements of physician-assisted suicide,[138] and might have offered a
salutary perspective.

Further, Judge Reinhardt's opinion repeatedly disguises the paucity
of evidence supporting the idea that suicide was not abhorred by
summarizing that evidence quite inaccurately. Sometimes he does it
before presenting that evidence. For example, he slips the "Jews" into
one sentence, in a footnote that begins: "Other ancient peoples also
viewed suicide with equanimity or acceptance."[139] This sentence is
meant to summarize what immediately follows:

Hundreds of Jews killed themselves at Masada in order to avoid being
captured by Roman legions. The ancient Sythians [sic] believed it was an
honor to commit suicide when they became too frail for their nomadic way
of life. The Vikings believed that the next greatest honor, after death in
battle, was death by suicide.[140]

One must keep in mind that *Compassion in Dying* was no ordinary
Ninth Circuit opinion. It makes new law in an area that is, literally,
a matter of life and death. Surely this is a case where a decent respect
for the opinions of the major philosophers, religious traditions, and
legal history—the accumulated wisdom of the past, of all those who
have pondered the matter, of philosophers, religions, and legal
scholars—would lead to a certain hesitancy, circumspection, and
doubt. But there is nothing hesitant about the opinion's treatment of
historical attitudes toward suicide. If one could allow oneself to
believe that it was simply the product of undue haste, that would be
bad enough. But a close examination of this part of Judge Reinhardt's
opinion shows no sifting of the sources, no distinguishing of those
sources that are famous polemical defenses of suicide (Alvarez's *The
Savage God* and Durkheim's *Suicide*), and those that are serious efforts
at summarizing historical attitudes toward suicide. Most disturbing of
all, when we examine the court's use of a single law review article on

which the historical summary largely rests, we find what can only be described as systematic distortion and obfuscation.

Recently, Professor Alan Watson discussed some of the problems that arise for students in understanding the justifications that judges offer for changes in the law, noting that "when a judge argues from the facts of history, the watchword is *Beware*. False history is probably as often adduced to support a proposition as is plausible or even accurate history."[141] False history is bad.[142] When false history seems to be the result not of carelessness but of premeditation, it is something worse.

NOTES

1. "Ce n'est jamais qu'à cause d'un état d'esprit qui n'est pas destiné à durer qu'on prend des résolutions définitives." Marcel Proust, *A la recherche du temps perdu* (Paris: Bibliothèque de la Pléiade, 1954) 578-79. Translation supplied by the authors.

2. *Griswold v. Connecticut*, 381 U.S. 479 (1965).

3. *Ibid.* at 484.

4. See *Planned Parenthood of Southeastern Pa. v. Casey*, 505 U.S. 833 (1992); *Roe v. Wade*, 410 U.S. 113 (1973).

5. See *Carey v. Population Services Int'l*, 431 U.S. 678 (1977); *Moore v. City of East Cleveland*, 431 U.S. 494 (1977); *Eisenstadt v. Baird*, 405 U.S. 438 (1972).

6. *Bowers v. Hardwick*, 478 U.S. 186 (1986).

7. *Cruzan v. Director, Mo. Dep't. of Health*, 497 U.S. 261 (1990).

8. *Ibid.* at 280.

9. *Cruzan*, 497 U.S. at 294-95 (Scalia, J., concurring)(citations omitted).

10. See *Compassion in Dying v. Washington*, 79 F.3d 790 (9th Cir. 1996) (*en banc*), *cert. granted sub nom.* Washington v. Glucksberg, 117 S. Ct. 37 (1996). See also *Quill v. Vacco*, 80 F.3d 716 (2d Cir. 1996) (holding that New York's statute prohibiting assisted suicide is unconstitutional under the Fourteenth Amendment's Equal Protection Clause because it lacked a rational basis when applied to the terminally ill, but noting that the prohibition would be upheld under the Due Process Clause), *cert. granted*, 117 S. Ct. 36 (1996). But see *People v. Kevorkian*, 527 N.W.2d 714, 733 (Mich. 1994) (holding that the Fourteenth Amendment provides no due process fundamental right to physician-assisted suicide), *cert. denied*, 115 S. Ct. 1795 (1995).

11. The original three-judge panel had upheld the statue 2-1. See *Compassion in Dying v. Washington*, 49 F.3d 586 (9th Cir. 1995).

12. *Bowers*, 478 U.S. at 191.

13. *Bowers*, 478 U.S. at 191-92 (citing *Palko v. Connecticut*, 302 U.S. 319, 325, 326 (1937) and *Moore v. City of East Cleveland*, 431 U.S. 494, 503 (1977) (Powell, J., for plurality)).

14. *Palko*, 302 U.S. at 325 (quoting *Snyder v. Massachusetts*, 291 U.S. 97, 105 (1934)). Justice Holmes had a similar understanding of the importance of history. For example, in his famous *Lochner* dissent, Holmes suggested that legislation might give way when "a rational and fair man necessarily would admit that the statute proposed would infringe fundamental principles as they have been understood by the tradition of our people and our law." *Lochner v. New York*, 198 U.S. 45, 76 (1905) (Holmes, J., dissenting). As he later wrote, "If a thing has been practiced for two hundred years by common consent, it will need a strong case for the Fourteenth Amendment to affect it...." *Jackman v. Rosenbaum*, 260 U.S. 22, 31 (1922).

15. *Bowers*, 478 U.S. at 192.

16. *Ibid.* at 192-94 (citations omitted).

17. *Ibid.* at 194-95.

18. *Compassion in Dying v. Washington*, 49 F.3d 586, 591 (9th Cir. 1995), *rev'd en banc*, 79 F.3d 790 (9th Cir. 1996), *cert. granted sub nom.* Washington v. Glucksberg, 117 S.Ct 37 (1996).

19. See *Quill v. Vacco*, 80 F.3d 716, 724 (2d Cir. 1996) ("Indeed, the very opposite is true."), *cert. granted*, 117 S.Ct. 36 (1996).

20. See *Compassion in Dying*, 79 F.3d at 806.

21. *Ibid.* At 805 (emphasis added).

22. See *ibid.* At 806-10.

23. *Ibid.* at 806 (quoting *Compassion in Dying*, 79 F.3d at 591).

24. *Compassion in Dying*, 79 F.3d at 806. The full quote reads: "As we have pointed out at p. 803, our inquiry is not so narrow. Nor is our conclusion so facile. The relevant historical record is far more checkered than the [three-member panel's] majority would have us believe." *Ibid.* Because there is no such discussion on p. 803, the court must have intended to refer to p. 801.

25. *Ibid.* At 801.

26. See *ibid.* at 801. The use of history in the abortion cases has been widely criticized. See, e.g., John Finnis, "'Shameless Acts' in Colorado: Abuse of Scholarship in Constitutional Cases" in 7 *Academic Questions* 10, 10-19 (1994).

27. See Hippocrates, *Oath*, reprinted in 1 *Hippocrates* 299 (tr. W.H.S. Jones, 1923) ("I will use treatment to help the sick according to my ability and judgment, but never with a view to injury and wrong-doing. Neither will I

administer a poison to anybody when asked to do so, nor will I suggest such a course.").

28.] *Compassion in Dying*, 79 F.3d at 807 (citing *Roe v. Wade*, 410 U.S. 113, 131 (1973)). The majority opinion observes that the *Roe* Court "noted that the Pythagorean school represented a distinctly minority view." *Ibid. Roe* had also claimed that:

> with the end of antiquity a decided change took place. Resistance against suicide and against abortion became common. The Oath came to be popular. The emerging teachings of Christianity were in agreement with the Pythagorean ethic. The Oath "became the nucleus of all medical ethics" and "was applauded as the embodiment of truth." Thus, suggests Dr. Edelstein, it is "a Pythagorean manifesto and not the expression of an absolute standard of medical conduct."
>
> This, it seems to us, is a satisfactory and acceptable explanation of the Hippocratic Oath's apparent rigidity.

Ibid. at 132 (citing Ludwig Edelstein, *The Hippocratic Oath* (1943) 64).

29. *Roe*, 410 U.S. at 131.

30. *Compassion in Dying*, 79 F.3d at 829 ("Clearly, the Hippocratic Oath can have no greater import in deciding the constitutionality of physician assisted-suicide than it did in determining whether women had a constitutional right to have an abortion.")

31. *Compassion in Dying*, 79 F.3d at 855 (Beezer, J., dissenting) (emphasis added).

32. Thomas J. Marzen, Mary K. O'Dowd, Daniel Crowe, & Thomas J. Balch, "Suicide: A Constitutional Right" in 24 *Duquesne Law Review* 1 (1985).

33. *Compassion in Dying*, 79 F.3d at 806.

34. *Ibid.* at 806 (quoting Alfred Alvarez, "The Background" in *Suicide: The Philosophical Issues*, eds. M. Pabst Battin & David J. Mayo (1980) 7, 18.

35. *Ibid.*

36. *Ibid.*

37. *Ibid.* at 808 n.25 (quoting Marzen, *supra* note 32, at 19).

38. *Ibid.* at 807 n.24 (quoting Marzen, *supra* note 32, at 20).

39. To attribute a particular significance to the facts of Masada, one would have to adduce evidence as to the reaction to the event by the Jews of the time. The bald statement of those facts permits no conclusion about the accepted view of suicide among the ancient Hebrews, any more than the facts of Jonestown allow us to conclude anything about American society's attitude towards such mass suicides.

40. Marzen, *supra* note 32, at 18-19.

41. *Ibid.* at 19-20, citing Battin, "Ethical Issues in Suicide" (1982) 31.

42. *Ibid.* at 20, quoting Jacques Choron, *Suicide* 13-14 (1972) 13-14.

43. *Ibid.* at 20, quoting Norman L. Farberow, "Cultural History of Suicide" in *Suicide in Different Cultures,* ed. Norman L. Farberow (1975) 1, 4.

44. *Ibid.*

45. Compare *Compassion in Dying v. Washington,* 79 F.3d 790, 808 n.25 (9th Cir. 1996)(*en banc*), *cert. granted sub nom.* Washington v. Glucksberg, 117 S. Ct. 37 (1996), with *ibid.* at 845 (dissent).

46. Anthony Fisher, "Theological Aspects of Euthanasia" in *Euthanasia Examined: Ethical, Clinical and Legal Perspectives,* ed. John Keown (1995) 315-16.

47. 2 *Samuel* 1:11-12.

48. 2 *Samuel* 1:16.

49. The Amelikite's crime was more serious than murder, as it was technically regicide, the murder of an anointed king. However, if, as Judge Reinhardt imagines, that society condoned suicide and assisted suicide, then the fact that the king had requested the mercy killing ought to have mitigated the Amelikite's offense. Yet David characterized this "assisted suicide" as tantamount to murder.

50. Fisher, *supra* note 46, at 316.

51. *Exodus* 20:13; *Deuteronomy* 5:11.

52. Moshe Weinfeld, *Deuteronomy* 1-11, at 314 (Anchor Bible Vol. 15, 1991). The Anchor Bible commentary, by Protestant, Catholic, and Jewish scholars, is the most detailed modern commentary on the Bible, and now runs to more than 60 volumes.

53. Baruch A. Brody, "A Historical Introduction to Jewish Casuistry on Suicide and Euthanasia" in *Suicide And Euthanasia: Historical And Contemporary Themes,* ed. Baruch A. Brody (1989) 39.

54. *Ibid.* at 40.

55. *Ibid.* at 64. What makes Brody's summary even more persuasive is that he also argues that traditional Judaism "is not committed to a belief in the sanctity of human life," which he defines as a "belief that mere physical existence is in the patient's best interest or... a belief that residual life in pain has infinite worth." *Ibid.* at 40. It is curious that Judge Reinhardt makes no mention of Brody's essay, of which he can hardly have been unaware, for he cites another essay from the same book in which Brody's study appears. *Compassion in Dying v. Washington,* 79 F.3d 790, 808 n.30 (9th Cir. 1996)(*en banc*), *cert. granted sub nom.* Washington v. Glucksberg, 117 S. Ct. 37 (1996).

56. *Compassion in Dying,* 79 F.3d at 808, n.25.

57. Raymond G. Brown, *The Death of The Messiah* 1:644 (1994) (citations omitted).

58. *Compassion in Dying,* 79 F.3d at 807.

59. Emile Durkheim, *Suicide: A Study in Sociology*, ed. George Simpson, trans. John A. Spaulding and George Simpson (1951) 329-30.

60. *Ibid.* at 329-30 (bracketed word added) (citations omitted).

61. Anton J. L. Van Hoof, *From Autothanasia to Suicide: Self-Killing in Classical Antiquity* (1990) 168.

62. *Compassion in Dying*, 79 F.3d at 807 (quoting *Roe v. Wade*, 410 U.S. 113, 131 (1973)) (citation omitted).

63. *Ibid.*

64. *Ibid.*

65. *Ibid.* (Quoting Alvarez, *supra* n. 34, at 19).

66. Marzen, *supra* n. 32, at 22 (citations omitted).

67. *Ibid.* at 23 (emphasis added) (citations omitted).

68. *Ibid.* at 24 (emphasis added).

69. Robert P. George and William C. Porth, Jr., "Death, Be Not Proud" in *National Review* (June 26, 1995) at 49.

70. Marzen, *supra* n. 32, at 24 (quoting Aristotle, *Ethics* 200-201, tr. J. Thompson, 1976).

71. *Ibid.* at 24 (citing Aristotle, *supra* n. 70, at 128-29).

72. *Ibid.* (citing Aristotle, *supra* n. 70, at 130).

73. *Ibid.* at 24.

74. *Compassion in Dying v. Washington*, 79 F.3d 790, 807 (9th Cir. 1996)(*en banc*) (quoting Alvarez, *supra* note 34, at 22-23), *cert. granted sub nom.* Washington v. Glucksberg, 117 S. Ct. 37 (1996).

75. *Lex Cornelia de sicariis et veneficis* in *Dig.* 48.8.1.1, 48.8.3 (Marcian, *Institutes* 14).

76. *Ibid.* at 50.16.236 (Gaius, *XII Tables*, 4).

77. Judge Reinhardt, however, states in a footnote:
We note that even in ancient times many physicians did not interpret the oath literally. As three commentators said, "It is well established that Greek and Roman physicians, even those who were Hippocratic, often supplied their patients with the means to commit suicide, despite the injunction against suicide embodied in the Hippocratic oath."
Compassion in Dying, 79 F.3d at 829 n.110 (quoting Rebecca C. Morgan, Thomas C. Marks, Jr., and Barbara Harty-Golder, "The Issue of Personal Choice: The Competent Incurable Patient and the Right to Commit Suicide" in 57 *Missouri Law Rev.* 3, 46 (1992)). The "three commentators" turn out to be the three co-authors of that law review article. Their source for that assertion is a letter to a medical journal, which in turn cites Sherwin Nuland's book. See Morgan at 46 n.290 (citing Steven Beeson, Letter to the Editor, "Euthanasia and the American College of Physicians Ethics Manual"

in 111 *Ann. Int. Med.* 952-53 (1989) (quoting Sherwin B. Nuland, *Doctors: The Biography of Medicine* 25 (1988)). However, there is no authority given in Nuland's book for this remark; he simply states: "[C]ertain of the Oath's prohibitions, such as those against abortion, cutting for stone, and aiding a suicide, fly in the face not only of the usual medical practices of the time, but specifically of those in which some of the Hippocratics are known to have engaged." Nuland at 25. How this undocumented assertion "establishes" that "Greek and Roman physicians...often supplied their patients with the means to commit suicide" is a puzzlement. One celebrated ancient source provides us, almost in passing, with evidence quite to the contrary. The source is *The Golden Ass* by Apuleius, a pagan novelist of the second century.

A physician, we are told, was asked for a fast-acting poison, allegedly "for a sick man in the throes of an inveterate, intractable disease who longed to escape the torture of his life," in reality for the purpose of murdering him. The physician sold a potion, but when later an innocent man was accused of murder, the physician revealed that the poison had only been a sleeping draught and not a deadly poison, "because he did not believe it proper for his calling to be instrumental in bringing death to anybody, and because he had been taught that medicine had been invented not for the destruction of man but for his welfare."

Owsei Temkin, "The Idea of Respect for Life in the History of Medicine" in Owsei Temkin, William K. Frankena, and Sanford H. Kadish, "Respect for Life in Medicine, Philosophy, and the Law" in 1, 4 (1977) (quoting Apuleius, *Metamorphoses* [the Latin title of *The Golden Ass*] 10.9-12).

78. O. F. Robinson, *The Criminal Law of Ancient Rome* (1995) 44.

79. *Ibid.* (citing *Dig.* 48.8.15 (Ulpian, *Lex Julia et Papia*, book 8), which says, "It makes no difference whether someone kills or provides the occasion of death." [*Nihil interest, occidat quis an causam mortis praebeat.*]).

80. *Compassion in Dying*, 79 F.3d at 838 n.140.

81. *J.Inst.* 4.18.6.

82. *Compassion in Dying*, 79 F.3d at 845 (Beezer, J., dissenting) (citing Marzen, *supra* n. 32, at 27).

83. *Compassion in Dying*, 79 F.3d at 808 (citing Alvarez, *supra* n. 34, at 27).

84. St. Augustine, *The City Of God*, tr. Henry Bettenson (Penguin 1972) 31: "It is significant that in the sacred canonical books there can nowhere be found any injunction or permission to commit suicide either to ensure immortality or to avoid or escape any evil. In fact we must understand it to be forbidden by the law 'You shall not kill'...."

85. *Ibid.* at 27. Significantly, this passage from St. Augustine was included in Gratian's *Decretum*, the collection of authoritative canon law texts, edited around the year 1140. Second Part, C.23, q. 5, c.9, ed. Emil Friedberg (Leipzig 1879).

86. *Compassion in Dying*, 79 F.3d at 808 (citing Marzen, *supra* n. 31, at 26).

87. St. Augustine, Sermon 328, in III-9 *Sermons*, tr. Edmund Hill (New City Press, 1994) 179. There are at least a dozen appearances in Augustine's works of this phrase, or one virtually identical.

88. "[W]e see little, if any, difference for constitutional or ethical purposes between providing medication with a double effect and providing medication with a single effect, as long as one of the known effects in each case is to hasten the end of the patient's life." *Compassion in Dying*, 79 F.3d at 824. The court had previously recognized that "[p]hysicians routinely and openly provide medication to terminally ill patients with the knowledge that it will have a 'double effect'—reduce the patient's pain and hasten death. Such medical treatment is accepted by the medical profession as meeting its highest ethical standards." *Ibid.* at 823.

89. The distinction between intention and foresight is traditional. Abraham Lincoln, for example, had insisted in another context: "I simply expressed an *expectation*. Cannot the Judge perceive the distinction between a *purpose* and an *expectation*. I have often expressed an expectation to die, but I have never expressed a *wish* to die." Abraham Lincoln, Speech at Springfield, Illinois (July 17, 1858), in Abraham Lincoln, *Speeches And Writings 1832-1858*, ed. Don E. Fehrenbacher ed., 1989) at 470.

90. *Compassion in Dying*, 79 F.3d at 808 (citing Thane Josef Messinger, "A Gentle and Easy Death: From Ancient Greece to Beyond Cruzan Toward a Reasoned Legal Response to the Societal Dilemma of Euthanasia" in 71 *Denver Univ. Law Rev.* 175, 185 (1993)).

91. Gerard B. Wegemer, *Thomas More on Statesmanship* (1996) 92.

92. Thomas More, *Utopia*, ed. & tr. H.V.S. Ogden (1949) 82-83: "I admit that not a few things in the manners and laws of the Utopians seemed very absurd to me.... I cannot agree with everything that he said."

93. Gerard B. Wegemer, *Thomas More: A Portrait Of Courage* (1995); Gerard B. Wegemer, *Thomas More on Statesmanship* (1996).

94. E-mail correspondence from Gerard B. Wegemer to Dwight G. Duncan (Mar. 13, 1996).

95. "In 562 A.D., the Council of Braga denied funeral rites to anyone who killed himself. A little more than a century later, in 693 A.D., the Council of Toledo declared that anyone who attempted suicide should be excommunicated." *Compassion in Dying*, 79 F.3d at 808 (citing Marzen, *supra* note 32, at 27-28). (In fact, there is no mention of the Council of Toledo in Marzen, and Marzen's discussion actually occurs on page 29.)

96. Gratian quotes St. Augustine, St. Jerome, and the Council of Braga as expressing virtually unqualified disapproval of suicide. See Gratian, *supra* note 85, at C. 23 q.5 cc.9-12. He introduces the canons by saying that "it is permitted by no authority of law for anyone to do away with himself." *Ibid.* at c.10. Translation by the authors of this Article.

97. *Ibid.* at c. 12. Translation by the authors of this article.

98. *Compassion in Dying*, 79 F.3d 808. Obviously, one could expound at length on the medieval authorities' condemnation of suicide. Judge Beezer's dissent quotes St. Thomas Aquinas as saying it is contrary to love of self, opposed to the community, and opposed to God. *Ibid.* at 845-46 (citing St. Thomas Aquinas, *Summa Theologiae*, eds. Fathers of the English Dominican Province (1947) 2:1465 *et seq.* Nor did such a view end with the Middle Ages. In the late eighteenth century Blackstone, whom Judge Beezer also quotes, treats suicide in a virtually identical manner. See *ibid.* at 846 (citing 4 William Blackstone, *Commentaries* *189).

99. *Compassion in Dying*, 79 F.3d at 808-09 (quoting Marzen, *supra* note 31, at 58-59, in turn quoting 2 Henry de Bracton, *On the Laws and Customs of England*, tr. Samuel E. Thorne, ed. George E. Woodbine (1968) 366, 424 (bracketed words added).

100. *Ibid.* at 807 (quoting Alvarez, *supra* n. 34, at 22-23).

101. *Ibid.* at 809.

102. Marzen, *supra* n. 32, at 57-58 (quoting *The Civil Law*, tr. Samuel P. Scott (1932) 9:129).

103. *Ibid.* at 58 (quoting Bracton, *supra* n. 99, at 423-24).

104. Marzen, *supra* n. 32, at 59 (emphases added).

105. *Ibid.*

106. See *Compassion in Dying*, 79 F.3d at 807; Marzen, *supra* n. 32, at 58.

107. *Dig.* 48.21.3.4 (Marcian, Accusers).

108. *Ibid.* at 48.21.3.

109. Marzen, *supra* n. 32, at 58 (quoting Scott, *supra* n. 102, at 129).

110. *Compassion in Dying*, 79 F.3d at 809.

111. *Ibid.* at 809.

112. *Cruzan v. Director, Mo. Dep't. of Health*, 497 U.S. 261, 294 (1990) (Scalia, J., concurring).

113. *Compassion in Dying*, 79 F.3d at 809.

114. *Ibid.*

115. Blackstone, *supra* n. 98, at *189-90 (first emphasis added).

116. See Stanley N. Katz, "Introduction" to *William Blackstone, Commentaries* (Univ. of Chicago Press, 1978) 1:1.

117. Bernard Bailyn, *The Ideological Origins of the American Revolution* (1992) 27.

118. See Forrest McDonald, *Novus Ordo Seclorum: The Intellectual Origins of the Constitution* (1985) at ix: "That the central argument of the Declaration is based mainly upon John Locke's *Second Treatise* is indisputable...."

119. *Ibid.* "Jefferson, as is well known, departed from Locke's trinity... and substituted 'the pursuit of happiness' for Locke's 'estate'."

120. *The Declaration of Independence*, para. 2 (U.S. 1776).

121. John Locke, *Two Treatises of Government*, ed. Peter Laslett (1988) 270-71 (third emphasis added).

122. *Ibid.* at 284.

123. *Ibid.* at 271.

124. *Ibid.* at 357.

125. *Ibid.* at 284.

126. Abraham Lincoln, Speech on the *Dred Scott* Decision (Springfield, Illinois) (June 26, 1857), in Lincoln, *supra* n. 89, at 396-400. Lincoln's insistence on equality in the inalienable right to life should be compared with the Ninth Circuit's remark that "even though the protection of life is one of the state's most important functions, the state's interest is dramatically diminished if the person it seeks to protect is terminally ill or permanently comatose and has expressed a wish that he be permitted to die.... When patients are no longer able to pursue liberty or happiness and do not wish to pursue life, the state's interest in forcing them to remain alive is clearly less compelling." *Compassion in Dying*, 79 F.3d at 820. The Second Circuit was even more blunt: "But what interest can the state possibly have in requiring the prolongation of a life that is all but ended? Surely, the state's interest lessens as the potential for life diminishes." *Quill*, 80 F.3d at 729. Note that the state's prohibition on helping to kill people at their actual or constructive request is described by these courts as "forcing them to remain alive" or "requiring the prolongation of a life."

127. Locke, *supra* n. 120, at 284.

128. *Compassion in Dying*, 79 F.3d at 809.

129. Marzen, *supra* n. 32, at 68-69 (quoting Zephaniah Swift, *A System of the Laws of the State of Connecticut* (n.p.: 1795-96) 305). Swift's use of the words "crime," "offender," "such crimes," and "this crime so abhorrent" make his attitude clear.

130. *Compassion in Dying*, 79 F.3d at 809.

131. *Compassion in Dying*, 79 F.3d at 809 n. 42 (citing Marzen, *supra* n. 32, at 76).

132. Marzen, *supra* n. 32, at 75-76.

133. *Compassion in Dying*, 79 F.3d at 809-10, citing *Campbell v. Supreme Conclave Improved Order Heptasophs*, 49 A. 550 (N.J. 1901).

134. Marzen, *supra* n. 32, at 84.

135. *Ibid.*

136. Burke Balch also writes under the name Thomas J. Balch, the name he used as a co-author of Marzen, *supra* n. 32.

137. Burke Balch, "Court Suicide Decision Distorts American History" in Nat'l Right To Life News (May 7, 1996) at 22 (citing *State v. Ehlers*, 119 A. 15 (1922). Judge Reinhardt mistakenly assumed that Marzen's reference to a 1901 New Jersey decision by "the state's highest court" meant the New Jersey Supreme Court; it did not. The highest court at that time was called the Court of Errors and Appeals.

138. This is not surprising, as that experience is not an advertisement for assisted suicide but more like a cautionary tale. On Oct. 7, 1933, in Berlin,
    [t]he Ministry of Justice in a detailed memorandum explaining the Nazi aims regarding the German penal code today announced its intention to authorize physicians to end the sufferings of incurable patients.
       The memorandum, still lacking the force of law, proposed that "it shall be made possible for physicians to end the tortures of incurable patients, upon request, in the interests of true humanity." ...According to the present plans of the Ministry of Justice, incurability would be determined not only by the attending physician, but also by two official doctors who would carefully trace the history of the case and personally examine the patient.... The legal question of who may request the application of euthanasia has not been definitely solved. The Ministry merely has proposed that either the patient himself shall "expressly and earnestly" ask it, or "in case the patient no longer is able to express his desire, his nearer relatives, acting from motives that do not contravene morals, so request."
Associated Press, "Nazis Plan to Kill Incurables to End Pain; German Religious Groups Oppose Move" in *N.Y. Times* (Oct. 8, 1933) at 1. One ought always to be diffident about invoking the Nazi example. In defense of the Ninth Circuit's omission, it could be argued that the Nazis are simply outside the Western tradition. Nevertheless, once the "taboo" against the direct taking of innocent human life is violated, the violation may not be so easy to cabin.

139. *Compassion in Dying*, 79 F.3d at 807 n.24.

140. *Ibid.* It is interesting that Judge Reinhardt does not mention the Eskimos, where suicide among the aged was once encouraged in order to preserve scarce resources. For clearly Reinhardt is not unsympathetic to such considerations: "[W]e are reluctant to say that, in a society in which the costs of protracted health care can be so exorbitant, it is improper for competent, terminally ill adults to take the economic welfare of their families and loved ones into consideration." *Ibid.* at 826.

141. Alan Watson, "Introduction to Law for Second-Year Law Students?" in *Journal of Legal Educ*ation 46 (1996) 430, 442.

142. John Finnis has demonstrated some of the ways in which, in recent constitutional adjudication, history and the truth have been abused. In *Roe*, the majority opinion relied on two historical articles that were

"demonstrably false," *see* Finnis, *supra* note 26, at 11; in *Webster*, 281 historians signed an amicus brief supporting a version of American attitudes towards abortion that was contradicted by the best evidence, including a book written by one of the signatories, see *ibi.* at 12-13; in the trial of *Evans v. Romer*, one well-known scholar offered highly misleading philological evidence as to classical Greek attitudes towards homosexuality. See *ibid.* at 19-35. Finnis regards these abuses of scholarship as "nothing less than attempts to get the American people to constitute themselves around conceptions of their own past, and the past of their civilization, that are profoundly untrue—worlds not of reality, which we in principle can share, but of fantasy, which can provide no lasting basis for community." *Ibid.* at 35. Finnis thinks it does matter whether or not constitutional rulings "are being promoted by means of deeply corrupt scholarship." *Ibid.* So do we.

FACING UP TO INFANTICIDE

J. Bottum

FOR OVER TWENTY YEARS the legality of abortion in America has been defended with an ethical system that most Americans now recognize as philosophically incoherent—a system based on taking the constitutionally acknowledged right to possess private property and translating it into rights of personal privacy and possession of the body. The system may have been forced upon abortion supporters originally by the Supreme Court's use of it in *Roe v. Wade*, but it has proved false in both the ways in which ethical systems prove false: as being both externally and internally inconsistent, that is, both contradicting what we know about human reproduction and contradicting itself.

And for these same twenty years defenders of unborn children have battled abortion primarily by pointing out the inconsistencies of the ethical system on which abortion defenders rely: the notion of the body as a possession is meaningless; the fact that a fetus is a human life is medically demonstrable; the language of rights, extended to the taking of life, simply contradicts itself.

As the American public's faith in the "rights-talk" of radical, Me-Generation individualism decreases, the pro-life movement has steadily advanced. Many Americans may still inhabit "the mushy middle," as it was called by Norma McCorvey (the "Jane Roe" of *Roe v. Wade*, who defected to a pro-life position). But that middle has substantially shifted toward the limiting of abortions, and some abortion proponents have begun to change their ground, seeking a new ethical system with which to defend unlimited abortion.

What the pro-life movement must face is that they may find what they're looking for. Though it is true that there are not many possible ethical systems, the history of philosophy reveals that there are more than one. And in the stern philosophies of the ancient world—a world that accepted slavery, infanticide, and gradations of human life—the pro-abortion movement may find the coherent ethics it currently lacks.

Since the 1970s abortion rhetoric has been dominated by euphemisms whose dishonesty and disingenuousness increase with each new medical technique for saving prematurely born children. By displaying sonograms, heart-beat monitors, and even the corpses of aborted children, pro-life activists have been able to employ the simple strategy of exposing the truth beneath "pro-choice" euphemisms. And though this relentless exposure is called pornography by pro-abortion activists, it has had its intended effect of leaving abortion rhetoric sounding increasingly heartless in response to America's million and a half abortions a year.

Some liberal writers and analysts have begun at last to recognize this. In an essay in the October 1995 issue of the *New Republic*, the well-known feminist Naomi Wolf asserted that abortion activists, by sticking to the old rhetorical lines, condemn their followers to "three destructive consequences—two ethical, one strategic: hardness of heart, lying, and political failure."[1] Only a month earlier, Peter Singer (the radical activist for animal rights) suggested in the London *Spectator* that we acknowledge that "the fetus is a living human being."[2]

Such suggestions are not entirely new. In the late sixties and early seventies, several liberals argued that true liberalism requires the rejection of abortion. But there were few on the Left willing to listen to such an argument in 1967, and there are fewer now, when support for abortion has became *the* test for liberal credentials. And if the tatters of the Left have inescapably tied themselves to the abortion license, general American culture may have as well. Supreme Court Justice Sandra Day O'Connor, though denounced by pro-life activists for her part in the 1992 *Planned Parenthood v. Casey* decision, was at least right when she observed that in the years since *Roe v. Wade* an entire generation has grown up expecting to be able to rely upon abortion to terminate not merely pregnancies resulting from rape or incest and pregnancies that threaten the life of the mother, but also pregnancies resulting from inattention or contraceptive failure and pregnancies that threaten a deformed child, an unwanted child, or even a child of the wrong gender.

This current entanglement with abortion is finally what distinguishes the essays by Naomi Wolf and Peter Singer from attempts in the late sixties and early seventies to speak honestly about abortion. Unlimited abortion is now the reality, and honesty about abortion's murderousness no longer necessarily means its rejection. Some supporters of abortion, having rejected the old, incoherent ethical system of privacy rights, are now willing to acknowledge that abortion kills babies. But they are willing to claim the necessity for allowing abortion anyway.

The traditional pro-life strategy of exposing pro-abortion euphemism relies on the tacit assumption that under any Jewish, Christian, or even post-Christian ethical system, the knowledge that it kills a living baby would suffice to end the practice of abortion. That assumption may no longer be true. Wolf tells the story of arguing, while she was pregnant, against an opponent of abortion and snapping at last in frustration, "Of course it's a baby. . . . And if I found myself in circumstances in which I had to make the terrible decision to end this life, then that would be between myself and God." Her opponent, as she tells the story, was silenced because she had at last said something that made sense to him. But the truth is more likely that she had at last said what penetrates to so fundamental a clash between ethical systems that any sort of argument becomes impossible. In his *Spectator* article entitled "Killing Babies Isn't Always Wrong," Peter Singer writes, "Pope John Paul II proclaims that the widespread acceptance of abortion is a mortal threat to the traditional moral order.... I sometimes think that he and I at least share the virtue of seeing clearly what is at stake in the debate."

If we are so entangled with the practice that legal and common abortion is now inescapable, and if we acknowledge that abortion kills, then we live in the tragic, redemptionless sort of world imagined by the Ancients from the Greek tragedians to the Roman Stoics—a world which had at various times, we must admit, an ethical system consistent both externally and internally, both with the commonly accepted facts of the universe and with itself. In moves that ought to have been predictable, Wolf and Singer both begin to seek a way to accept infanticide by re-creating, consciously or unconsciously, the stern philosophies of the ancient, pre-Christian world.

Wolf argues that pro-abortion rhetoric, by denying life to the unborn child and gravity to the act of killing it, has deprived women of a "moral framework" with which to understand abortion—and thus driven middle America to embrace the pro-life movement that has monopolized all moral discourse. Feminists need to admit, she asserts, many of the perfectly true points they are foolishly committed to disputing: that the fetus is a child, that the current abortion rate is a terrible social evil, that "pregnancy confounds Western philosophy's idea of the autonomous self, [for] the pregnant woman is in fact both a person in her body and a vessel." The blind adherence to privacy rights and "the refusal to use a darker and sterner and more honest moral rhetoric" have robbed women of a "sense of sin," and consequently of the possibility of atonement, grief, and healing.

Some philosophical and theological naivety seems inevitable even in otherwise well-educated writers nowadays—Wolf herself bemoans contemporary "religious illiteracy"—and it is perhaps unfair to complain about skewed uses of terms like "soul," "sin," "guilt," and "atonement" in what is admittedly a popular essay. And yet, all the elements are present in Wolf's analysis for a full-blown philosophical Stoicism and a Stoic acceptance of infanticide: not just the ethical elements of self-possession, resignation to a tragic world, and stern moral rhetoric, but all the metaphysical elements as well. When Wolf writes first of "what can only be called our souls," but then later in her essay calls it "'God' or 'soul'—or if you are secular and prefer it, 'conscience,'" she is not simply confounding philosophical terms, but aiming in an untrained way at the metaphysical equations that stand behind the Stoic worldview.

Peter Singer similarly aims toward Stoicism. The recognition that there are "living human beings whose lives may intentionally be terminated" means that abortion activists can "at last properly engage with the arguments of those opposed to abortion," he observes. The real question proponents of abortion should ask is, "Why—in the absence of religious beliefs about being made in the image of God, or having an immortal soul—should mere membership of the species *Homo sapiens* be crucial to whether the life of a being may or may not be taken?"

The sleight-of-hand in such a question is one that Americans have encountered so often, it almost doesn't bear mentioning: by fiat, religious belief—alone among beliefs—is prohibited from public discourse; by fiat, religious believers—alone among believers—are prohibited from employing in rational discourse the facts they hold about the universe. In Singer's question, however, there is also something Americans haven't often encountered, for he sees clearly that the Judeo-Christian prohibition against baby-killing is a tattered, incoherent, and indefensible ethical remnant, in the absence of Judeo-Christian religious belief. We must stoically resign ourselves, Singer argues, to an unredeemed and overpopulated world in which we have to kill useless and unwanted human beings.

The strategy of refusing euphemism has, in one sense, won the day. The facts about abortion are now acknowledged even by solidly liberal and feminist writers, and the incoherence and social disaster of a general ethics based on the right of privacy are now taken for granted by thoughtful analysts. The pro-life movement must not imagine, however, that it has thereby won the abortion debate. There exist philosophically coherent ethical systems that grant no sanctity to all grades of human life, ethical systems to which ancient history repeatedly testifies.

The proponents of abortion seeking a new ethics seem to imagine that admitting the facts will allow a real discussion to begin between the pro-abortion and pro-life movements. Without such honesty, Singer concludes his essay, "people on both sides of the debate will continue to argue past each other." But the truth is rather that an agreement that we share no fundamental ethical positions would mean the end of public discourse. The pro-life movement is undoubtedly still correct that most Americans consider infanticide something worse than a stern necessity. But the longer we live with abortion, the closer the day comes when all the supporters of abortion emerge from their fog of euphemism and incoherence to announce a fundamental rupture between ethical systems in America. The urgency to ban abortion is, of course, an urgency to save the four thousand babies it kills every day. But it is also an urgency to preserve an ethics that holds infanticide to be wrong.

NOTES

1. Naomi Wolf, "Out Bodies, Our Souls" in *New Republic* (Oct. 16, 1995) 26-35.
2. Peter Singer, *The Spectator* (Sept. 16, 1995).

MORE PEOPLE, GREATER WEALTH, MORE RESOURCES, HEALTHIER ENVIRONMENT

Julian L. Simon

INTRODUCTION

This is the economic history of humanity in a nutshell. From 2 million or 200,000 or 20,000 or 2,000 years ago until the 18th century there was slow growth in population, almost no increase in health or decrease in mortality, slow growth in the availability of natural resources (but not increased scarcity), increase in wealth for a few, and mixed effects on the environment. Since then there has been rapid growth in population due to spectacular decreases in the death rate, rapid growth in resources, widespread increases in wealth, and an unprecedently clean and beautiful living environment in many parts of the world along with a degraded environment in the poor and socialist parts of the world.

That is, more people and more wealth has correlated with more (rather than less) resources and a cleaner environment—just the opposite of what Malthusian theory leads one to believe. The task before us is to make sense of these mind-boggling happy trends.

The current gloom-and-doom about a "crisis" of our environment is all wrong on the scientific facts. Even the U.S. Environmental Protection Agency acknowledges that our air and water have been getting cleaner rather than dirtier in the past few decades. Every agricultural economist knows that the world's population has been eating ever-better since World War II. Every resource economist knows that all natural resources have been getting more available rather than more scarce, as shown by their falling prices over the decades and centuries. And every demographer knows that the death rate has been falling all over the world—life expectancy almost tripling in the rich countries in the past two centuries, and almost doubling in the poor countries in just the past four decades.

63

POPULATION GROWTH AND ECONOMIC DEVELOPMENT

The picture also is now clear that population growth does not hinder economic development. In the 1980ˢ there was a complete reversal in the consensus of thinking of population economists about the effects of more people. In 1986, the National Research Council and the National Academy of Sciences completely overturned its "official" view away from the earlier worried view expressed in 1971. It noted the absence of any statistical evidence of a negative connection between population increase and economic growth. And it said that "The scarcity of exhaustible resources is at most a minor restraint on economic growth."[1] This U-turn by the scientific consensus of experts on the subject has gone unacknowledged by the press, the anti-natalist environmental organizations, and the agencies that foster population-control abroad.

LONG-RUN TRENDS POSITIVE

Here is my central assertion: Almost every economic and social change or trend points in a positive direction, as long as we view the matter over a reasonably long period of time.

For proper understanding of the important aspects of an economy we should look at the long-run trends. But the short-run comparisons—between the sexes, age groups, races, political groups, which are usually purely relative—make more news. To repeat, just about every important long-run measure of human welfare shows improvement over the decades and centuries, in the United States as well as in the rest of the world. And there is no persuasive reason to believe that these trends will not continue indefinitely.

Would I bet on it? For sure. I'll bet a week's or month's pay—anything I win goes to pay for more research—that just about any trend pertaining to material human welfare will improve rather than get worse. You pick the comparison and the year.

Let's quickly review a few data on how human life has been doing, beginning with the all-important issue, life itself.

THE CONQUEST OF TOO-EARLY DEATH

The most important and amazing demographic fact—the

greatest human achievement in history, in my view—is the decrease in the world's death rate. Figure 1 portrays the history human life expectancy at birth. It took thousands of years to increase life expectancy at birth from just over 20 years to the high twenties about 1750. Then about 1750 life expectancy in the richest countries suddenly took off and tripled in about two centuries. In just the past two centuries, the length of life you could expect for your baby or yourself in the advanced countries jumped from less than 30 years to perhaps 75 years. What greater event has humanity witnessed than this conquest of premature death in the rich countries? It is this decrease in the death rate that is the cause of there being a larger world population nowadays than in former times.

FIGURE 1: HISTORY OF HUMAN LIFE EXPECTANCY
AT BIRTH (3000 B.C.E.—2000 C.E.)

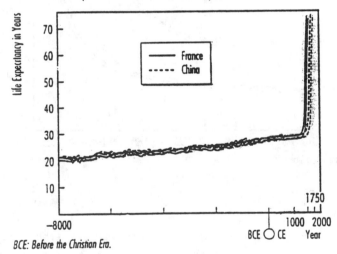

BCE: *Before the Christian Era.*

Then starting well after World War II, the length of life you could expect in the poor countries has leaped upwards by perhaps fifteen or even twenty years since the 1950⁵, caused by advances in agriculture, sanitation, and medicine. (See Figure 2)

Let's put it differently. In the 19th century the planet Earth could sustain only one billion people. Ten thousand years ago, only four million could keep themselves alive. Now five billion people are living longer and more healthily than ever before, on average. The increase in the world's population represents our victory over death.

FIGURE 2: FEMALE EXPECTATION OF LIFE AT BIRTH

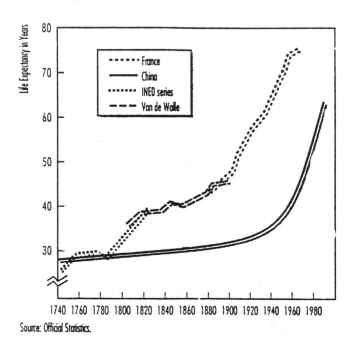

Source: Official Statistics.

Here arises a crucial issue of interpretation: One would expect lovers of humanity to jump with joy at this triumph of human mind and organization over the raw killing forces of nature. Instead, many lament that there are so many people alive to enjoy the gift of life. And it is this worry that leads them to approve the Indonesian, Chinese and other inhumane programs of coercion and denial of personal liberty in one of the most precious choices a family can make—the number of children that it wishes to bear and raise.

THE DECREASING SCARCITY OF NATURAL RESOURCES

Throughout history, the supply of natural resources always has worried people. Yet the data clearly show that natural resource scarcity—as measured by the economically-meaningful indicator of cost or price—has been decreasing rather than increasing in the long run for all raw materials, with only temporary exceptions from time to time. That is, availability has been increasing. Consider copper, which is representative of all the metals. In Figure 3 we see the price relative to wages since 1801. The cost of a ton is only about a tenth now of what it was two hundred years ago.

FIGURE 3: COPPER PRICES INDEXED BY WAGES

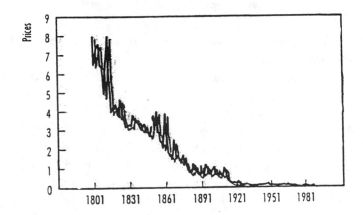

This trend of falling prices of copper has been going on for a very long time. In the 18th century B.C.E. in Babylonia under Hammurabi—almost 4000 years ago—the price of copper was about a thousand times its price in the U.S. now relative to wages. At the time of the Roman Empire the price was about a hundred times the present price.

In Figure 4 we see the price of copper relative to the consumer price index. Everything that we buy—pens, shirts, tires—has been getting cheaper over the years because we know how to make them cheaper, especially during the past 200 years. Even so, the extraordinary fact is that natural resources have been getting cheaper even faster than consumer goods.

FIGURE 4: COPPER PRICES DIVIDED BY CPI

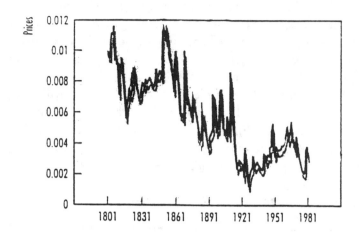

So by any measure, natural resources have getting more available rather than more scarce.

Regarding oil, the shocking price rises during the 1970ˢ and 1980ˢ were not caused by growing scarcity in the world supply. And indeed, the price of petroleum in inflation-adjusted dollars has returned to levels about where they were before the politically-induced increases, and the price of of gasoline is about at the historic low and still falling. Concerning energy in general, there is no reason to believe that the supply of energy is finite, or that the price of energy will not continue its long-run decrease forever. I realize that it sounds weird to say that the supply of energy is not finite or limited; for the full argument, please see my book, *The Ulimate Resource.*[2] (Science is only valuable when it arrives at knowledge different than common sense.)

FOOD—"A BENIGN TREND"

Food is an especially important resource. The evidence is particularly strong for food that we are on a benign trend despite rising population. The long-run price of food relative to wages is now only perhaps a tenth as much as it was in 1800 in the U. S. Even relative to consumer-products the price of grain is down, due to increased productivity, just as with all other primary products.

Famine deaths due to insufficient food-supply have decreased even in absolute terms, let alone relative to population, in the past century, a matter which pertains particularly to the poor countries. Per-person food-consumption is up over the last 30 years. And there are no data showing that the bottom of the income-scale is faring worse, or even has failed to share in the general improvement, as the average has improved.

Africa's food production per person is down, but by 1996 almost no one any longer claims that Africa's suffering results from a shortage of land or water or sun. The cause of hunger in Africa is a combination of civil wars and collectivization of agriculture, which periodic droughts have made more murderous.

Consider agricultural land as an example of all natural resources. Though many people consider land to be a special kind of resource, it is subject to the same processes of human creation as other natural resources. The most important fact about agricultural land is that less and less of it is needed as the decades pass. This idea is utterly counter-intuitive. It seems entirely obvious that a growing world population would need larger amounts of farmland. But the title of a remarkable prescient article in 1951 by Theodore Schultz tells the story: "The Declining Economic Importance of Land."[3]

The increase in actual and potential productivity per unit of land have grown much faster than population, and there is sound reason to expect this trend to continue. Therefore, there is less and less reason to worry about the supply of land. Though the stock of usable land seems fixed at any moment, it is constantly being increased—at a rapid rate in many cases—by the clearing of new land or reclamation of wasteland. Land also is constantly being enhanced by increasing the number of crops grown per year on each unit of land and by increasing the yield per crop with better farming methods and with chemical fertilizer. Last but not least, land is created anew where there was no land.

THE ONE SCARCE FACTOR

There is only one important resource which has shown a

trend of increasing scarcity rather than increasing abundance. That resource is the most important of all—human beings. Yes, there are more people on earth now than ever before. But if we measure the scarcity of people the same way that we measure the scarcity of other economic goods—by how much we must pay to obtain their services—we see that wages and salaries have been going up all over the world, in poor countries as well as in rich countries. The amount that you must pay to obtain the services of a barber or a cook has risen in India, just as the price of a barber or cook—or economist—has risen in the United States over the decades. This increase in the price of people's services is a clear indication that people are becoming more scarce even though there are more of us.

About pollution now: Surveys show that the public believes that our air and water have been getting more polluted in recent years. The evidence with respect to air indicates that pollutants have been declining, especially the main pollutant, particulates. (See Figure 5). With respect to water, the proportion of monitoring sites in the U.S. with water of good drinkability has increased since the data began in 1961. (Figure 6).

Every forecast of the doomsayers has turned out flat wrong. Metals, foods, and other natural resources have become more available rather than more scarce throughout the centuries. The famous Famine of 1975 forecast by the Paddock brothers—that we would see millions of famine deaths in the U.S. on television in the 1970s—was followed instead by gluts in agricultural markets. Paul Ehrlich's primal scream about "What will we do when the [gasoline] pumps run dry?" was followed by gasoline cheaper than since the 1930s. The Great Lakes are not dead; instead they offer better sport-fishing than ever. The main pollutants, especially the particulates which have killed people for years, have lessened in our cities. (Socialist countries are a different and tragic environmental story, however!)

FIGURE 5: NATIONAL AMBIENT CONCENTRATIONS OF POLLUT-
ANTS: USA, 1960-90

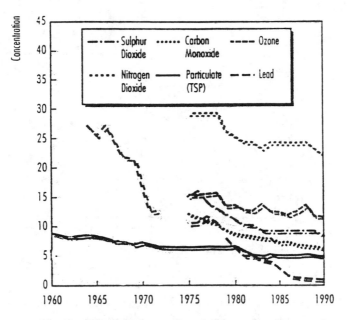

Source: *Council on Environmental Quality,* Environmental Quality, 22nd Annual Report, 1992,
p. 276. Council on Environmental Quality, Environmental Quality 1981, 12th Annual Report,
1981, p. 243. Sulphur: 1964 thru 1972: EPA (1973): 32 stations.

DAMAGE OF WRONG FORECASTS

The wrong forecasts of shortages of copper and other metals
have not been harmless, however. They have helped cause
economic disasters for mining companies and for the poor
countries which depend upon mining, by misleading them
with unsound expectations of increased prices; similarly with
airplane design, U.S. government-mandated mileage-per-gallon
standards (CAFE) have misdirected valuable resources. But
nothing has reduced the doomsayers' credibility with the press
or their command over the funding resources of the federal
government.

FIGURE 6: NATIONAL AMBIENT WATER QUALITY IN RIVERS AND STREAMS, USA, 1973-90: FECAL CALIFORNIA BACTERIA (200+ CELLS PER 100 ML)

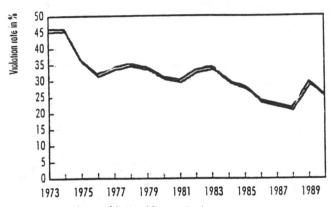

Source: *Statistical Abstracts of the United States, various issues.*

Let's dramatize these sets of changes with a single anecdote. The trend toward a better life can be seen in most of our own families if we look. For example, I have mild asthma. Recently I slept in a home where there was a dog, and in the middle of the night I woke with a bad cough and shortness of breath. When I realized that it was caused by the dog-dander, I took out my twelve-dollar pocket-inhaler, good for 3000 puffs, and took one puff. Within ten minutes my lungs were clear. A small miracle. Forty years ago I would have been sleepless and miserable all night, and I would have had to give up the squash-playing that I love so much because exercise causes my worst asthma in the absence of an inhaler. ...Or diabetes. If your child had diabetes a hundred years ago, you had to watch helplessly as the child went blind and died early. Now injections, or even pills, can give the child almost as long and healthy a life as other children. ...Or glasses. Centuries ago you had to give up reading when your eyes got dim as you got to be 40 or 50. Now you can buy magnifying glasses at the drugstore for nine dollars. And you can even wear contact lenses for eye-problems and keep your vanity intact. Is there not some condition in your family that in earlier times would have been a lingering misery or a tragedy, that nowadays our increasing knowledge has rendered easily bearable?

With respect to population-growth: A dozen competent statistical studies, starting in 1967 with an analysis by Nobel prizewinner Simon Kuznets, agree that there is no negative statistical relationship between economic growth and population-growth. There is strong reason to believe that more people have a positive effect in the long run.

Population-growth does not lower the standard of living—all the evidence agrees. And the evidence supports the view that population-growth raises it in the long run.

Incidentally, it was those statistical studies that converted me in about 1968 from working in favor of population-control to the point of view that I hold today. I certainly did not come to my current view for any political or religious or ideological reason.

The basic method is to gather data on each country's rate of population-growth and its rate of economic growth, and then to examine whether—looking at all the data in the sample together—the countries with high population-growth rates have economic growth rates lower than average, and countries with low population-growth-rates have economic growth rates higher than average. All the studies agree in concluding that this is not so; there is no correlation between economic growth and population-growth in the intermediate run.

Of course one can adduce cases of countries that seemingly are exceptions to the pattern. It is the genius of statistical inference, however, to enable us to draw valid generalizations from samples that contain such wide variations in behavior. The exceptions can be useful in alerting us to possible avenues for further analysis, but as long as they are only exceptions, they do not prove that the generalization is not meaningful or useful.

POPULATION-DENSITY FAVORS ECONOMIC GROWTH

The research-wise person may wonder whether population-density is a more meaningful variable than population-growth. And indeed, such studies have been done. And again, the statistical evidence directly contradicts the common-sense conventional wisdom. If you make a chart with population-density on the horizontal axis and either the income-level or the rate of change of income on the vertical axis, you will see that higher density is associated with better rather than poorer economic results.

You can check for yourself: fly over Hong Kong—just a few decades ago a place seemingly without prospects because of insoluble resource-problems—and you will marvel at the astounding collection of modern high-rise apartments and office buildings. Take a ride on its excellent smooth-flowing highways for an hour or two, and you will realize that a very dense concentration of human beings does not prevent comfortable existence and exciting economic expansion—as long as the economic system gives individuals the freedom to exercise their talents and to take advantage of opportunities. And the experience of Singapore demonstrates that Hong Kong is not unique. Two such examples do not prove the case, of course. But these dramatic illustrations are backed by the evidence from the aggregate sample of countries, and hence do not mislead us.

(Hong Kong is a special thrill for me because I first saw it in 1955 when I went ashore from a U. S. Navy destroyer. At the time I felt great pity for the thousands who slept every night on the sidewalks or on small boats. It then seemed clear to me, as it must have to almost every observer, that it would be impossible for Hong Kong to surmount its problems—huge masses of impoverished people without jobs, total lack of exploitable natural resources, more refugees pouring across the border each day. But upon returning in 1983, I saw bustling crowds of healthy, vital people full of hope and energy. No cause for pity now.

The most important benefit of population-size and growth is the increase it brings to the stock of useful knowledge. Minds matter economically as much as, or more than, hands or mouths. Progress is limited largely by the availability of trained workers. The more people who enter our population by birth or immigration, the faster will be the rate of progress of our material and cultural civilization.

Here we need a qualification that tends to get overlooked: I do not say that all is well everywhere, and I do not predict that all will be rosy in the future. Children are hungry and sick; people live out lives of physical or intellectual poverty, and lack of opportunity; war or some new pollution may finish us off. What I am saying is that for most relevant economic matters I have checked, the aggregate trends are improving rather than deteriorating.

Also, I don't say that a better future happens automatically or without effort. It will happen because women and men will struggle with problems with muscle and mind, and will probably overcome, as people have overcome in the past—*if the social and economic system gives them opportunity to do so.*

THE EXPLANATION OF THESE AMAZING TRENDS

Now we need some theory to explain how it can be that economic welfare grows along with population, rather than humanity being reduced to misery and poverty as population grows.

The Malthusian theory of increasing scarcity, based on supposedly-fixed resources—the theory that the doomsayers rely upon—runs exactly contrary to the data over the long sweep of history. Therefore it makes sense to prefer another theory.

The theory that fits the facts very well is this: More people, and increased income, cause problems in the short run. Short-run scarcity raises prices. This presents opportunity, and prompts the search for solutions. In a free society, solutions are eventually found. And in the long run the new developments leave us better off than if the problems had not arisen.

To put it differently, in the short-run, more consumers mean less of the fixed available stock of goods to be divided among more people. And more workers laboring with the same fixed current stock of capital mean that there will be less output per worker. The latter effect, known as "the law of diminishing returns," is the essence of Malthus' theory as he first set it out.

But if the resources with which people work are not fixed over the period being analyzed, then the Malthusian logic of diminishing returns does not apply. And the plain fact is that, given some time to adjust to shortages, the resource-base does not remain fixed. People create more resources of all kinds.

When we take a long-run view, the picture is different, and considerably more complex, than the simple short-run view of more people implying lower average-income. In the very long run, more people almost surely imply more available resources and a higher income for everyone.

I suggest you test this idea against your own knowledge: Do you think that our standard of living would be as high as it is now if the population had never grown from about four million human beings perhaps ten thousand years ago? I don't think we'd now have electric light or gas heat or autos or penicillin or travel to the moon or our present life-expectancy of over seventy years at birth in rich countries, in comparison to the life-expectancy of 20 to 25 years at birth in earlier eras, if population had not grown to its present numbers.

SCARCITY AND DISCOVERY

Consider this example of the process by which people wind up with increasing availability rather than decreasing availability of resources. England was full of alarm in the 1600s at an impending shortage of energy due to the deforestation of the country for firewood. People feared a scarcity of fuel for both heating and for the iron industry. This impending scarcity led to the development of coal.

Then in the mid-1800s the English came to worry about an impending coal crisis. The great English economist, Jevons, calculated that a shortage of coal would bring England's industry to a standstill by 1900; he carefully assessed that oil could never make a decisive difference. Triggered by the impending scarcity of coal (and of whale oil, whose story comes next) ingenious profit-minded people developed oil into a more desirable fuel than coal ever was. And in 1990 we find England exporting both coal and oil.

Another element in the story: Because of increased demand due to population-growth and increased income, the price of whale oil for lamps jumped in the 1840ˢ, and the U.S. Civil War pushed it even higher, leading to a whale oil "crisis." This provided incentive for enterprising people to discover and produce substitutes. First came oil from rapeseed, olives, linseed, and camphene oil from pine trees. Then inventors learned how to get coal oil from coal. Other ingenious persons produced kerosene from the rock oil that seeped to the surface, a product so desirable that its price then rose from $.75 a gallon to $2.00. This high price stimulated enterprisers to focus on the supply of oil, and finally Edwin L. Drake brought in his famous well in Titusville, Pennsylvania. Learning how to refine the oil took a while. But in a few years there were hundreds of small refiners in the U.S., and soon the bottom fell out of the whale oil market, the price falling from $2.50 or more at its peak around 1866 to well below a dollar. And in 1993 we see Great Britain exporting both coal and oil.

Here we should note that it was not the English government that developed coal or oil, because governments are not effective developers of new technology. Rather, it was individual entrepreneurs who sensed the need, saw opportunity, used all kinds of available information and ideas, made lots of false starts which were very costly to many of those individuals but not to others, and eventually arrived at coal as a viable fuel—because there were enough independent individuals investigating the matter for at least some of them to arrive at sound ideas and methods. And this happened in the context of a competitive enterprise system that worked to produce what was needed by the public. And the entire process of impending shortage and new solution left us better off than if the shortage problem had never arisen.

THE ROLE OF ECONOMIC FREEDOM

Here we must address another crucial element in the economics of resources and population—the extent to which the political-social-economic system provides personal freedom from government-coercion. Skilled persons require an appropriate social and economic framework that provides incentives for working hard and taking risks, enabling their talents to flower and come to fruition. The key elements of such a framework are economic liberty, respect for property, and fair and sensible rules of the market that are enforced equally for all.

The world's problem is not too many people, but lack of political and economic freedom. Powerful evidence comes from an extraordinary natural experiment that occurred starting in the 1940ˢ with three pairs of countries that have the same culture and history, and had much the same standard of living when they split apart after World War II—East and West Germany, North and South Korea, Taiwan and China. In each case the centrally planned communist country began with less population "pressure," as measured by density per square kilometer, than did the market-directed economy. And the communist and non-communist countries also started with much the same birth rates.

The market-directed economies have performed much better economically than the centrally-planned economies. The economic- political system clearly was the dominant force in the results of the three comparisons. This powerful explanation of economic development cuts the ground from under population-growth as a likely explanation of the speed of nations' economic development.

THE ASTOUNDING SHIFT IN THE SCHOLARLY CONSENSUS

So far we have been discussing the factual evidence. But in 1996 there is an important new element not present twenty years ago. The scientific community of scholars who study population-economics now agrees with almost all of what is written ahove. The statements made above do not represent a single lone voice, but rather the current scientific consensus.

The conclusions offered earlier about agriculture and resources and demographic trends have always represented the consensus of economists in those fields. And now the consensus of population-economists also is now not far from what is written here.

In 1986, the U.S. National Research Council and the U.S. National Academy of Sciences published a book on population-growth and economic development prepared by a prestigious scholarly group. This "official" report reversed almost completely the frightening conclusions of the previous 1971 NAS report. "Population growth at most a minor factor...." "The scarcity of exhaustible resources is at most a minor constraint on economic growth," it now says. It found benefits of additional people as well as costs.[4]

A host of review-articles by distinguished economic demographers in the past decade have confirmed that this "revisionist" view is indeed consistent with the scientific evidence, though not all the writers would go as far as I do in pointing out the positive long-run effects of population-growth. The consensus is more toward a "neutral" judgment. But this is a huge change from the earlier judgment that population-growth is economically detrimental.

By 1996, anyone who confidently asserts that population-growth damages the economy must turn a blind eye to the scientific evidence.

SUMMARY AND CONCLUSION

In the short run, all resources are limited. An example of such a finite resource is the amount of space allotted to me. The longer run, however, is a different story. The standard of living has risen along with the size of the world's population since the beginning of recorded time. There is no convincing economic reason why these trends toward a better life should not continue indefinitely.

The key theoretical idea is this: The growth of population and of income create actual and expected shortages, and hence lead to price run-ups. A price-increase represents an opportunity that attracts profit-minded entrepreneurs to seek new ways to satisfy the shortages. Some fail, at cost to themselves. A few succeed, and the final result is that we end up better off than if the original shortage-problems had never arisen. That is, we need our problems though this does not imply that we should purposely create additional problems for ourselves.

I hope that you will now agree that the long-run outlook is for a more abundant material life rather than for increased scarcity, in the United States and in the world as a whole.

Of course, such progress does not come about automatically. And my message certainly is not one of complacency. In this I agree with the doomsayers—that our world needs the best efforts of all humanity to improve our lot. I part company with them in that they expect us to come to a bad end despite the efforts we make, whereas I expect a continuation of humanity's history of successful efforts. And I believe that their message is self-fulfilling, because if you expect your efforts to fail because of inexorable natural limits, then you are likely to feel resigned; and therefore to literally resign. But if you recognize the possibility—in fact the probability—of success, you can tap large reservoirs of energy and enthusiasm.

Adding more people causes problems, but people are also the means to solve these problems. The main fuel to speed the world's progress is our stock of knowledge, and the brakes are (a) our lack of imagination, and (b) unsound social regulations of these activities. The ultimate resource is people—especially skilled, spirited, and hopeful young people endowed with liberty—who will exert their wills and imaginations for their own benefit, and so inevitably they will benefit not only themselves but the rest of us as well.

NOTES

1. National Research Council, Committee on Population, and Working Group on Population Growth and Economic Development. *Population Growth and Economic Development: Policy Questions* (Washington, D.C.: National Academy Press, 1986).

2. J. L. Simon, *The Ultimate Resource 2* (Princeton: Princeton Univ. Press, revised edition, 1996 [1981]).

3. T. W. Schultz, "The Declining Economic Importance of Land" in *Economic Journal* 61 (1951) 725-40.

4. National Research Council, *op. cit.*

THE VALUE OF LIFE

James W. Carey

IN THE EARLY 1960S Julian Simon convinced me that the dire conclusions of population "experts," including the belief that we were at sometime in the future likely to squeeze one another to death, had little scientific foundation and no economic warrant. I had come to a similar belief, namely, that we were being seriously led astray by tracts such as Paul Ehrlich's *The Population Bomb*,[1] on the basis of moral and spiritual considerations. Consequently, I was greatly disturbed by our attempt to bring these arguments before Catholic students at the Newman Club at the University of Illinois. Our presentation on the value of life, argued on both economic and moral grounds, met much resistance, even some hostility. Moreover, the response was thoughtlessly prejudicial, made without reference to scientific evidence and without consideration of what I took to be traditional Catholic doctrine and belief. This dismaying conclusion led me to try to set out a simple enunciation of what you might call lay Catholic beliefs in ways that partially paralleled Julian Simon's scientific arguments. My contention went (and still largely goes) roughly as follows.

We have been subjected, courtesy of Planned Parenthood, the Zero Population Growth movement, and other such groups, to a concerted campaign of population-control designed to constrain the size of the population of the United States and of other counties. That campaign has had a strong impact on Americans generally as well as on American Catholics. In presenting their case against population-growth these groups rely upon some exceedingly shaky scientific evidence. But, more to the point, they call into question the notion that life itself is a value, a value superordinate to other values that animate social life. This value—the value of life itself, unmodified and uncompromised—has been the center of Catholic experience, Catholic belief, and Catholic liturgy. The Church, as a community of people, can perform a spiritual as well as a social service in these times by preaching to Catholics and to non-Catholics alike the value of life as the central value in human affairs.

But is life the central value in Catholic thought? I always presumed that it was. The admonition to "be fruitful and multiply" was part of a shared heritage of Judaism and Christianity, and it is more than an incitement to copulation or domination. Life is the greatest gift of God to man. The ability to create life is God's noblest bestowal upon us, and, in turn, the creation of life the greatest gift we can return to God. It is, I think, the central belief of Catholicism: not only did the Word become flesh, but in return the flesh became word. However mean or dispirited in a material sense, life remains the source of awe, mystery, and joy.

And it is precisely this sense of life that the population-control movement attempts to undercut. By playing on a modern reversal of meanings, such movements find that life, as it is ordinarily lived, is awful rather than awe-full. In the literature of this movement, there is a frequent metaphor in which life consists of "worms in a bucket." People in groups and crowds are described as "massed" and "teeming." They are depicted as consuming the earth: eating, fornicating, defecating, and despoiling. Such people are rarely seen as spiritual creatures, creatures capable of love, nobility, and friendship, capable of contributing to a shared life. This image and this metaphor have taken over the discussion of population: an image of massed humanity and a metaphor of animality. Its implicit commitment is to the belief that life is only really lived in American communities at a particular standard of living; others, living at "lower" standards of living are less alive, less spiritual, less human. This image and metaphor, and the beliefs that they harbor, are contrary to Catholic experience and values.

I am hardly one to discuss the Church's doctrine on these matters. But I have looked at John Noonan's histories of Catholic attitudes toward contraception and abortion, and I believe that his work is consistent with the mainstream of Catholic thought. Discussions of contraception, abortion, and infanticide arose within a Catholic community living amidst the Roman Empire, where these were widespread practices. "By these signs they shall know us." Christians distinguished themselves from the Roman community by the reverence they expressed for life. Early Christians opposed these ordinary practices of Roman life, not only because they were morally repugnant in themselves but because they sinned against a larger conception of human nature and human value. It should be remembered that the central iconography of the early Church was not the crucifixion. It should also be remembered that an emphasis on death does not preclude—in fact, it often discloses—an intense interest in life: metaphorically, through death into life. Not until the tenth century does the crucifixion move from a marginal to a central place in Christian iconography. Early Christian art is concerned with healing, miracles, and hopeful aspects of the faith such as the Ascension and the Resurrection. In this respect, the focus of church art and liturgy was a direct expression of the force of life itself: growth, healing, exfoliation. To many modern minds, including some Catholics, this belief now seems naive and parochial.

The early Church, the doctrinal Church, was drawn to a stand on contraception and abortion because these practices pointed beyond themselves toward a value at the root of the Christian community: the value of life itself and the supreme position of this value relative to those other clamorous values with which it has always struggled: wealth, power, success, domination. But to discover the value of life in Catholic experience and belief, one needs to look beyond the doctrinal Church to the living community. In an exchange of letters between John Henry Cardinal Newman and Sir James Stephens, Stephens implores Newman to take up the attack against the Utilitarians, "the most subtle enemy which Christianity has ever had." Newman replies something to the effect that Stephens had it wrong: the Utilitarians attacked the doctrines of the Church, but the Church was not principally her doctrines. It is in the Church of sacraments and tradition, the Church as community, that one encounters the value of life. No one, let us remember, ever joined the Church and only few leave it because of a conflict over abstract doctrine. One joins and stays with the Church because of what one encounters sacramentally: the actual physical exchange through taste, touch, and ear with the Godhead, that sacramental realization and promise that one will come to know life in spiritual community. These central sacramental symbols are precisely about life itself. To put it this way—the only way possible in discursive prose—is immediately to distort the matter. The "idea of life" is never experienced as an "idea" about anything. The Church is not about ideas. Life is experienced through touch, taste, and sight as an immediately apprehensible truth and reality. It is not a doctrine to be debated or a truth to be realized by the methods of formal philosophy.

There are two ways of losing sight of the central place that life holds as a value in the Church. The first is to become preoccupied by the connection of the central symbols of ritual to death. On Passion Sunday, on Ash Wednesday, and on Good Friday one is directly reminded of the power of death. But one cannot be interested in life without also being interested in death. (It is the attempt to deny both that is so troubling in modern culture.) One is merely the reverse of the other. Those who find life the ultimate value will also, at least in general, be intensely interested in death: in the special meanings and possibilities that the shadow of death casts back upon life.

The second way to miss the point of the living Church is to assume that life is a central value only insofar as it is spiritual life that we are discussing, to assume that spiritual life has no direct, intrinsic connection and linkage to human, corporeal life. Yet, the most attractive figure in the modern Church, St. Francis, contradicts such a view, and his immense influence stems from his capacity to blend the spiritual and the natural. His joyful prayers and canticles celebrate the world he so happily abjured.

Whenever life is presented in the liturgy of the Catholic community, spiritual life and human life are happily interfused. One does not live spiritually by casting up a world of forms independent of the concretely human. In the liturgy, therefore, there is a constant, reiterated presentation of the spiritual and the natural fused, but not transcended, in metaphor: "it will become for us the bread of life," "by rising from the dead he destroyed death and restored life," "the resurrection of the dead and the life of the world to come," "the Lord and Giver of life."

The same emphasis is found in the liturgical calendar, which fixed the beginning of the year in Advent, like the beginning of life in pregnancy. Life is seen as human and divine at Christmastide, and as if to punctuate the relation of humanity and divinity, the Annunciation is placed nine months before the birth of Christ. The entire liturgical year pivots about this central event of birth.

These values, of course, were never exclusively Catholic. The Church in its early years attempted to vivify pagan celebrations of life by deepening and widening their spiritual significance. The ancient practices of bouncing seeds off the buttocks of a woman during planting or throwing the same seeds at the womb of a bride testifies eloquently to the longstanding reverence for life and the capacity for so-called primitive peoples to see life in a spiritual context. Contemporary people are so often divorced from this structure of feeling that they can see in the central symbols of primitive art—the representation of female genitals—only superstition or eroticism or nascent pornography. But if one is part of a people who revere life, who find it the central, mysterious principle of existence, who see it manifest in the regenerative, creative power of nature, the primal linkage of the self and the world, then how better to represent this mystery and belief in potent and dramatic form than in the sexual organs. The breast engorged with milk is the gift of nature that sustains the gift of life.

Catholic tradition infused these pagan practices with the personage of Christ and Mary: Mother as creator and child as the gift of life. From the personage derives the central core of Catholic belief: that it is good to increase life, to share it with as many as can partake of its banquet. The value is not thoughtless; it incorporates a prudential world of limitation and complication. Yet, within that recognition is a commitment to the vocation of life.

A brief passage from a book at once intensely Catholic and deeply agnostic, one of the greatest books written in English in contemporary times, William Gibson's *A Mass for the Dead*,[2] brings home this commitment to life in unusually vivid terms. Gibson wrote his "mass" as a substitute for offering one, and the sections of the book bear such titles as "*Sanctus*," "*Pater Noster*," "*Confiteor*," "*Dies Ira[e]*," and "*Ite, Missa Est*." In a section entitled "*Kyrie*" he writes of his dead uncle and of the relationship of his uncle to his own children:

It is my uncle's shadow that falls upon my boys. The sense of mortality irks them at odd moments, and sleepless at bedtime one boy invites me to "figure out a way" he need not die, and I think how the animal wants to live; sitting at his hip I say he will be immortal in his son as I am in mine, which satisfied neither of us....

But when he is asleep, and I am out on the hill for my nightly count of stars, I think, is this townful of roofs not a miracle? I can tell my son how we have dug for the forgotten hands and surmised a million centuries that crept by the beast living isolate in caves; only yesterday he perceived that in bands he might overcome the mammoth and changed wilderness into cities;

and he did not rape, homicide, plunder, incest, cannibalism; he laid down another imperative, it was the tool he invented chief of all tools, and it moved the earth. He called it conscience, a knowing together, and I can tell my boy it is our warranty of human life, which houses us under the hopes of these roofs.

Tonight the wind is contaminated; on other roofs in each country men are measuring the fall of the shadow, strontium, carbon, cesium, across the loins of every child.... Murder enough is around me on this hill, mole, snake, owl, and I make this eleison to the stars.... Now, as before it is outgrow or die.... And faint in the roar of the foundries I hear again the feet of my father walking the streets of the city that year, with his brother dead, when... he marked on the calendar for the wife and kids his vow to outgrow, and taught me the animal wants to live.

It is his eleison I make. Have mercy upon my increase. And thus saith God himself that formed the earth and made it; he hath established it, he created it not in vain, he formed it to be inhabited.

Not in vain, but to be inhabited, to be filled with life; this is the essence of Catholic life as I understand it. An essence consistent, as Julian Simon has argued, with the laws of economics, but more to the point, consistent with the essence of the Christian admonition: "I have that you may have life and have it abundantly."

As a Catholic I am worried that this essence is draining out of the Catholic community, partly because it has been under savage assault from those who find life an affront to nature and mechanics and, paradoxically enough, from those as well who center on the problem of abortion and on the Right to Life movement. We are the ultimate heirs, the contemporary proprietors, of a grand and noble vision of the value of life and that is what we must keep firmly in mind. Life is the issue, social, moral, and theological—not the selling of condoms in Connecticut or the performance of abortion in New York. Abortion is only a concern in terms of the larger theological commitment to what is behind and transcendent to it: life itself in all its enigma and complexity. Abortion may, I fear, stand in the same relationship to Catholic history as did the temperance movement to Protestant history: an episode in which a people win a battle but lose a culture. Protestants, too, tried to reform a community not by witness and humility, but by assertiveness and constitutional amendment. In struggling so hard with the dragon, they became a kind of dragon themselves. In order to secure legislative and congressional acceptance, Catholics may have to redefine their entire culture so much that they forget the historical meaning and experience that animates their concern and thus win a merely pyrrhic victory. Catholics must largely accept the secular definitions of life in order to struggle politically for the "right to life." But the right to life is not just a constitutional right, not a legal right, not even a natural right in the Western political sense. Life, its growth and development and enhancement, as a gift from God and for God is the Catholic value, and no court, only a community of faith and belief, will adequately protect it.

The great contribution which the Catholic community has to make to contemporary life is not to struggle in the courts and legislatures about technical definitions of whether or not the fetus is protected by the first ten amendments, although in simple justice I think that it should be. Its real contribution comes from the commitment, as witnessed presentation, that life is the central value in human experience. Catholics are the only group (the Latter Day Saints excepted) in which this value, this sense, is a known remnant of historical experience and living theological concern. The nurture of this sense is the contribution of Catholics to themselves and to the wider community in which they live.

NOTES

1. Paul Ehrlich, *The Population Bomb* (Rivercity Press, 1968).

2. William Gibson, *A Mass for the Dead* (Pleasantville: Akadine Press, 1996).

HEALTH-CARE REFORM:
A HUMAN RIGHTS ISSUE

Marie A. Conn

PROLOGUE

Whether they realized it or not, those responsible for putting Measure 16 on the Oregon ballot in 1994 underscored the futility of debates over health-care reform which lack an ethical focus.

As Art Caplan, Director of the Center for Biomedical Ethics at the University of Pennsylvania, observed, "Measure 16, or what Oregonians are calling the Death with Dignity Act, permits physicians to prescribe lethal does of medicine to patients who want to end their lives."[1] Although the proposal was well thought-out, had many safeguards, and put the responsibility for ending a life on the individual, it was nevertheless dangerous in a society that has no right to basic health-care. Ultimately, the choice to end a life can only be informed and voluntary if the terminally ill individual has other options from which to choose. For Americans who lack money and insurance, these other options may not be available. This means, in effect, that money becomes the major factor in decisions of life and death. Caplan went on to insist that people should not have to ingest a fatal dose of pills because of a lack of health insurance or because they could not qualify for home care. In his words, "A society that is not ready to offer a decent package of comprehensive health-care to all its citizens is a society that is not ready to offer them death by prescription."[2]

Until recently Representative Jim Moran (D-Va) was doubtful about the call for universal health-care. Then, on August 13, 1994, he and his wife learned that their three-year-old daughter, Dorothy, was suffering from a deadly form of brain cancer. Realizing his own health-care coverage was tied to winning re-election (which he did), Moran vowed to fight for universal coverage for children.[3]

INTRODUCTION

It is clear that debates over health-care reform have become arguments over costs, procedures, and policies, and have lost sight of the single most important issue, namely, the people behind the statistics. Health-care is, in the end, all about people. And any issue that affects human life and development is an ethical issue. There is no such thing as a decision that is simply political or simply economic: all decisions that have impact on human life have an ethical dimension. Health-care reform, therefore, is more than just a medical and economic challenge; health-care reform is also part of the struggle for universal human rights. A purely technological or economic approach to health-care reform ignores families who lack insurance, the sick who lack options, and children who lack proper care.

Adequate health care is a basic human need; therefore, every person has a right to such care. Yet today, in the United States, more than 35 million people have no guaranteed access to health care. Uninsured Americans are forced to let problems go untreated until routine health-incidents become medical emergencies. In addition to those who are currently uninsured, thousands more are in danger of losing insurance through job-changes or layoffs. By one estimate 45,000 New Jersey residents and 85,000 Pennsylvanians lose their insurance each month.[4]

Washington's failure to pass a health-care reform package leaves us with a problem that won't go away, a problem which will, in fact, grow only more burdensome and complex. Health-care costs will continue to rise and some 17% of Americans will continue to be denied access to quality care. Is it any wonder that a 17-year old high school senior shared her discouragement with a local journalist? "Everyone should have health-care. It should be one of the basic human rights. It's sad. I'm only 17 years old. My peak of idealism is supposed to be now, and it's over already."[5]

The statistics are readily available: one out of three Hispanics and one out of five African-Americans are uninsured. Some 39 million Americans, or one in five, are now officially poor. Over 22% of American children live in poverty, the highest level since 1964. Some 40% of all people living in poverty are children.[6] Our infant mortality-rates, especially in inner-city and rural communities, are shockingly high, rivaling those of some Third World countries. The U.S. also has a high percentage of babies born at dangerously low birth-weights. So, while the U.S. spends nearly 50% more per person on health-care than any other country, we don't compare favorably with them in terms of measurable health-outcomes.[7]

Obviously, then, existing patterns of health-care in the U.S. do not meet the demands of social justice.[8] Our nation's health-care system serves too few and costs too much.[9] And, the experts warn, health-care costs are continuing to grow at such a rate that costs by the year 2000 will be more than double those of 1980.

Reform, then, is imperative. Nor only are millions without adequate health-care, but rising costs deplete resources needed in other vital areas, such as housing and education. And, in all of this, it is the poorest who are most adversely affected; health-policies and efforts at health-care reform, then, must be examined in light of their effect on the poor and weak among us. We must believe, truly believe, that every American, indeed every human being, has the right to quality health-care. "The needs of the frail elderly person, the unborn child, the person living with AIDS, and the undocumented immigrant must be addressed by healthcare reform."[10]

SOME ASSUMPTIONS

Any attempt to address health-care reform in the U. S. must also realistically acknowledge several underlying attitudes or assumptions that affect bioethical thought.[11] One of the most pervasive of these attitudes is the denial of our mortality. It is a basic fact of human life that death is a certainty, and yet Americans seem determined to prolong life at any cost. "Health-care has much more important things to offer than the false hope of immortality."[12]

The attempt to deny our own mortality leads to the conviction that no one must die who can be saved, no matter the cost or ultimate futility of the treatment. Intensive care units, which often function more like high-tech hospices, are over-used, while around 30% of Medicare's money goes to patients with less than a year to live.[13] It is also widely accepted that doctors are trained to cure diseases, not to address the place of suffering in human life. Curing is, in effect, more highly valued than caring. Medicine has, to a large extent, been divorced from values. Being a physician is becoming increasingly a service-oriented profession, with doctors forced to spend more and more time on the business aspects of medicine, such as utilization-review.

Americans, who tend to consider morality as something purely personal, also fail to see the social dimension of issues like reproductive technology and positive eugenics. Yet, anything that affects an individual's life affects the life of society. In an era of increasingly sophisticated prenatal diagnosis in a culture which considers abortion an acceptable form of health-care, the danger of applying a consumer-mentality to human reproduction is unfortunately quite real. Although no one would deny parents the right to use all means available to assure the healthiest child possible, the leap to discarding children who do not meet certain subjective standards of perfection is not unthinkable.

This eugenic mentality leads further to a denial of the aging process. A good deal of surgery is performed, not because it is medically indicated, but to allow people to conform to their own, or society's notion of acceptability. "Contemporary medicine is increasingly treating the desires of people in a move toward a discomfortless society and in the process medicalizing some basic human problems."[14]

Another assumption currently driving developments in health-care is that of patient-autonomy. Although the move away from the "Doctor knows best" (or "Doctor God") paternalism of earlier days was a positive change, reaction to it has become over-reaction: patient-autonomy is now viewed as absolute. "The offshoot of this absolutization is that very little attention is given to the values that ought to guide the use of autonomy. The sheer fact that the choice is the patient's is viewed as the sole right-making characteristic of the choice."[15] The result of assumptions such as these is an over-emphasis on longevity, which leads to an over-valuing of technology. When a society undervalues the social dimension of medical choices and refuses to acknowledge human mortality, it is difficult to move people to the kind of sacrifice which true health-care reform involves.

SOME BACKGROUND

What has been missing in the health-care reform debates, then, is attention to the deeper issues. Instead of quarreling over policies and procedures, Americans should be called to examine their attitudes toward life and death. We must ask ourselves what we mean by "health" and assess the real goals of medicine.[16] Until now much of the public debate has centered on costs, not justice. Since 1968 the percentage of the GDP (gross domestic product) devoted to health-care has nearly doubled, from 7.6% to 14%. Obviously, the increased money targeted for health-care is taken away from programs like drug-control, crime-prevention, and so on.[17] Furthermore, as we have already seen, even such a large increase in health-spending has not resulted in a system that works for vast numbers of Americans.

In 1986 the Catholic bishops of the United States made an observation that has even more urgency today: "By bringing healthcare cost inflation down, we could cut the federal deficit, improve economic competitiveness, and help stem the decline in living standards for many working families."[18] Resources have to be freed up to address other problems that have impact on health.

Real reform can be jeopardized by special-interest groups and powerful lobbies who have a major stake in maintaining the status quo. Partisan politics likewise works against true reform. Health-care reform has come up in every administration since World War II. In 1948 President Harry S. Truman introduced proposals for national insurance. Under pressure from political opponents Truman cut the proposals, but the plan was never enacted. During the 1950s the impetus for reform waned as much of the middle class gained private health coverage. Federal medical coverage, at least for the elderly, was part of John F. Kennedy's "New Frontier." President Richard M. Nixon, Senator Edward Kennedy, and Representative Wilbur Mills worked for reform in the early 1970s but a compromise plan fell victim to Watergate, Chappaquidick and special-interest forces. President Jimmy Carter's efforts in the later part of the 1970s met with similar frustration. In every case partisan politics or the wishes of the affluent and those with special interests have blocked attempts at reform. During the Reagan/Bush years there was a definite move toward applying market principles to health-care.[19]

In the first ten months of 1993 the health-care industry gave $8.4 million to members of Congress, an increase of 27% over 1992. Members of the Senate Finance Committee received an average of $393,000 in donations from the health and insurance industries between 1987 and 1993, as compared to $232,553 for other senators.[20] It is easy to see why the health-care reform debate has focused on the needs of special-interest groups rather than on the broader ethical issues about government-responsibility in the area of health-care.

Health-care in America, then, is marked by ever-rising costs, increasing gaps in health-insurance coverage, and persistent inequities in access to health-care. The American model of health-care relies on treatment rather than on prevention, and it invests more in high technology than in basic health-care. Policy-making must address these disturbing trends and conceptualize health-care as a human right while reforming the system.[21]

A RIGHTS-BASED APPROACH TO HEALTH-CARE REFORM

The U.S. is the only Western democracy that does not recognize a right to health-care. While other countries consider health-care a social, public good, in the U.S. health-care is considered a private good, a commodity. The fundamental basis of a reformed health-care system must, therefore, be a recognition of the right to adequate health-care. Furthermore, this belief in a right to health-care must be rooted in the wider context of a commitment to improve the health of the general public. This commitment in turn must be translated into specific steps, taking into account our society's resources.[22]

Ethically, health-care is a basic right. In other words, a basic standard of health-care is a human right for all people.[23] Obviously, it is important to have a clear understanding of the meaning of *rights* and *human rights* as these terms are being used here. After all, too much insistence on *my rights* can make it difficult to establish a framework for reform. Rights-language must be related to the common good and must be balanced by the language of duties and responsibilities.[24]

There does exist a good for a society as a whole which respects but is ultimately more important than the good of any individual. In the context of health-care reform, health-services must truly foster this common good. Nor are material concerns enough: a holistic notion of the common good considers all facets of who we are as human persons. Such a notion demands that we not limit considerations of health-care reform to questions of cost and number served. Reform must yield a true sense of participation and partnership in health-care; it must enhance the quality of human life and interpersonal relationships; it must foster values; and it must be realistic about the limitations of human life.[25]

Ethically, a right is an entitlement to some good or service. If the entitlement is universal, i.e., based solely on one's status as a human being and not tied to gender, race, nationality, or economic and social status, it is referred to as a human right. Human rights generally include the minimum conditions necessary for a person's life, growth, and development. Society recognizes these rights and accepts responsibility for their promotion and protection.[26] A right to health-care implies an entitlement to a basic and adequate standard of health-care consistent with a society's resources. In our country "basic and adequate" health-care must include both preventative and curative services, as well as access to rehabilitation, mental health-care and related supports. Just as crises in health are common to all humans, so too should access to health-care be.[27]

Since health-care is a social good rather than a commodity, health-care reform must be based on the principles of justice, equity, and social obligation. A rights-based approach to health-care reform respects the dignity of each individual and thus satisfies the demands of justice by focusing special attention on the poor, on minorities, and on children.[28] In other words, such an approach rightly emphasizes the ethics of health-care reform over the economics of reform. Quantifiable questions are important, but so is a more complete vision of the meaning of human life. Only in this way can quantifiable issues be approached with justice. An individualist mentality makes real health-care reform virtually impossible.[29]

This human rights approach to health-care reform has other advantages. It provides standards and goals which can be useful not just for the immediate process of reform but also for the ongoing evaluation and revision of the system. It goes beyond individual interests and links health-care to our nation's concept of the social covenant binding government and society. (Of course, groups who profit from the expansion and commercialization of health-care will resist such fundamental changes since their income and profits would potentially be affected.)

A human rights approach to reform protects the benefits of the "haves" while giving priority to improving the health-status of the "have-nots." It does this by going beyond the provision of health-insurance in order to address inadequacies and structural deficiencies in the health-care system as a whole. Such an approach translates human rights into moral norms which are themselves translated into laws, thus institutionalizing the social covenant and creating a framework for a national consensus. Government recognizes the entitlement to basic health-care for all; individuals accept limits on the scope of publicly provided health-care. Here the need for wide public input becomes clear since citizens are expected not to demand a standard of care for themselves that would not also be available to all other members of society and affordable within specified, agreed upon budgetary limits.[30]

The goal of a human rights approach to health-care reform is not equality of well-being but a decent minimum level of health. In reality, a second tier of services would be available to those who could afford it, but that second tier must not be permitted to jeopardize the prior right of those not getting the decent minimum, for example, by tying up the best physicians or monopolizing research-facilities.[31]

JUSTICE

Justice demands that we give all persons the goods and services that they rightly expect. Justice is about duties and responsibilities and building a good community. Justice concerns what we must do for others on the basis of our common humanity. Even more central to the health-care debate is the question of distributive justice or allocation.[32] "The litmus test... is the extent to which the rights of the most vulnerable and disadvantaged individuals... are assured.... A human rights standard assumes a special obligation or bias in favor of the needs and rights of the poor, the disadvantaged, the powerless, and those at the periphery of society."[33] Decisions must be judged in light of what they do to and for the poor, and what they enable the poor to do for themselves.[34] We must see reasonable access to health-care as a social responsibility. As long as over 35 million Americans are uninsured, we are failing to meet the demands of distributive justice. Cost, the market, tax burdens, these are all necessary issues, but they are not central.

What is central in health-care reform is to discover criteria for reform that satisfy the demands of social justice. Criteria based on consideration of merit, social usefulness, or the ability to pay must be rejected, since judgments in these areas would both be arbitrary and hard to reach, and they would work against children, the elderly, and those of limited means. Level of need is an appropriate criterion, but it is not enough. Perhaps the most fitting standard to satisfy distributive justice is similar care for similar cases.[35] In other words, we as a society should determine what we consider a minimum standard of health-care and then pledge ourselves to provide that standard to everyone, without regard to merit, social usefulness, and so on.[36] It should be noted that such a standard requires an acceptance of death as part of life. The extension of life is not always an absolute need, especially if the common good ultimately outranks the individual good.

HEALTH-CARE RATIONING

Once a society has agreed that every person has a right to guaranteed access to health-care, a recognition of the limitations of that society's resources leads naturally to the question of health-care rationing. We have to face head-on the question of what we must do for all people in terms of supplying them with access to health-care. The goal, once a decent minimum standard has been set, is to give everyone whatever health-care it takes to bring them to that level.[37] We must be honest about the existence of *de facto* rationing caused by variations in income, insurance, geographical location, or even type of disease or condition. No one can deny that under the present system the rich have access to a number of advanced medical procedures which are unlikely to be made available to the poor. There are natural limits, too, to individual life and health; and as we have seen, it is possible to spend money on health-care that might be spent more effectively in some other area, such as education.

So, the question is not whether we should ration health-care, but how we should do it. Covert or secret rationing must be exposed to the light of ethical examination, and criteria governing the morality of its use must be developed and applied. Rationing, defined as the decision not to develop or not to provide people with potentially beneficial medical treatments, should be considered a last resort, used only after all alternatives have been explored. Society must determine what constitutes "futile" measures and apply the same standard universally, so that beneficial treatment is not withheld from some in order to provide others who can afford it with futile treatment. Further, that universal standard must be high enough that most people agree to it, while recognizing that the cost and resources involved in some elaborate medical procedures can take away from the common good.

An honest approach to rationing must also deal with questions of gender-based and age-based discrimination. Some treatments may be specific to one sex and not to the other, and while age-discrimination is generally not acceptable, there may be treatments which are not age-appropriate. Gender and age, then, may be valid factors in rationing decisions, but only in a holistic examination of all the circumstances involved in a particular case. Finally, while the patient always has the option of refusing treatment, treatment may only be withheld because of factors arising from the treatment itself, such as cost or disproportionate use of resources, and never because of any personal judgment about the patient.[38]

Furthermore, while some rationing will be unavoidable, our society is actually affluent enough to provide more than a minimum level of care for all its citizens. Government and the private sector must work together so that all Americans, most of whom support universal health care in the abstract, will become convinced of the justice of the concrete measures needed to make such universal care a reality. All of us have a responsibility to be sure that society has the resources it needs to provide a basic set of health-care services to all people. The level of services would be the same for all, but the poor and marginalized may need extra assistance and training to be sure they fully understand their right to access to just health care.[39]

CRITERIA FOR REFORM

The central question is how much inequity in the distribution of health-care we as a society can tolerate. Current levels of disparity are significant, costly, and unjust.[40] The best health-care system would be one that combines universal access to health-care with cost-control, quality-care for the poor, and respect for human life and dignity. To achieve such a goal, government as the instrument of the common good must work together with all parts of the private sector to develop and promote policies and procedures that satisfy the demands of fundamental human justice. "Linking the healthcare of poor and working class families to the healthcare of those with greater resources is probably the best assurance of comprehensive benefits and quality care."[41] Health-care is collective in nature: sick and healthy, poor and wealthy, all must participate with equal freedom and access.

Success or failure in the area of health-care reform will have a lot to say about who we are as a nation and about what kind of nation we will be in the 21st century. A single-payer plan (similar to Canada's), in which all citizens have guaranteed access to a comprehensive standard benefits package, is most consistent with a human rights approach, because such a system is best capable of achieving universality, assuring social equity, and holding down health-costs.[42]

Since the single-payer system faces stiff opposition from both the health-insurance industry and health-care providers, however, managed competition is likely to provide the framework for reform. How can managed competition be improved from a human rights perspective? Audrey R. Chapman (Program Director, Science and Human Rights, American Association for the Advancement of Science) suggests the following recommendations.

Recognize the right of all citizens and residents to basic and adequate health-care. Reduce stratification in the present system and limit regional price-differentials. Develop stronger monitoring of regional health-alliances to prevent the exclusion of certain categories of the population. Incorporate older Americans into regional health-alliances at benefits equal to those granted younger citizens to avoid age-discrimination. Place greater emphasis on protection and prevention, including environmental and lifestyle concerns. Facilitate the adoption by states of a single-payer system, to avoid penalizing states for attempting to provide greater equity. Give regional health-alliances both the responsibility and the resources to provide health-care services to under-served populations. Give highest priority in the allocation of resources to low-income persons and those with disabilities and special needs. Utilize taxes on things like cigarettes, alcohol, and guns and ammunition, to finance health-care reform. Control costs by setting funding priorities and imposing price-controls on fees, procedures, and pharmaceuticals. Promote public participation in shaping health-care reform. Develop an effective monitoring system that will be able to assess the impact of health-care reform on an ongoing basis.[43]

AN INTERESTING EXPERIMENT

In Buckpoint, Maine, several full-time employees of MacLeod's Restaurant are participating in a unique program called "First Sunday," which allows them to operate one day a month for their own profit and pay health-insurance premiums with pre-tax earnings. George MacLeod, the restaurant's owner, estimates that his outlay (rent, utilities, licenses, and so on) is just 15% of what it would cost to provide insurance for his employees. In other words, MacLeod has made it possible for any employee who is willing to work one eight-hour shift on a day when the restaurant would otherwise be closed to have adequate health-insurance which they could not otherwise afford. This program could serve as one model for providing employee-coverage at minimal cost to the employer.[44]

CONCLUSION

"The injustice of the mansion next to the ghetto is dwarfed by the prospect of an uninsured mother with poor prenatal care giving birth to a child four weeks premature while, several floors below in the same hospital, an endocrinologist is evaluating a boy for synthetic growth hormone to improve his self-esteem."[45] We can equalize the system and still allow for individual freedom and technological advances.

The moral force of a right to health-care should sustain continuing efforts to provide equitable health-care for all. Only then will our nation have achieved true health-care reform.

NOTES

1. A. Caplan, "Let's get universal health care before granting the right to die" in *The Philadelphia Inquirer* (Sept. 27, 1994) A 19.

2. Ibid.

3. J. Moran, "Moment of Crisis" in *People* (Oct. 31, 1994) 129-30, 132. Inquiries to Rep. Moran concerning his pursuit of this goal have gone unanswered.

4. S. Burlind, R. Smith and S. Vedantam, "Lost in the health debate: People who need insurance" in *The Philadelphia Inquirer* (Aug. 21, 1994) E 1-2.

5. M. Dribben, "Politics enough to make you sick" in *The Philadelphia Inquirer* (Sept. 1, 1994) B 1.

6. R. A. Zaldivan, "Poverty rate rises despite growth in the economy" in *The Philadelphia Inquirer* (Oct. 7, 1994) A 1, 12.

7. S. FitzGerald, "U.S. is the top spender on health" in *The Philadelphia Inquirer* (Oct. 6, 1994) A 1, 17.

8. Comments and statistics like these are available in many sources. See, for example, the U. S. Bishops, "A Framework for Comprehensive Healthcare Reform" in *Health Progress* (Sept. 1993) 20-23.

9. Bishops 20.

10. Bishops 22.

11. See R. A. McCormick, "Value Variables in the Health-Care Reform Debate" in *America* 168/19 (May 29, 1993) 7-13.

12. C. F. Koller, "An Open Letter: Four Things to Keep in Mind" in *Commonweal* (April 23, 1993) 5-6.

13. McCormick 8 (statistic from *The New England Journal of Medicine*, April 15, 1993).

14. McCormick 10.

15. Ibid.

16. W. Gaylin, "Faulty Diagnosis: Why Clinton's health-care plan won't cure what ails us" in *Harper's Magazine* (Oct. 1993) 57-64.

17. Ibid. 58.

18. U. S. Bishops, *Economic Justice for All* (Washington, D.C.: USCC 1986) 23.

19. A. Chapman, "Introduction in *Health Care Reform: A Human Rights Approach*, ed., A. R. Chapman (Washington, D.C.: Georgetown Univ. Press 1994) 1-32, here 23-25.

20. These figures are from a study by Citizen Action and are cited in Chapman 27.

21. Chapman 1-4.

22. Chapman 1, 11.

23. P. S. Keane, *Health Care Reform: A Catholic View* (New York: Paulist Press 1993) 128.

24. Keane 126-27. See also M. A. Glendon, *Rights Talk: The Impoverishment of Political Discourse* (New York: The Free Press, 1991).

25. Keane 130-31.

26. Chapman 4-5, 7.

27. Keane 128.

28. V. A. Leary, "Defining the Right to Health Care" in Chapman 87-105.

29. Keane 133.

30. Chapman 5, 17.

31. R. M. Veatch, "Egalitarian Justice and the Right to Health Care" in Chapman 106-23, here 112.

32. Keane 133.

33. Chapman 7.

34. U. S. Bishops, *Economic Justice for All*, esp. paragraphs 23-24 and 61-95.

35. Keane 139-42.

36. For an extended treatment of what constitutes a decent minimum standard of health-care, see M. A. Baily, "Defining the Decent Minimum" in Chapman 167-85.

37. Veatch 112.

38. Keane 144-47.

39. Keane 143.

40. Koller 6.

41. U. S. Bishops, "A Framework" 22.

42. A. R. Chapman, "Policy Recommendations for Health Care Reform" in Chapman 308-14, here 308.

43. Chapman 309-14.

44. N. Matza, "Cooling up an idea for health care" in *The Philadelphia Inquirer* (Dec. 26, 1994) A 1, 4.

45. Koller 6.

PROBLEMS OF COOPERATION
IN AN ABORTIVE CULTURE

John J. Conley, S.J.

UNTIL THREE DECADES AGO the moral problem of abortion in American society was relatively straightforward. The conscientious citizen faced two principal questions. The first concerned whether the individual could perform or procure an abortion. The second concerned whether the state should tolerate abortion under certain circumstances. Although public opinion divided on the proper moral and public-policy posture concerning a minute number of "therapeutic" abortions (predominantly those tied to maternal life-endangerment and felonious intercourse),[1] American society maintained a firm moral and legal censure against the practice of abortion in general.[2] The conscientious citizen experienced little difficulty in distancing himself or herself from an abhorrent practice which remained occult and illegal.

In the intervening years, the moral and public policy dilemmas of abortion remain, in a far more agitated state than that of the hushed debate over therapeutic abortion in the early 1960s. A new moral dilemma, however, has emerged for the citizen opposed to abortion. No longer must this citizen face only the personal issue of whether to perform or procure an abortion. The citizen must now face the question to what extent he or she may cooperate in an abortive culture, that is, a society where abortion is actively promoted, not merely tolerated, by key institutions.

In the current American climate the individual citizen is often forced to finance abortion through taxes and insurance premiums.[3] Individual health professionals or social workers may find themselves pressured to provide referrals for abortion. Judges may find themselves facing cases where judicial authorization for abortion is sought.[4] In an academic setting, teachers, administrators and students must confront the issue of the recognition, funding and facilitation of groups which promote abortion.[5] At the present moment, medical schools find themselves under increasing pressure to provide instruction in abortion-techniques or, in lieu of such instruction, to

103

provide referrals to programs which give such education.[6] These
pressures to legitimize abortion, however indirectly, indicate the
social coercion barely masked beneath the slogans of "choice." They
also pose acute problems of conscience for the individual who wants
to refuse any sanction for abortion but who must live in a society
which relentlessly promotes abortion and increasingly entraps the
private citizen in this promotion.

In order to examine this dilemma, it can be useful to explore certain
principles of the manualists, the natural-law ethicians of mid-century,
who analyzed the issue of cooperation with evil. The works of
Austin Fagothey,[7] Andrew Varga,[8] Martin O'Keefe[9] and Germain
Grisez[10] are especially helpful in this area. The manualists attempted
to sketch certain principles for demarking acceptable and unacceptable cooperation with evil, especially in work-related settings.
Realistic in their appraisals of the possibilities of social reform, they
balanced the rights and duties of the conscientious person to refuse
participation in evil with the need of the person to live peacefully in
a society where certain evils are pervasive and obdurate. Many of
these manualists warn that the issue of cooperation with evil,
especially that of material cooperation, is one of the thorniest
questions in all of moral philosophy. The line-drawing on such an
issue is inevitably vague. As valuable as these principles may be in
illuminating the quandary of participation in an abortive culture,
they cannot substitute for the prudential judgment of the individual
conscience attempting to combat abortion in a particular setting.

In the manualist perspective the key distinction in the area of
cooperation with evil lies in the difference between formal and
material cooperation. In the case of formal cooperation, one
positively wills and assists the evil act, although one does not
personally perform it. "There is formal cooperation when one not
only helps another to do evil but also joins in his evil intention."[11]
In the case of material cooperation, one assists another in an evil act,
although one personally opposes the act. "There is material
cooperation when, without approving another's wrongdoing, one
helps him perform his sinful act by an action of one's own that is
not of its nature sinful."[12] The distinction between the two kinds of
cooperation lies primarily in the posture of the will (the intention)
toward the evil act in question.

The manualists concur that formal cooperation can never be

justified, since it involves the agent in approval of an evil action. "Formal cooperation is always morally wrong and cannot be justified under any circumstances."[13] Establishing the limits of formal cooperation in the area of abortion, however, can be more complicated than this categoric condemnation suggests. Germain Grisez suggests the numerous actions which may involve a moral agent in formal cooperation. "A person who commands, directs, advises, encourages, prescribes, approves or actively defends doing something immoral is sometimes said to cooperate in the immoral act."[14] As Grisez indicates, all such actions can involve the moral agent in instigating or provoking an evil act. In the area of abortion, formal cooperators would include those who counsel in favor of abortion or provide abortion-referrals. They cannot elude responsibility for the evil by claiming that they do not personally perform the abortion. The more deliberate and the more coercive the prescription, the graver the cooperation in abortion manifested by these moral agents.

In *Evangelium Vitae* Pope John Paul II suggests that the sphere of formal cooperation in abortion is even broader. It includes all those, especially within the elite fields of law, journalism and academe, who create an ideological climate which favors abortion. "Responsibility likewise falls on he legislators who have promoted and approved abortion laws, and to the extent that they have a say on the matter, on the administrators of health-care centers where abortions are performed. A general and no less serious responsibility lies with those who have encouraged an attitude of sexual permissiveness and lack of esteem for motherhood, and with those who should have ensured—but did not—effective family and social policies in support of families, especially larger families and those with particular financial and educational needs. Finally, one cannot overlook the network of complicity which reaches out to include international institutions, foundations and associations which systematically campaign for the legalization and spread of abortion in the world."[15] Since formal cooperation is distinguished by the posture of the will, those who shape the will in a positive attitude toward abortion share in the evil of the act of abortion. Behind the individual decision of a woman to procure and of a health-care professional to perform an abortion stands a network of persons shaping the values and ideologies which inform the moral decision-making of a particular culture.

As the citation from *Evangelium Vitae* suggests, one particular problem in the area of formal cooperation concerns the role of abortion-related legislation. One commonly hears the argument that a legislator or, in the case of a referendum, the individual citizen personally opposes abortion but supports its legalization. Since the individual claims to abhor the practice and might even personally dissuade others from the practice, the person's actions in the legislative arena might appear divorced from formal cooperation in abortion.

In fact, while the issue of moral responsibility for abortion *via* legislative or judicial action is complicated, legislative action on behalf of abortion would often appear to provide *prima facie* evidence of formal cooperation. In American society, abortion has recently been presented as a legal right of the citizen. A "right," properly speaking, involves a title which justifies a moral agent in demanding immunity or assistance from the community of moral agents for the exercise of a putative claim.[16] To support "abortion rights," as the media currently (and usually accurately, even if the term is an oxymoron) labels many legislative and judicial decisions in this area, is to claim that the pregnant woman and the attending medical personnel are justified in performing the act. If such an action is justifiable, it is difficult to understand why one would be "personally opposed" to it. Such opposition would appear to a matter of personal pique or a credal conviction as sectarian as the refusal to eat meat on Good Friday. The supposed moral repugnance of the agent to abortion is either feigned or simply based upon ignorance of the actual nature of the legislation or judicial principle one claims to support. This disjunction between moral opposition to and political support for abortion becomes especially grave when, in the wake of *Roe v. Wade*, the citizen supports a program of unrestricted abortion-on-demand. The current campaign to bolster abortion as a right—or even worse, as an entitlement to be funded by the state—involves a citizen in a more difficult cooperation with evil than do other polities, still extant in parts of Europe and Latin America, which limited their legislation to the toleration of abortion as a restricted evil.[17] The claim to oppose abortion morally when one acclaims it as a right and engenders a political culture favorable to abortion is implausible. While ignorance and prejudice may mitigate the personal responsibility of the citizen in such a contradictory posture, enthusiastic support for a putative right to abortion would usually indicate tacit consent to such a practice.

While formal cooperation in evil is categorically condemned, since the upright agent may neither approve moral evil nor willingly help to bring it about, the issue of material cooperation in evil is more complicated. Following the tenets of the principle of double effect,[18] the manualists argue that one may tolerate certain participations in acts which indirectly help another to bring about a moral evil which one personally opposes. On the one hand, one must void a scrupulosity which, by refusing any association with evil acts, simply paralyzes the agent in the face of social interaction. On the other hand, to avoid moral laxness, one must carefully discern the circumstances under which such cooperation is reasonably tolerable.

The natural law tradition has focused upon three principles by which one can measure the reasonableness of the material cooperation with evil which might confront the moral agent. First, one must evaluate the gravity and amount of evil that others might be permitted to perform through the agent's cooperation. Second, one must evaluate the gravity and amount of evil that will probably occur to oneself if one refuses this cooperation. Third, one must evaluate the proximity of one's cooperative act to the evil act which one opposes.[19] Following the framework of the principle of double effect, such considerations permit the moral agent to ponder the proportionate balance of good over bad effects in a congeries of acts, while carefully refusing any endorsement of an intrinsically evil action and any effort to use such an evil act as the means to bring about good.

In the current cultural context of abortion, these principles can illumine the boundaries between acceptable and unacceptable material cooperation. The first principle, that concerning the gravity of the evil act, underlines the seriousness of any material cooperation with abortion. The evil one contemplates is the act of homicide. It is the killing of the innocent. The massive number of such homicides in American society (approximately 1.5 million a year) and the levity of the reasons for which abortion is commonly performed only heighten the evil of the act in which one may consider cooperation. Although material cooperation in evil, especially in complex urban cultures, is inevitable, cooperation with an evil of this gravity requires far stronger justification than cooperation than the majority of evils in daily life. Even remote connection to abortion in the actions one performs demands strict scrutiny of the nature of the assisting material acts.

The second principle, that of evaluating the evil one must bear if one refuses material cooperation, underlines the limits of refusing material cooperation to all instances of abortion. One cannot demand the heroic of oneself and of others in opposing abortion. One cannot ignore legitimate demands of livelihood, family-life and other social obligations in evaluating the possibility of material cooperation in a given case. If we were to refuse any material cooperation to the act of abortion, we would all be meeting at the D.C. jail. We would refuse to pay taxes, since the government uses them to fund abortion. We would be an illiterate lot, since we would not patronize newspapers, magazines, radio-stations or television-channels which show pro-abortion bias. And we would be an unemployed lot, since we would refuse to work in schools, hospitals or businesses which show the slightest trace of pro-abortion sentiment. While such heroism may be appealing in moments of idealistic fervor, and while we may on occasion be called to such heroism, such a stance would seem to deny other pressing obligation toward God, others and ourselves. Such a strategy would also seem to promise little in terms of effective challenge to the wave of abortion which has over-whelmed our society in the past generation. Conscientious objection to abortion, and the practical lines drawn on material cooperation, must reflect prudently the variety of obligations and resources which the individual agent brings to this complex work of resistance.

The third principle, that which evaluates the proximity or remoteness of one's act to another evil act, can be especially helpful in discerning the limits of material cooperation in the workplace. A hypothetical case can illustrate this utility. In a certain American city, an abortion-clinic is is operation. Certain staff members are obviously guilty of formal cooperation. This would include the staff-doctors who actually perform the abortions and the majority, if not all, of the other medical personnel and counseling-staff who serve the clinic. One could imagine the case of a secretary who works at the clinic. She sincerely opposes abortion. She would never procure one for herself and she has actually discouraged two friends from having abortions through her personal counsel. It is difficult to imagine, however, how her clerical work at the clinic could ever be justifiable material cooperation. She draws her livelihood from the practice of abortion. Her answering of the phone, her direction to clients, her care of files and her scheduling of appointments facilitate the performance of numerous abortions. This massive participation in a business whose sole purpose is the practice of abortion indicates that this a proximate, intimate cooperation in grave evil. Either the secretary is insouciant of the gravity of this evil or the secretary is deluding herself on how intimately and massively her work fuels the daily killing of the innocent. Such massive, integral cooperation in abortion could not balanced by other concerns, such as the higher salary the work in the clinic would bring her family.

The material cooperation of other workers involved with this clinic, however, could be far more remote. The building might have a night guard, for example, who must protect all the building's offices, of which the clinic is only one out of fifty. The guard's work does benefit the practice of abortion by securing the property of the abortionist. However, the guard's mission is to protect the property of the entire building. Only incidentally does the abortion-industry benefit. A conscientious guard might seek comparable employment where even this minor connection to abortion can be severed. His work does, after all, provide material assistance to the abortion industry. However, one could imagine a situation (such as the need to sustain his family and the paucity of other employment-opportunities) where such material cooperation would be minimally acceptable.

An even more remote instance of cooperation would be presented by the mail-carrier who delivers mail to the offices of the building, including the office of the abortion-clinic. There is no doubt that the delivered mail helps to further the work of the abortionist. Information is disseminated. Appointments for abortion might be made or confirmed. However, the mail-carrier's concern is simply to provide correspondence to all those on the route. The clinic is incidentally served by the carrier's work, which involves hundreds of other clients each day. Given the gravity of abortion's evil, even such minor cooperation may well prove disturbing to the conscientious agent. However, such slight material cooperation would not seem to necessitate a change of work.

It is not surprising that the workplace is the privileged area where many of the manualists explore the issue of material cooperation. These ethicians repeatedly argue that the standard of material cooperation in evil which one is willing to tolerate varies according to one's professional duties in a particular area. To cite one of the clichéd examples from the manualist literature, a thief's attempted robbery of a bank requires different standards of material response. The guard has a greater obligation to refuse material cooperation (such as opening the bank-vault) than does the bank-clerk who, in turn, has a greater obligation than does than the bank-patron who just happened to be making a transaction at the moment of the attempted robbery. While the obligation regarding formal cooperation is uniform for all—no one may legitimately will the act of theft—the obligations concerning material cooperation vary according to the nature of one's work, the demands of one's contract, even the physical and psychic capacities of the individual worker.

This focus upon the workplace as the privileged locus for exploring material cooperation in abortion can clarify certain of the dilemmas we face in our own workplace, the university. Obviously, the first duty is to avoid the actual performing of abortions in a university-hospital and to avoid the dangerously proximate form of cooperation of providing referrals for abortion. More problematic is the question of working in a hospital-setting where abortions are performed or in a counseling-situation where referrals for abortion are provided. One would need to ask questions regarding the frequency of abortion, how much of the enterprise is devoted to abortion, the proximity of the abortions to one's actual work and how great a cost to the welfare of one's family and oneself the abandonment of this work would entail. One must also ask whether one's presence in the institution, especially when one's refusal of abortion is public, might discourage abortion in certain instances and provoke qualms of conscience on the part of one's colleagues.

More typically, the issue of material cooperation for academics concerns their institutions' formal and material cooperation in abortion outside of the medical setting. Such evidence of cooperation might be manifested in a counseling-service's abortion-referrals, bias against pro-life faculty in hiring and tenure-decisions, bias against pro-life students in the recognition and funding of clubs, official statements by university-officials in favor of abortion, persistent official honors to pro-abortion politicians and the denial of such to pro-life politicians, the funding of abortion through university insurance-policies. Since the individual faculty-member both benefits the university through his or her services and benefits from the university through salary and medical insurance, there is a moral problem of material cooperation with an institution which indirectly legitimizes abortion through any of the preceding practices.

The development of responsible frontiers of acceptable and unacceptable material cooperation in the area of university-related abortion demands prudential judgments which will vary from one setting to another. To cite an obvious variation, the realistic possibilities of the faculty-member in a secular university and a religious one to oppose institutional embrace of abortion will differ. In certain secular universities, simply succeeding in providing equitable treatment for "pro-life" and "pro-choice" groups and programs may represent a minor, but real, victory for opposition to abortion. The development of a conscience-clause in the university health-insurance and United Way contributions, whereby the individual faculty-member may refuse to fund abortions, may be a substantial improvement over the standing insurance-policy which demands that everyone subsidize abortion as the cost of medical insurance. On the other hand, in a university which claims support by a particular religious confession, especially when that confession explicitly condemns abortion, the possibilities of effective resistance are far greater. One can more easily demand that the university refuse recognition of pro-abortion groups and programs, that it refuse to honor prominent pro-abortion dignitaries and that its health-care and counseling-policies follow in practice the pro-life positions which its sponsoring denomination proclaims in theory.

In discerning the boundaries of material cooperation with abortion in the setting of academe, two extremes must be avoided. The first is the path of insouciance, the confidence that one's personal refusal of formal cooperation with abortion excuses one from further consideration of one's tacit alliance with the abortionist. It is tempting in academe, for example, to refuse even to raise questions concerning policies of health-care, insurance, counseling, club-recognition and university honors. The evidence of complicity with abortion would often prove too overwhelming and the call to resist such material cooperation too excruciating. The courage to seek the truth regarding the presence of the evil of abortion, and the various complicities of one's institution with that evil, represents the first step in facing one's material cooperation with abortion and the quandaries of rejecting or tolerating specific instances of such cooperation.

The other extreme involves a rigorism which attempts to refuse all material cooperation, however indirect, with abortion. In the academic setting, such a rigorism could only lead one to resign from teaching in the contemporary university. The principle of academic freedom, for example, endorsed in its famous AAUP form by the vast majority of American universities,[20] guarantees that some teachers will promote pro-abortion theories and, tragically, tip certain students toward the choice of abortion in certain moments of crisis. While such actions do represent a material cooperation in abortion, they are incidental to the practice of academic freedom, which defends the right of other academics to oppose abortion and which defends an enormous host of academic speeches and books which have no connection whatsoever with abortion. It is legitimate that many faculty opponents of abortion choose to remain in universities with a decidedly pro-abortion tilt in certain activities because, on balance, the good achieved by the faculty-member's work in this setting (which might include the scholarly refutation of pro-abortion claims and the personal encouragement of pro-life groups) outweighs the evils of the material cooperation with abortion which the faculty-member must reluctantly tolerate.

Particularly thorny problems of material cooperation with abortion arise in the political arena. Citizens must currently confront laws which demand cooperation with abortion. Clearly, a conscientious citizen must refuse to obey any law which demands that the citizen actually perform an abortion. No consideration of one's personal welfare or respect for the law (in this case, an illegitimate law) could justify such complicity in the act of killing an innocent human being. One must also refuse cooperation which usually signifies endorsement of abortion, such as providing referrals to abortion-clinics, since such proximate cooperation cannot cohere with a principled opposition to abortion as an unjustified act of homicide. As a citizen shaping public policy and as a legislator, one is obliged to refuse all state-sanction and material support to the facilitation of abortion. One should earnestly refuse state-funding of abortion, of abortion-facilities and of groups and programs which promote abortion. Using the weapons of democratic reform, the citizen should make every effort to identify and reject all material and symbolic facilitation of abortion as crucial steps in opposing abortion, especially when immediate overturn of legal toleration of abortion is not imminent.

The limits of resistance to material cooperation with abortion as a citizen bound to obey laws, however, would appear to be more restricted than one's theoretical resistance as a citizen to current or proposed public policy. The fact that a small part of state-revenue is used to finance abortion or abortion-related activities does not necessarily justify the refusal to pay taxes in whole or in part. In contemporary American society, the bulk of tax-revenue is used to fund a variety of projects intrinsic to the promotion of the common good. While the citizen has every obligation to attempt to influence state-policy away from direct or indirect subsidy of abortion, the fact that a small part of revenue may tragically fund such actions does not free the citizen from financial obligation to the state. In any society, especially one as complex and pluralistic as contemporary America, certain state-funds will inevitably fuel programs which particular groups of citizens sincerely consider profoundly immoral. The ordinary means for correcting such material injustice is the vigorous use of the rights of petition, assembly, free speech, free press and election. In a democracy, one rarely exhausts such peaceful means of protest and social transformation. Recourse to civil disobedience, such as the use of tax-resistance, can only function as a type of last resort when the orderly means of protest have been exhausted. While such means have a legitimate currency in authoritarian regimes where such civil liberties have withered or in regimes (such as imperial India or the segregated South) where an entire class of citizens is disenfranchised, their justification is rarer in an authentic democracy. Consistently applied, the rigorist refusal to finance a state because some of the state-subsidized actions are patently evil can easily foster social anarchy. It can also divert the citizen from the patient work of properly political protest and organization which can identify the nature of the state's cooperation with evil, criticize this complicity and pressure the state to reverse its policies of cooperation.

In all such discernment of the limits of cooperation with abortion, the social dimension of the evil should be squarely recognized. For decades the issues of conscience in this realm have no longer confined themselves to the simple question of personal participation in abortion. Resistance to the homicidal evil of abortion requires scrutiny of the taxes one pays, the churches where one worships, the newspapers one reads, the schools where one sends one children. And it demands the anguished study of what material cooperation with this abortive culture may be tolerated for other goods and what material cooperation must be refused in the name of the rights of the innocent. For those of us with an academic and intellectual vocation, this discernment of material cooperation with an abortive culture arises in a distinctive setting. Our particular task often lies in research and teaching which carefully refutes the abortionist's propaganda and obfuscation in the areas of biology, philosophy, theology, law and history. It involves the construction of an alternative account of abortion based upon certain facts of biology, the rights of person-hood and the proper function of the law. It is precisely the lectern and the library which are the central tools proper to our particular resistance to abortion as academics. Our vocation also involves careful scrutiny of the complicity between abortion and academic culture. The intellectual's resistance to abortion involves the identification of the evil of abortion and grip of that evil upon the academy through the institution's teaching, biases, programs, clubs and awards. In collaboration with others committed to the defense of life, the conscientious intellectual identifies those institutional cooperations with abortion which must be resisted. And in those inevitable moments when one must regrettably tolerate material cooperation with abortion, one must still name it as an evil which is nothing less than the killing of the innocent.

NOTES

1. For a typology of the various legal approaches to abortion dominant before *Roe v. Wade*, cf. John M. Finnis, "Abortion: Legal Aspects" in *Encyclopedia of Bioethics*, ed. Reich, Vol.1 (New York: Free Press, 1978) 26-32.

2. For overviews of the history of the American attitude toward abortion, cf. Marvin N. Olasky, "Abortion News in the Late 1920's" in *Journalism Quarterly* 66/3 (1989) 724-26; "The Crossover in Newspaper Coverage of Abortion from Murder to Liberation" in *Journalism Quarterly* 63/1 (1986) 31-37; "Opposing Abortion Clinics" in *Journalism Quarterly* 63/2 (1986) 305-10.

3. On the problem of cooperation with unjust abortion-related laws, cf. William E. May, "Unjust laws and Catholic Citizens: Opposition, Cooperation and Toleration" in *Homiletic and Pastoral Review* 46/2 (Nov. 1995) 7-14.

4. Cf. Judge Joseph W. Moylan, "No Law Can Give Me the Right to Do What is Wrong" in *Life and Learning V*, ed. J. Koterski (Washington, D.C.: Univ. Faculty for Life, 1996) 234-42.

5. For a discussion of this dilemma in Catholic higher education, cf. "GU Choice Group" in *Origins* 22/1 (May 14, 1992) 14-15; Father Joseph O'Hare, S.J., "How Student Groups Impact the University's Catholicism" in *Origins* 22/9 (July 23, 1992) 163-66.

6. The decision of the Accreditation Council for Graduate Medical Education (February 15, 1996) to require abortion-training in all medical schools is illustrative of the coercive tendency. Cf. James Barron, "More prospective obstetricians will be taught abortion skills" in *The New York Times* (15 February 1995) A 1, 5.

7. Cf. Austin Fagothey, *Right and Reason*, 2nd ed. (St. Louis: Mosby, 1959) 338-41.

8. Andrew C. Varga, *On Being Human* (New York: Paulist, 1958) 95-96.

9. Martin D. O'Keefe, *Known from the Things that Are* (Houston: Center for Thomistic Studies, 1987) 65-70.

10. Cf. Germain Grisez, *The Way of the Lord Jesus*, Vol. I (Chicago: Franciscan Herald Press, 1983) 300-04.

11. Fagothey 338.

12. Fagothey 338.

13. Fagothey 338.

14. Grisez 300.

15. Pope John Paul II, *Evangelium Vitae* (Boston: St. Paul, 1995) #59, pp. 96-97.

16. For a theory of rights and title, cf. Varga 117-18.

17. Cf. Mary Ann Glendon, *Abortion and Divorce in Western Law* (Cambridge: Harvard, 1987), for a discussion of the extremism of the American legal position in comparison with European positions on the legal status of abortion.

18. Cf. Fagothey 152-56; O'Keefe 50-56.

19. Cf. Fagothey 339.

20. Cf. American Association of University Professors, "1940 Statement of Principles on Academic Freedom and Tenure" in *Academic Freedom and Tenure*, ed. Joughin (Madison: Univ. of Wisconsin Press, 1967) 33-39.

THE ESTRANGEMENT OF PERSONS FROM THEIR BODIES

John F. Crosby

"GOD DOES NOT CARE what we do with each other's bodies; He only cares whether we treat each other as persons." Frances Kissling is of course not a thinker of any significance, and yet she did manage with this sentence to give expression to a certain personalist sensibility. And at first glance it may seem to be nothing other than the personalism so often expressed by John Paul II. Recall the firestorm he created in the world press in 1981 when he said in an address that the "adultery in the heart" condemned by Christ can be committed *even within marriage.* It is not enough if the man and the woman are married; they may, he said, still not be respecting each other as persons, they may be only using each other for their gratification. In that case the moral substance of their marital intimacy is "adulterous." John Paul will hear nothing of the idea that the mutual using is legitimated by openness to offspring. It is morally intolerable, no matter how many children the man and the woman bring into the world and raise. Persons must simply never use each other. People like Frances Kissling are glad to hear this.

And yet she said that "God does not care what we do with each other's bodies" by way of expressing her rejection of many of the moral norms based on the fifth and sixth commandments. How is this? We might understand such a rejection coming from a hedonist, but her succinct little utterance does not express hedonism. As I say, there are some sexual things she thinks you ought not do; you must never *use* persons in the exercise of your sexuality, however pleasurable. How does it happen that this worthy concern with respecting persons can get turned against Christian morality? Is there something depersonalized about this morality? But John Paul is a prophet of Christian personalism. How does it happen that he affirms the person in such a way as to rethink and enrich traditional moral teachings on sexuality and respect for life, whereas she affirms the person in such a way as to make shipwreck of these teachings?

117

1

In the last few centuries the personhood of human beings has been experienced and understood as never before. Karol Wojtyla has captured the truth found in this rising personalism in his seminal essay "Subjectivity and the Irreducible in Man." He says that for centuries the image of man in Western thought was one-sidedly "cosmological." Man was thought to fit snugly into nature. Some of the Roman jurists spoke of the "law of nature" as one law that comprises both the moral law governing human beings and those natural laws describing animal instincts. They ran together in one of order of law what for us are two radically incommensurable orders of law (the one prescriptive, the other descriptive). When one approached cosmologically the sexual union of man and woman, what one primarily noticed was the procreative power of their union, a point in which human sexuality strongly resembles animal sexuality. This is why Wojtyla says that cosmologically man was seen too much "from without" and too little "from within," that is, too little in terms of his self-experience, or his subjectivity.

Wojtyla goes on to say that the cosmological view of man began to yield to a more personalist view when people began to notice in a new way their subjectivity, or interiority. With this they experienced each person not as a snugly fitting part of nature but as a "world for himself," his own center, existing in a sense as if the only person. The familiar personalist idea that each person is his own end and no mere instrumental means is born of this awakening to the inwardness of personal subjectivity. People experienced in a new way what it is to act through oneself in freedom, to possess oneself, to determine oneself. They could no longer live in certain archaic forms of social solidarity; each began to think and act in his own name. In the sexual union of man and woman they began to see not only procreative power but also the more specifically personal enactment of a self-surrendering love. And they began to see this because they were looking at man and woman more "from within," paying a new kind of attention to the evidence of spousal subjectivity.

This shift from the cosmological to the personalist view was bound to have consequences for our understanding of the moral life. It is again Wojtyla who points in the personalist direction—in moral philosophy no less than in the underlying anthropology. We have already mentioned the personalist inspiration of his teaching on "marital adultery." If now we look into that rich early work of his, *Love and Responsibility*, we find, among many other things, the most original personalist rethinking of the meaning of chastity. In one place he enters imaginatively into the shame a woman feels when she receives the look of aggressive male sexuality, sensing that in it she becomes only an object of his selfish sexual consumption. Wojtyla says that she shrinks back in a kind of shame because she feels violated as person; she subdues all that could be sexually provocative, not in a puritanical cramp, but in the attempt to remove the occasion for the look which reduces her to an object. Her practice of chastity, Wojtyla concludes, is not in the first place a matter of temperance, nor is it in the first place a matter of placing procreation in its true context: it is above all else a matter of respect for herself as person.

Here is another example of the kind of moral deliberation that we get once the cosmological image of man begins to be modified in a personalist direction. Well known are the old "physicalist" arguments that were sometimes made in the past by way of explaining the wrong of things like contraception. There was, for example, the argument that intercourse performed at a fertile time tends "naturally" to conception and that you act "unnaturally" and hence wrongly by interfering with this tendency. Wojtyla has nothing to do with such "physicalist" or "naturalist" arguments, and in fact he explicitly warns against them in his encyclical, *Veritatis splendor*. He thinks that they are cut from the cosmological cloth and are inadequate to the truth about the person. His own preferred argument on contraception is altogether personalist; he says that the self-donation of the spouses is inevitably perverted into a selfish using of each other when the marital act is sterilized. Whatever one makes of the argument, it is in any case not based on maintaining the intactness of physiological processes or on making natural use of bodily organs, but on what it takes for spouses authentically to live their love for each other. To understand the argument, we have to look at spousal love from within, that is, at the way spouses live their bodily self-surrender one to another.

One sees that Wojtyla's recourse to subjectivity in his personalism has nothing to do with *subjectivism*. In personal subjectivity he hopes to read the structures of personal being, which are for him objective structures underlying objectively valid ethical norms. There is no reason why we have to dissolve truth in a subjectivist way simply because we are doing greater justice to the interiority of man and thus to his personhood. On the contrary, Wojtyla affirms the objectivity of truth in proclaiming in his personalism "the truth about man," as he calls it.

But with all of this we have still not addressed the question we put above. We can put it again like this: why do many moral philosophers who call themselves personalists reject Wojtyla's understanding of chastity, why do they contest his position on contraception and even on abortion? Why does Wojtyla's personalism renew the traditional Christian morality, whereas theirs subverts it?

2

"God does not care what we do with each other's bodies; He only cares whether we treat each other as persons." Is it true that God does not care how we treat each other's bodies? Are we not embodied persons? When we show respect for another, do we not show it for him or her as embodied person? Are there not certain things done to the body of another which are inconsistent with showing him or her respect? Here is the reason why many a personalism gets derailed and becomes an enemy of Christian morality: it does not know how to do justice to the embodiment of human persons, nor does it understand the place of the body in moral action. We have to connect personalism with a proper understanding of embodiment; then, but only then, does it serve the renewal of authentic morality.

Those who fail to do justice to personal embodiment think that the body is in itself something *merely physiological*. Of course, they grant that the human body can take on a more than physiological meaning; it can be drawn up into the world of the person, taking on human and personal meaning. But all such meaning is conferred by persons, just as word-meanings are conferred on word-sounds by the speakers of a language. The human and personal meaning of the body is thus not rooted in the very nature of man as embodied person. In itself the body is just a raw material for the meaning-conferring activities of human persons; only from them does it receive any more-than-physiological meaning. A personalism based on this understanding of embodiment—I call it "spiritualistic personalism"—can only wreak havoc with traditional morality.

For example, according to this personalism the sexual union of man and woman is first of all something merely physiological, not so very different from what is found in some sub-human animals. But man and woman can give their sexual union personal meaning. Perhaps they decide to reserve this union for marriage and to let it express a spousal commitment; perhaps they even decide to leave open its procreative possibility so as to enhance this expressive power. So they may decide; but they may also decide very differently. The man and woman might just as well decide to give their sexual union the meaning of light entertainment, of casual fun with no responsibilities. In this case they will of course sterilize the procreative potential of their union; bringing a new human being into existence is utterly incongruous with the kind of lighthearted fun they have in mind. And there are undoubtedly other meanings besides these two that they might choose. Thus the man and the woman may decide to deprive their sexual union of any intrinsic meaning at all, conferring on it a merely instrumental meaning; this is what happens when they think of it as a mere means for procreation. With this meaning, of course, there can be no question of sterilizing their sexual union.

Now what characterizes the spiritualistic personalism is not that one interprets sexual intimacy as light entertainment. Within the framework of this position one may after all interpret it as spousal commitment. *One thinks as a spiritualist when one thinks that any of these meanings is eligible, that any can be conferred on sexual union, that any can be revoked, and that such union does not inherently, by its very nature, have any personal meaning.*

In thinking this, one may still understand oneself as a personalist, insisting that persons must never be used as mere instruments. Of course, it might seem as if any pretense to personalism had been given up; are man and woman not degraded to the status of a means when, say, their sexual union is said to be an instrument for procreation? But the spiritualist will respond that in this case only the bodies of the man and woman serve as instruments to be used; the persons who use the bodies respect each other as persons by freely collaborating for a common goal. He might explain himself saying that, since we are free to take a stance toward our bodies to the point of making them mere instruments, then it is no more disordered for us to use them instrumentally than to use a hammer. The using refers only to the bodies and does not extend to the persons. And if the spiritualist wants to bring God into it, then he, or she, might add, "God does not care what we do with each other's bodies; He only cares whether we treat each other as persons."

Indeed, the spiritualist goes one step farther and says that you fall away from personalism precisely when you take the personal meaning of sexual union to be a meaning intrinsic to it. For then you make personal meaning follow upon physical facts, and this is as bad as attempting any of those "physicalistic" or "naturalistic" arguments mentioned above. He might add that it is a too cosmological view of man to claim that personal meaning is intrinsic to certain bodily activities; the only truly personalist view is the one that recognizes the freedom of persons to confer and to revoke personal meaning in relation to the body.

3

What is it to take personal embodiment seriously and to hold what we might call an "incarnational personalism"? Let us stay with the example of the sexual union of man and woman. This personalist would say that sexual union intrinsically has an incomparable personal intimacy. In it man and woman expose their most intimate personal selves. Their sexuality extends with its roots into certain depths of their personal being; these depths are stirred up in any sexual encounter between them. If they encounter each other in a trivial way, not meaning anything personally deep or significant by their encounter, then there arises a conflict between the intimate depth in themselves which is engaged by genital sex, and the triviality of their subjective intention. They commonly feel, and the woman typically feels keenly, that they have somehow squandered themselves as persons. They lose self-respect, as one can see unmistakably in the face of every sexually promiscuous girl. They have said too much with their bodies, they have said far more than they mean; they have committed themselves objectively beyond anything that they intend subjectively—hence the dishonesty which shows itself to anyone who thinks closely about casual sex.

The all-important point to be made against the spiritualistic personalism is that man and woman cannot get rid of this dishonesty by deciding to change the meaning of sexual union. They cannot redefine this meaning so that it coincides with their trivial intention. They are impotent to disengage depth and intimacy from sexual union. They cannot repress the intimacy and let sexuality be merely physiological, or be only a medium for light entertainment. This act goes deep by its very nature; it either expresses spousal love and commitment, or it effects a self-squandering, a self-desecration. But it will not be neutralized, will not be rendered harmless. There is a sexual embodiment of the intimate center of each person which we did not ask for and cannot undo; it is a personal meaning of the body that no human person or human society conferred on the body and that no one can remove from it. It is the basis of all kinds of objective norms of sexual behavior, including the norm prescribing that sexual intimacy be reserved for the setting of an enduring spousal commitment.

The point I want to make here is that we cannot understand these norms merely by knowing that persons should always be respected as their own ends and never be used. *We must also know about the embodied personhood of man and woman.* Then it becomes clear that God does indeed care how we treat each other's bodies, *and He cares for the very reason that He requires us to respect each other as persons.*

Wojtyla would add that we do not fall into an excessively cosmological view of man by affirming the natural sexual embodiment of our intimate selves. He would say that our embodiment was well understood in the cosmological view and has to be preserved in any personalist development of the image of man. He would say that he never advocated *replacing* the cosmological with the personalist; it is only a question of *completing* the cosmological, but always only on the basis of preserving all its truth.

4

Men and women who take for granted the spiritualistic personalism have no scruples at all about the procedure of *in vitro* fertilization followed by artificial implantation. They see no personalist problem in using their reproductive systems to supply biological materials to a lab technician who assembles the materials so as to bring about conception. On the contrary, they think that this makes eminent personalist sense because it corrects a deficiency in nature for the sake of bringing into being a new person.

But men and women imbued by incarnational personalism think and feel differently. They instinctively feel the great value of embodied love serving as the cause of conception. They are distressed at how this incomparable way of living their embodiment gives way to an instrumental using of their bodies when these are taken simply as a source of gametes, which are extracted and brought together *in vitro*. They cannot believe that these are just two different methods for achieving conception and that they are to be judged simply on the basis of their effectiveness in achieving it: they feel sure that there must be some moral differences between them. They instinctively feel that with the *in vitro* method they are trying to step out of their bodies, objectifying and using them in a way that violates the truth of their embodiment. It is not that they profess more respect for persons than the other kind of personalists; it is rather that their sense of our embodied personhood leads them to draw different consequences from the imperative to respect persons. It is certainly not that they idolize the "natural" way of achieving conception and have some irrational aversion to the artificiality of the *in vitro* method of achieving it, as if they were hankering after the simplicity of the pre-technological world. No, if the artificial method did not interfere with some great value of their embodiment, they would have no moral qualms about it.

5

Consider the distinction so commonly drawn today between a human being as "biologically human" and a human being as "personal." One says, for example, that the very young human embryo is undeniably human in the biological sense but is not yet a person. To kill it is indeed to kill a human being but not a human person; it is therefore not the kind of killing that violates the imperative to respect persons. In fact, those who speak in this way go on to say that it is even de-personalizing to claim that every biological human being is a person; they say that this is to make the higher thing of personhood to follow upon the lower thing of biological life of a certain kind, and that this is akin to that ethical naturalism, mentioned above, which consists in making moral norms follow on physiological tendencies. They say that it expresses the old cosmological view to see a human person in every human being, whatever its stage of development, and that it is a far more personalist view to be more discriminating about which human beings really count as persons. Perhaps they will venture to take God's point of view and to say, "God does not much care what we do with biological humans; He only cares how we treat persons."

This idea of a biologically human being which is not a person is, of course, a creature of the spiritualistic personalism. If the human body gets raised above the merely physiological and gets invested with personal meaning only by the person conferring such meaning on it, then it seems to follow that the human embryo, in which we can find no meaning-conferring person, is not yet the body of a person: it is still something merely physiological, merely biological. Of course, a more adequate understanding of embodiment will recognize that, just as the sexual embodiment of our intimate personal self is a work of nature, so also the more fundamental thing of being embodied at all, of inhabiting a body, is a work of nature. Neither the one nor the other requires any conscious personal activity on the part of the embodied person. Thus there is no absurdity in the human embryo embodying a human person and therefore being more than biologically human.

This respect for "nature" has nothing to do with naturalism, nothing to do with an excessively cosmological self-understanding: but it has everything to do with respecting the truth of our embodiment. It also has to do with avoiding the delusion that we are capable of a kind of self-creation whereby we effect our own embodiment, embodying ourselves as much or as little as we like, and in whatever way we like, and for as long as we like.

6

The spiritualistic personalism also takes a great toll at a more fundamental level, at the level not just of sex ethics and of the life issues, but of moral first principles. It may at first sound surprising if I say that it underlies the ethical consequentialism that we see all around us: but it is not hard to show a certain spiritualism at the heart of consequentialism. Or to say it the other way around: it is not hard to understand why John Paul II, in the course of rejecting ethical consequentialism in his encyclical, *Veritatis splendor*, found it necessary to affirm repeatedly the unity of the person with his body.

By consequentialism I mean the ethical thesis that the right and wrong of any moral action derives exclusively from the consequences

of the action. Thus an action is right if it will be more productive
of good results or, more exactly, will give a better balance of good
over bad results than any other action open to me when I perform
that action. What, you will ask, is conspicuously spiritualistic here?
Notice that the consequentialist, or proportionalist, speaks here only
of the *right and wrong of moral actions.* But he knows that there is
more to morality than actions; he also has a teaching concerning the
good and bad of inner responses and attitudes. He typically holds that
this moral goodness and badness has nothing to do with results and
consequences; it comes from intentions, motives, ultimate loves,
fundamental options, and the like. He thus posits two almost
incommensurable spheres of morality: an intimate sphere of willing
and loving, and an external sphere where our actions are hardly more
than causes in nature and are measured exclusively by their
consequences.

And now his spiritualism ceases to be hidden. *He thinks that he can
take such a distance to his body that his moral actions become nothing
but an instrumental means for achieving good results.* He thinks he
can place the center of his moral existence in a kind of acosmic
inwardness and can detach from this personal center his external
actions, almost to the point that their norm is nothing more than
their technical efficiency. If you try to object to him that at least
certain actions are so inherently disordered that no good motive can
possibly redeem them morally, he will retort that you must not let
the exterior actions limit the interior act in this way—that this is
akin to the depersonalizing attempt of naturalism to let physiological
tendencies bind us morally—that you are thinking cosmologically
where you should be thinking more personalistically. He might even
say, "God does not care what we do in our external actions; He only
cares whether in our heart of hearts we are loving persons."

If, however, we take seriously our personal embodiment, then we
will not for a minute think that in our moral actions we merely use
the body as an instrument. We readily recognize in the acosmic
inwardness just mentioned a radical estrangement of the person from
his body. We know that being present in the body, incarnate in it,
we are far more than natural causes; we are acting persons, subject
not just to laws of technical efficiency, but to moral norms. We
incarnational personalists know that certain bodily actions, such as
those having the form of using persons, can never be brought into

moral order by good motives; they are inalienably, incurably disordered. If a man and a woman become one flesh apart from any spousal commitment to one another, we know all we need to know to determine the wrong they do; we do not have to examine first the fundamental option of their lives. It is not that we think that a physical event implies a moral condemnation; it is rather that the moral action of an embodied person is not only a physical but also a personal and moral event. We will assert our incarnational personalism by saying, "God cares very much about the form of certain bodily actions *for the very reason* that He cares whether we are loving persons."

People like Frances Kissling and other modern pagans think that the Church hates the human body and especially the sexuality of men and women. It should now be clear that it is in fact these people who hate the body, who chafe under their embodiment, who impotently try to undo it, who would rather use the body instrumentally than be embodied in it, who would cultivate a disembodied moral existence that does not befit human beings. It is only the Christian tradition for which John Paul speaks that knows how intimately the body is incorporated into the human person and what dignity it has as a result. He is *the* defender of the human body against its modern detractors. In raising his voice in witness of the "truth about man," he protests not only against materialism, but no less against this spiritualism.

His personalism, then, is an incarnational personalism. It is a personalism that knows the whole man, the embodiment of man no less than his personhood. It underlies the authentic personalist ethics. But the spiritualistic, or gnostic, personalism, recognizing only personhood and doing little justice to embodiment, works with a caricature of man. Little wonder that it develops an ethics constantly in conflict with the ethics of authentic, integral personalism.

INTENTIONS IN MEDICAL ETHICS

J. L. A. Garcia

INTRODUCTION

In Western medical ethics, the center has not held and things are fast falling apart. Some practices long recognized as barbarous in themselves and opposed to the nature and aims of medicine are now routine, others are fast winning acceptance, and even those still beyond the pale have an air of inevitability. Abortion is now one of the most common medical procedures; assisted suicide enjoys broad public support and has won some contests in courts, legislatures, and popular referenda; infanticide and passive euthanasia are increasingly widespread practices, for which some demand legalization and moral legitimation. Flood tides of social change erode our long-held conception of medicine and its associated restraints and pull us into a sea of medical homicide. A new ethic, really a reinvigorated ethic from the Enlightenment, has emerged to grant its moral and intellectual *imprimatur* to medicine's lethal new agenda. In it medical technology is to proceed largely unconstrained by any fear that we degrade humanity when we consider the sick and dying merely as providers of recyclable organs, or when we treat people as objects of manufacture and their parts as commercial goods, or when we experiment on embryos *in utero* or in test-tubes or on the terminally ill. Indeed, in the emerging ethic, modern medicine's technological imperative increasingly meets its match only when it runs afoul of the new agenda of death and dehumanization. For these "ethicists" technology systematically loses out only to the fear lest it be used to preserve life our elites deem unworthy, nonautonomous, or undignified, especially the lives of those relegated to their new, Orwellian category of human "unpersons": the brain-damaged, the irreversibly comatose, the unborn, and so on.

The Hippocratic tradition famously deplored several of these now accepted, even fashionable, practices, most notably, euthanasia and abortion. However, it acknowledged that some medical procedures it deemed legitimate could sometimes go wrong, prematurely ending a patient's life or pregnancy, while others were known to cause pain or loss of function as side-effects of measures taken to restore health

or preserve life. The medical code came to limit its condemnation
to the "intentional termination of life," a formulation still sometimes
employed. One reason for this is straightforward. Medicine is, as we
say today, a part of *health*-care. Its primary goal, and that of its
practitioners, is the patient's health, understood as the integrated
functioning of her systems as an organism. Dying is the comprehensive breakdown and dissolution of this functioning. You do not get
any less healthy, any worse off as an organism, than death. So, as
the tradition recognized, it perverts medical skills to turn them to the
pursuit of death, whether as means or end, as happens when
physicians become executioners, suicide assistants, or—assuming the
unborn are human beings—abortionists.[1] Those "ethicists" who
celebrate the emerging medical order have made this restriction their
preferred target, identifying the traditional claim that life is sacred
with endorsement of just such a moral principle against the
intentional termination of human life.[2] Thus, Helga Kuhse labels
"the [Q]ualified Sanctity-of-Life Principle" the thesis that "it is
absolutely prohibited either intentionally to kill a patient or
intentionally to let a patient die, and to base decisions relating to the
prolongation and shortening of human life on consideration of its
quality or kind; it is, however, sometimes permissible to refrain from
preventing death."[3] She directs her book's arguments chiefly against
this thesis. The self-declared enemies of life's sanctity insist the
stricture against medical personnel acting with the intent that a
patient's life end stems from religious faith and lacks all justification
outside that context.[4]

In my view, these hostile critics of this element of traditional
medical ethics deeply misunderstand or ignore reasons supporting it.
In other essays I have tried to defend traditional moral absolutism
against general philosophical attacks, especially its emphasis on the
moral crucial role of the agent's intentions. Here I wish to rebut
some of the criticisms salient in the medical ethics literature,
concentrating on Kuhse's discussion, which is, as far as I know, the
most detailed and sophisticated attack on the moral importance of
intentions in medical ethics. I will defend what we can call
"intention-sensitivity" in medical ethics. More specifically, I will try
to show (i) that there is a genuine psychological difference between
intending something to result from one's behavior and merely
expecting it to, (ii) how it can matter to whether a health-care

worker acts in ways morally permissible that she intended (and does not merely foresee) certain aspects or results of her behavior, and (iii) that we can often have reasonable beliefs about whether an agent acted with an intention that should disqualify a course of action. My approach here will be secular in James Rachels' sense: I will not treat morality simply "as a matter of faithfulness to abstract rules or divine laws," but rather will treat "the point of morality [or, as I should prefer to say, one of the chief objectives of moral agents] as the good of creatures on earth."[5]

I. MUST SOMEONE INTEND TO DO ALL SHE EXPECTS TO DO?

Kuhse worries about efforts to limit the scope of the agent's intentions so that a physician might intend to turn off a patient's life-sustaining respirator without intending to kill her. She thinks there is no principled way of keeping this restricted notion of intention from contracting to the point where blatant malefactors are exonerated. If the physician can say she meant only to turn off the respirator but not to kill, why cannot the greedy and impatient heir say she did not mean to kill her rich uncle but only to shut his body down long enough for the authorities to think him dead and award her the inheritance? What Kuhse calls the Qualified Sanctity of Life doctrine requires some limitation in the scope of intentions, but then how do we keep things that common sense and traditional medical ethics classify as intended from turning into mere side-effects? If intended means can turn into side-effects so easily, is there a real difference between them?

I think Kuhse exaggerates the problem here, misled perhaps by misinterpreting a line of argument defenders of intention-sensitive ethics offer. It is true that to show that the physician injecting a medicine does not intend the pain she causes her patient, defenders sometimes point out that the physician's medical objective derives no advantage from the pain itself but only from the injection. This is true, but by itself it is not sufficient to show that the physician does not intend the pain. The physician may hate the patient, who has been uncooperative and rude, say, and may not only delight in the latter's pain but inject the medicine motivated in part by her desire for such revenge. The traditionalists who made this point relied on the fact that they were discussing a *physician*, presumed to be a person of good-will, not ill-will. Their point was that this injection did not itself compromise that good-will. They were not imagining an agent motivated by hate or revenge. The injection need not involve any intent to cause pain and they assumed that nothing else in the agent committed her to such an intention. Once this is seen, fears like those of Kuhse can be shown to be immaterial.

She points out that in certain kinds of abortion motivated by concern to save the pregnant woman's life, the fetus' death is not a "necessary means" to the medical end.[6] That is correct. However, the relevant psychological issue is not what an agent rationally *has to* intend in acting to achieve her end, but what she *does* intend. Even if fetal death is not a "necessary means" in many abortions, it may be true that it is an *actual* means, what the agent does intend, even if she could have acted similarly with other intentions. Where Kuhse talks about what needs to be included within the scope of the agent's intention on "any plausible interpretation of what the agent intends," what we need is not a merely "plausible" interpretation of her intention but an accurate one.[7] There is no reason to suppose that agents always intend only the bare minimum necessary to achieve their goals. Normally, people leave themselves a little margin for error in what they intend. Oftentimes, if we aim to attain the result $X + Y$, then we are more likely to ensure it is at least X. So often we set ourselves the wider aim. The detective detains all those present at the scene of the crime to ensure the one who killed does not escape. The frightened infantry soldier decides to kill all civilians in a village to make sure that no members of the guerrilla movement survive. The baseball manager has the relief pitcher warming up early so she will be ready if and when needed later on. The physician removes extra tissue beyond that known to be cancerous to make it more likely she gets all the diseased tissue. In all these cases, an agent, sometimes permissibly, sometimes not, intends more than she minimally needs for her goal.

This fact provides a response to Kuhse and others.[8] They maintain that the restricted conception of intention employed to exonerate the physician from the charge of intentionally harming when she gives the injection will similarly exonerate from any intention to kill the greedy heir who need only intend that her victim be judged dead long enough for her to collect, the terror-bomber who need only intend that her victims look dead long enough to demoralize the enemy leaders, as well as the physician who need only intend to collapse or remove the fetus' head to save the woman's life. These thinkers tend to welcome the last conclusion and to deplore the others, but their main point is that the distinction between what is intended and what merely foreseen becomes unstable, even incoherent, therein undermining its use in any acceptable ethics. However, it should now be clear that the more serious question is not whether the greedy heir, the terror-bomber, and the physician *need to* intend death but whether in fact they do. There is good reason to suppose so. First, few real-life agents are likely to have framed their practical deliberation and their decision-making in such sophisticated terms as those these enemies of intention-sensitive ethics place in the minds of their imaginary agents. For familiar Humean, associationist reasons, not every distinction of propositions the mind can be brought to recognize is one that it does (or is likely or able to) observe/utilize in actual practical deliberation and decision-making. Second, it is not the case simply that each agent had a certain limited objective and took action to achieve it. Each must also have adopted some scheme for connecting action to objective. To identify that we need to determine, as best we can, each agent's plan of action. We need to find out how these agents meant their actions to get them to their objectives. Surely, even if they are so sophisticated (indeed, sophistical) that they adopt such rarefied objectives as those of making it appear that their chosen victims are dead, nevertheless, the most likely, secure, and attractive scenario for getting from dropping the bomb on a city to demoralizing enemy leaders with the thought that its inhabitants are dead is to have the bomb actually kill them. That an agent adopts such an artificially narrowed objective does not preclude her also adopting a wider instrumental one as a way of securing it. Indeed, as we see, the broader objective is quite likely to be part of the intended path from the action to the narrower objective, just as the baseball manager may ask two pitchers to warm up as her way of ensuring that she will have ready the one she needs. That separates the imaginary, sophistical agents of the critics' examples from the familiar ones the tradition described, whose sensibly narrowed intentions (to heal but not to hurt, for example) were related to ordinary, recognizable human planning.

We should note another difficulty as well. Both Kuhse and her opponents may have mislocated the more important moral issue for an intention-sensitive ethics. I think that in such cases as those of abortions to spare the woman's body physical traumas from pregnancy—as distinct from those to save her (or others) from the difficulties of birth or child-rearing—the major question may lie elsewhere: not in whether the agent intends the death, but whether the intention she does act with (even if not to cause or allow death) is comparably illicit, as in intentionally crushing or removing someone's head. Foot claimed that occasionally two possible contents of intention, p and q, are so "close" that when someone intends p she intends q. Kuhse asks what this talk of "closeness" of possible intentional contents means and how it can matter to what an agent intends.[9] I think the insight to which Foot points is that p is *sometimes* so connected to q that it is either implausible to claim (i) that an agent intended p but did not intend q, or implausible to claim (ii) that the difference between her intending p and intending q makes an important moral difference. It is crucial to intention-sensitive ethics that this is not *always* true, of course. But to make such an ethics credible, its proponents do well to follow Foot in conceding that it is, in some circumstances, true for some propositional pairs, p and q.

"Closeness" can matter to what an agent intends ("psychological closeness") because, as we noted, that the mind can be brought to recognize a certain distinction of possible intentional contents does not imply that, on a given occasion, it utilizes that distinction in its actual practical deliberation and decision-making. Closeness can matter to the moral permissibility of what the agent intentionally does ("moral closeness"), because sometimes p and q will be so connected that intending p will be vicious for largely the same reasons that intending q is. Consider a much-discussed example from Foot, in which spelunkers use dynamite to blow up the body of an overweight comrade who has gotten himself caught in the cave's entrance and his company trapped inside. Perhaps they do not mean to kill him but "only" to destroy his body. However, it is reasonable to think that, given the nature of bodily integrity as a component of human well-being, the latter intention, like the former, will suffice to rule out the action as vicious. So, too, for the abortionist's intention to remove someone's head. There will, of course, be different accounts of what makes acting from one intention immoral in a way comparable to that of acting from a closely connected one. I think the best way to understand such matters is to say that each intention is about equally distant from the standard of some relevant moral virtues. Whether or not that is correct, intention-sensitive ethics is committed neither to the claim that absolutely every difference in intention matters morally nor to the claim that an agent's intentions must be in the clear morally if she does not intend anyone's death.

II. DISTINGUISHING INTENDED RESULTS FROM SIDE-EFFECTS

Even if there is in principle a relatively stable difference between intended results and side-effects, is it a difference sufficiently discernible to be of use to us in our moral deliberation or assessment? Can we *know* what we intend to do (as distinct from what we merely expect to do)? In general, there are several questions we can ask to help determine what we or others intend in action and, specifically, to determine whether a medical care-giver intends someone to die. (i) Does the patient's death figure in the agent's plan not just as a presupposition, or a probable result, but as an *objective* (an interim or ultimate goal), a thing to be attained? (ii) Is she *trying* to attain the patient's death? (iii) Does she do anything *in order to* attain death? (iv) Does she perform the lethal action *in order to* derive some objective (perhaps only an interim goal) *from the death itself*? (v) Does the death make her and her behavior at least a partial *success*? (vi) Would survival make her and her behavior at least a partial *failure*? When the answer to any of these questions is affirmative, the agent intends the death, for any affirmative answer places the behavior within a plan of action in the special role only intentions occupy.[10]

Other tests for distinguishing intended results from side-effects have sometimes been proposed, but they have misled some. So, it is said that we must welcome intended results but not expected side-effects, and must regret it when an intended result does not occur but not when a merely expected one fails to materialize. However, this is open to the argument that since the high-minded mercy-killer need not rejoice over the death of her victim/beneficiary and might even be cheered if the patient not only miraculously escaped death but fully recovered, then perhaps the mercy-killer does not intend to kill.[11] I suppose the mercy-killer might be pleased by a miraculous cure, but what matters is that, in the event of such a miracle, she and her action would have been *failures* in the effort to get the patient dead. Welcoming the recovery involves abandoning and repudiating her plan to kill, and that distinguishes her mental stance from that of someone who expected to shorten life but did not intend to. (Of course, she can still stand ready to reactivate the homicidal plan should the patient relapse, but she renounces the plan for the time being.)

Similarly, some defenders of intention-sensitive ethics have relied upon what is called the counterfactual test for intention. According to it, on Kuhse's formulation, the key question for the agent is: "If you had believed your action would not have resulted in the patient's death, would you still have acted in the way you did?"[12] Partisans of intention-sensitive medical ethics have wanted to say that the physician who legitimately prescribes high doses of pain-killer to a patient for whom lesser doses would be ineffective, even though they may shorten the patient's life, can answer this question affirmatively. Similarly, a doctor can answer affirmatively who withdraws what are usually deemed "extraordinary means," such as dialysis and artificial respiration machines, from an irreversibly comatose patient for the sake of "avoiding 'the investment of instruments and personnel... disproportionate to the results foreseen.'"[13] However, according to traditional defenders of intention-sensitive medical ethics, the mercy-killer cannot "act the same way." The mercy-killer needs the patient's death for her plans for pain-relief to succeed, and must change her plans if she loses her belief that the patient will die from her conduct. The plans of the first two physicians, in contrast, do not depend on the patient's dying, so they need not change them and can continue to act "the same way," even if they think their patients will survive the high dosage of pain-killer and the withdrawal of treatment, respectively.

Problems attend this test as well. Kuhse rejects the usual interpretation of the test question, according to which only the expected results of the patient's death ("causally downstream factors"), but not its causes ("causally upstream factors"), are changed in the situation where we imagine that she will not die.[14] She argues that this interpretation is unfair and "misleading because it makes it easy to ignore causally upstream factors that are relevant to letting die but not to killing: whether, because of causally upstream factors, the agent's action or omission is under particular circumstances sufficient to bring about a patient's death. If it is, as it is in the cases mentioned, then we cannot leave out the causally upstream factors that make the agent's action what it is: an instance of letting die, or of refraining from preventing death, rather than an instance of 'turning off an iron lung.'"[15]

To the limited extent that I follow Kuhse's reasoning, it appears to me that she has misunderstood the test's point. The relevant issue is what is part of the agent's actual plan. What the proponent of intention-sensitive medical ethics has wanted to show is that death is not part of the agent's plan in permissible instances of letting die. The test helps show this because changing her expectation of death tends to change the mercy-killer's behavior because it forces a change in her plans to end her patient's pain, while it tends not to change the behavior of the other physicians (i. e., the ones who discontinue extraordinary means or who prescribe high dosages of pain-killers to relieve discomfort even at the risk of hastening death) because it forces no change in their plans, since their patients' deaths were not planned in the first place. These latter physicians "act the same way" even if they know their omissions will not now constitute instances of letting die. However, the mercy-killer has no reason to 'act the same way' when she finds her action will not be a killing, since she acts as she does *inter alia* in order to kill. To accept Kuhse's interpretation of the test question is to beg the question by rigging things so that the agent's plan-changes track death.[16]

Kuhse thinks "incoherent" common sense's moderate conception of intention, according to which an agent intends all her ends and means (objectives) but not the side-effects of her actions (the ones she merely foresees). We have seen that there is no basis for such a judgment. We intend what we plan to do and the tests I earlier proposed can usually identify what we intend, especially when the question is whether someone acts with a homicidal or other seriously evil-minded intention. Hence, we can reject both disjuncts in the dilemma with which Kuhse confronts defenders of intention-sensitive ethics and the Qualified Sanctity of Life thesis: "accept the broad conception of the intentional, according to which the agent terminates life intentionally whenever she could by an act or omission prevent a foreseen death and refrains from doing so; or... accept the narrow conception of the intentional, according to which an agent terminates life intentionally only when she intends the death in question as her end, for its own sake."[17]

It is absurd to think I intend to terminate your life even though I do nothing whatever aimed at making sure you are dead, so any broad conception of intent is unacceptable. It is counter-intuitive on its face and in its implications, and it goes contrary to our best current understandings of intention, which conceive of intention as what one plans, aims, or tries to do whether as end or means.[18] It also, quite absurdly, renders intentional even things the agent expects to do but tries to avoid, such as boring an audience or lisping. Kuhse and others who support such an excessively broad conception of intention at least owe us some general and persuasive account of intention to make such a view plausible. This is missing. Likewise, the extremely narrow conception of intention that includes only what the agent pursues "for its own sake" and excludes the agent's chosen means is absurd. There is little in life we pursue for its own sake. Many philosophers have thought there was only one such end, though they disagreed on what it was. The narrow conception of the intentional, whether meant to apply (quite arbitrarily) only to cases of intending death or as a general account, implies that we do almost nothing intentionally, depriving the notion of its crucial role in the explanation of human action. Thus, quite apart from their implications for morality, these extremely broad and narrow views of the intentional, at least insofar as they imply (as Kuhse's argument requires) comparably broad and narrow conceptions of what is *intended*, are unacceptable simply as theses in philosophical psychology, independently of their implausible implications for ethics.

III. CAN AN ACTION'S MORALITY DEPEND UPON WHAT THE AGENT INTENDS?

Even if there is an accessible, coherent, and moderate notion of intention, according to which an agent intends her means and ends but not the side-effects of what she does, does the morality of behavior ever hang on what the agent intended? More specifically, can it make a difference to whether an agent acted permissibly whether she intended a certain result or merely expected it as a side-effect? This is what proponents of intention-sensitive ethics affirm and its opponents deny. Let us consider some grounds offered for this denial.

Rachels charges that any theory that makes the morality of an agent's conduct thus depend on the agent's intentions must violate the principle of rationality and morality that similar cases be treated alike. To show this, he invites us to consider Jack and Jill, both of whom visit their "sick and lonely grandmother"—Jill in order to ingratiate herself to win inclusion in the old woman's will, Jack simply from the compassionate desire to cheer her up. "Jack's intention was honorable and Jill's was not. Could we say on that account that what Jack did was right but what Jill did was not right? No: for Jack and Jill did the very same thing, and if they did the same thing in the same circumstances, we cannot say that one acted rightly and one acted wrongly. Consistency requires that we assess similar actions similarly." He concludes, "the traditional view says that the intention with which an act is done is relevant to determining whether the act is right. The example of Jack and Jill suggests that, on the contrary, the intention is not relevant to deciding whether the act is right or wrong, but is instead relevant to assessing the character of the person who does it, which is another thing entirely."[19]

The relation between assessments of intentions and character assessment is a complex matter into which I will not now proceed. What should we make of Rachels' argument for his thesis that intention is irrelevant to whether conduct is right or wrong? Not much, I think. Such arguments blatantly beg the question. Consistency does not require that things in *any* way similar be treated alike, only that things *relevantly* similar be treated alike. Proponents of intention-sensitive ethics maintain that the intention with which an action is done is relevant to its moral permissibility. Rachels' argument merely presupposes that this is not true, it offers no reason to reject it. One could as easily "prove" that consistency rules out any moral theory, e. g., act utilitarianism. Suppose that, out of affection, Joe and Jane both visit their sickly and rather grumpy grandfather. Since the old man loathes Joe but loves Jane, Joe's visit brings about less pleasure than his staying home would, but Jane's act brings more pleasure into the world than anything she could have done. The act utilitarian judges Joe's action impermissible but Jane's right. However, they did "the very same thing" (visit grandfather) in the same circumstances (the sickness, e. g.), and so the utilitarians' judgment violates consistency. Obviously, this argument merely presupposes that the acknowledged difference in the effects of Joe's and Jane's actions makes no moral difference.   This consistency argument against utilitarianism does not prove false the utilitarian thesis that effects are relevant; it simply assumes it is false. In   just the same way, however, Rachels' consistency argument assumes that the acknowledged difference in the intentions behind Jack's and Jill's actions makes no moral difference. It presupposes that the thesis of intention-sensitivity is false, instead of showing it is false.[20]

The charge of inconsistency fails without support, but it may suggest a somewhat better argument against intention-sensitivity in ethics. If the rightness or wrongness of what I do depends on my intentions, then will not an intention-sensitive ethics normally be unable to answer the ordinary request for moral advice: Is it permissible morally for me to do *V*? Will not the intention-sensitive theorist have to duck any such straightforward question, and reply only, weakly, "Well, it depends (on what intentions you would have)?" And is this not a serious weakness insofar as a moral theory is supposed to guide practice?   These worries are less blatantly without merit, but on examination they pose no serious difficulty. Again, this can be brought out by comparing intention-sensitive ethics with other approaches to moral theory. Intention-sensitive medical ethics is no more at fault here than is either (direct or indirect) consequentialism or Kant's theory. All demand further information before answering such a question as "May I morally do *V*?" Before it can offer its own answer to the request for moral advice, each must await answer to its special question: With what intentions would you do *V*? With what total results? From what "maxims"?   Indeed, the answer to the question that inten-tion-sensitive medical ethics asks is likely to be contained in the term "*V*," at least, if "*V*"is a term from our familiar, ordinary moral vocabulary, such as "lie," "rape," or "kidnap," or from specialized medical ethics terminology such as "directly kill" or "directly abort."[21] The application of any of these terms requires that the agent have certain intentions, and these are precisely the kinds of intentions (to deceive, to coerce, etc.) to which intention-sensitive ethical theories have traditionally assigned morally determinative import. This is not the case for total results or "maxims." I cannot know that what I do would be a lie without knowing some of the morally pertinent intentions with which I would be acting, but I can know it would be a lie without knowing its total effects or the 'maxim' on which I would be acting. When it comes to giving a non-evasive response to a request for moral guidance couched in the terms of our ordinary moral discourse or in suitably specialized vocabularies, then, intention-sensitive ethical theory is at a considerable advantage over its chief rivals.

Now consider a different, stronger argument against intention-sensitive ethics. Many have rejected intention-sensitivity in ethics on the grounds that it threatens to evacuate moral norms of power and invites hypocrisy, because an agent can, it is said, always evade an intention-sensitive norm against what she wants to do simply by tinkering with her intentions but otherwise acting the same to similar effect. Glanville Williams considers it "altogether too artificial to say that a doctor who gives an overdose of a narcotic having in the forefront of his mind the aim of ending the patient's existence is guilty of sin, while a doctor who gives the same overdose in the same circumstances in order to relieve pain is not guilty of sin, provided he keeps his mind off the [inevitable] consequence...." He concludes that if intention-sensitivity "means that the necessity of making a choice of values can be avoided merely by keeping your mind off one of the consequences, it can only encourage a hypocritical attitude towards moral problems."[22]

Must intention-sensitivity make norms of action vacuous and encourage hypocrisy? I think not, though it seems to me that Williams and other critics of intention-sensitivity have a legitimate concern when they raise the danger of easy changes of intention by the mere "redirection" of one's will. We cannot plausibly maintain that intentions play a decisive moral role if they are so shallow in the person, phenomena so readily manipulable that they may, like some internal flashlight, be turned on or off, directed this way or that, with only the slightest and easiest of adjustments. The sorts of changes of mind and conduct that respectable norms of moral actions must require of an agent inclined toward evildoing must be real, and they must be *substantial*. When I say that changes of intention must be something real, I mean that they cannot consist solely in redescription, nor in pretense (lies), nor in self-deception. When I say that they must be substantial, I mean that they cannot consist simply in the agent's keeping this or that at the "forefront of his mind," and that they cannot be merely ceremonial (e. g., repeating to oneself "I'm only trying to do X, not Y").

Fortunately, there is little basis for regarding intentions as shallow phenomena. A real change of intentions is a genuine change in one's actual plans. It requires adopting a different set of objectives and instruments. It is to launch oneself on a different path to one's destination, at least, if not to set off for a different destination itself. This is not a merely linguistic matter, dressing things up in finer language, let alone concealing them behind a false front. Yet this is the picture Williams offers. Tellingly, he contrasts an agent's putting "in the forefront of his mind [one] aim" with "keep[ing] his mind off the consequence." However, if we examine it, we shall see that this passage runs together two contrasts, and runs them together in a way designed to make the discredit of the merely ceremonial one, a difference of emphasis, to rub off on and bias us against the other, which is important and substantive. The first contrast in the passage is that between what I keep at the mental forefront and what I manage to distract myself from. The second contrast is between what the agent aims to achieve and what she merely expects as a consequence of her action. This latter is an important psychological difference. Indeed, it contrasts two *types* of psychological stance, since expectation is a doxastic state and intention a volitional, and thus, conative, state. Doxastic states are evaluated for truth-value; the way the world is stands as the standard against which they are assessed. Conative states normally are not evaluated for truth-value. Rather, we tend to treat them as standards against which we assess the way the world is to determine which parts of it to change.[23]

Williams, of course, may think that the difference between something's being my aim and its being a consequence is the same thing as the difference between my having it in the forefront of my mind and my keeping my mind off it. However, this is a highly implausible account of intention, and I can see no advantage it has over the more sophisticated accounts we have today, which understand intentions in terms of what plays a certain peculiar role in one's practical planning. While it is highly implausible to maintain that it makes an important moral difference what I keep telling myself (or otherwise maintain at the front of my mind) and what I distract myself from, that is very different from the thesis of intention-sensitive ethics that it matters morally what I do or do not treat as good, that is, what I aim at, strive after, and favor as an *agendum*, a thing to be attained or done. Whether I keep something at the forefront or the background of my mind is a matter of no evident moral import and seems quite a fishy business in any case, an empty psychological ceremony or—worse—an opportunity for self-deception. However, whether I adopt something as a good, as a thing to be attained or, on the other hand, merely accept it as a probability that I make no special plans to oppose, is a matter of different responses to possible situations. Moreover, since some of these responses are desirable or undesirable, this distinction marks a difference between two contrasting forms of value-response. Modes of value-response constitute a long-acknowledged and highly plausible source of morality, most notably in Brentano and Scheler, but also more recently in Chisholm and Nozick.

Although Williams *et al.* have, as we saw, a valid (though overstated) concern here, we should note something ugly and disturbing in their criticism itself: the critics seem to assume a merely instrumentalist picture of human relationships. Hobbes provides a negative model of instrumentalism, in which other persons confront one primarily as rivals, dangers. Bentham and Epicurus, perhaps, provide a more positive model, in which others matter to one as potential sources of new benefits, not just as threats to the benefits one could acquire alone. What is important is that no such instrumentalism about human relationships is either appealing or plausible. People matter to one another not merely as potential *causes* of welcome or unwelcome results, but as *subjects*. I care about you as such, independently of and prior to my interest in what you can do for me (and my fear of what you may do to me). I care about how you feel about me, irrespective of whether you bring me additional benefits or burdens. Because of this, the contents of your heart—your desires for me, hopes, fears, and aims—take on human significance independent of their causal impact on me.

An appealing and human moral theory should assign such contents of the human heart and aspiration moral importance in their own right. One of the places where these critics go wrong is in their implicitly instrumentalist assumption that no "mere" change of heart can really matter to morality, let alone be its focus. I think a human morality makes what matters centrally in morality the same things that matter centrally to us as people. Those are not merely the probable effects on us of people's actions, but the contents of their hearts in their attitudes and aims (instrumental or ultimate) toward us. This is the essence of a properly intention-sensitive ethics, and it suggests that such a theory should be part of a broader theory centered on what people want, enjoy, aim at, and oppose—in short, on the virtues.

CONCLUSION. "THOU SHALT NOT KILL; BUT NEED'ST NOT STRIVE/OFFICIOUSLY TO KEEP ALIVE."
    A final observation. Glover, Kuhse, and other proud opponents of life's sanctity pour scorn on naive defenders of the tradition who have quoted A. H. Clough's satiric line from his "The New Decalogue," as if meant straightforwardly. They are, of course, right to remind us of the poet's irony. However, we should not be misled into thinking the poem is well interpreted as an endorsement of Rachels' thesis that killing and letting die are morally equivalent. The poem makes little sense read as bestowing a moral *imprimatur* on killing, especially medical killing, as today's ethicists are wont to do. Rather, Clough seems to satirize the legalistic abuse that looks for moral loopholes and supposes we are automatically in the clear if we can just avoid the behavioral extreme explicitly condemned. Intention-sensitive ethical theory, especially if virtues-based, nicely avoids that legalism while preserving the spirit, grounds and letter of the moral condemnation of typical killings as wrong because vicious in the attitudes toward human life they express. Letting die, like killing, can but need not also embody such vice. Whether it does will depend on the motivational inputs that inform their behavior or omission. An ethical theory that is insensitive to what, we must admit, are sometimes subtle matters of intention is condemned to insensitivity to the human heart and thus to the heart of medical ethics and of any genuinely human morality as well.

NOTES

1. See J. L. A. Garcia, "Better Off Dead?" in *American Philosophical Association Newsletter on Philosophy and Medicine* 92:1 (1993) 85-88 and responses in following numbers of that periodical.

2. See especially James Rachels, *The End of Life* (Oxford: Oxford Univ. Press, 1986) chs. 2, 6; Helga Kuhse, *The Sanctity of Life Doctrine in Medicine: A Critique* (Oxford: Oxford Univ. Press, 1987) chs. 1, 3 ; Peter Singer, *Rethinking Life and Death* (New York: St. Martin's Press, 1994, *passim*. "Celebrate" is not too strong a word. Singer, for example, sees medicine's recent turn toward death as great news, "a period of opportunity, in which we have a historic chance to shape something better... an ethic that is more compassionate and more responsive to what people decide for themselves." By this last, he means less fussy about killing those who despair or who are deemed unworthy of protection. Singer (6, 189) offers five "new commandments" to replace the old ones and enthusiastically heralds "another Copernican Revolution," in ethics this time.

I should make it clear at the outset that throughout I presuppose that an agent intentionally does only what she intends to do. This is sometimes denied both by defenders and opponents of intention-sensitive ethics, but I think it true, have defended it elsewhere and, since Kuhse (whose work I treat in some detail) also seems to presuppose it, it is best to work with it here. On the dispute, see, especially J. L. A. Garcia, "The Intentional and the Intended" in *Erkenntnis* 33 (1990) 191-209.

3. Kuhse 23.

4. "[T]he absolute prohibition of the intentional termination of life has its source in theology, and makes little sense outside that particular framework." (Kuhse 15)

Discussing some "assumptions" of traditional Western moral thought, including the principle "that we are responsible for what we intentionally do in a way that we are not responsible for what we deliberately fail to prevent," Singer writes, "Taken independently of their religious origins, both of the crucial assumptions are on very weak ground." (Singer 221)

The critics tend to remain silent on whether they think it justified even *within* a religious context, perhaps because they find such thinking too unfamiliar. Not all the apologists for medical homicide are so circumspect, however. Rachels writes, "We have now looked at three arguments [against the morality of euthanasia] that depend on religious assumptions. They are all unsound, but I have not criticized them simply by rejecting their religious presuppositions.... The upshot is that religious people are in the same position as everyone else. There is nothing in religious belief in general, or in Christian belief in particular, to preclude the acceptance of mercy-killing as a humane response to some awful situations." (Rachels 165)

5. Rachels 6, 38. This secular approach frees me from the need here to show how what I say squares with any religious or ethical tradition, let alone recent interpretations or extensions of it. On the other hand, I do not deny that such fidelity can be a useful corrective to our tendency to go astray when we try in Singer's terms to "rethink" complex matters *ab initio*. I suspect that Kuhse gets confused by taking the innovations of a dissident theologian such as Fr. Gerard Hughes as amply representative of his

tradition, and that Rachels makes a similar mistake in relying upon Daniel Maguire. I hope my approach here will also free me from that sort of danger. Of course, as Rachels notes, my taking a secular approach here does not commit me to a generally anti-theistic understanding of morality.

6. Kuhse 96.

7. Kuhse 108.

8. See Jonathan Bennett, "Morality and Consequences" in *Tanner Lectures on Human Values*, vol. 2, ed. Sterling McMurrin (Salt Lake City: Univ. of Utah Press, 1981) 47-116; Robert Holmes, *On War and Morality* (Princeton: Princeton Univ. Press, 1989); and the discussion of David Lewis' objection by Warren Quinn, "Actions, Intentions, and Consequences: The Doctrine of Double Effect" in *Philosophy and Public Affairs* 18 (1989) 334-51 at 343 n.16.

9. Philippa Foot, "The Problem of Abortion and the Doctrine of Double Effect" in *Oxford Review* 5 (1967) 5-15 [reprinted in Foot, *Virtues and Vices* (Berkeley: Univ. of California Press, 1978), ch. 1]; Kuhse 100ff.

10. These are discussed a bit further in J. L. A. Garcia, "On the Irreducibility of the Will" in *Synthese* 86 (1991) 349-60. On intentions and plans, see Michael Bratman, *Intentions, Plans, and Reasons for Action* (Cambridge: Harvard Univ. Press, 1990).

11. See Kuhse, secs. 3.43, 3.44, esp. p. 126.

12. Kuhse 131.

13. Kuhse 124ff.

14. Kuhse prefers to interpret the question as requiring us to suppose that everything causally connected to the death either as effect or as cause changes. She maintains that, so interpreted, not just the mercy-killer but also the physicians whose conduct partisans of intention-sensitive ethics have traditionally defended would answer the test question negatively. On her preferred interpretation of the test question, she says, the doctor in the "extraordinary means" case we mentioned, no less than the mercy-killer, "would also answer 'no' if asked the test question, because he too believes that there is no death, and hence must believe there will be no saving of disproportionate resources (for he believes the resources are needed to keep the patient alive)." She concludes that "the test question will not allow us to distinguish between the intentions of the doctors." (Kuhse 132f)

I confess that I cannot follow Kuhse's reasoning here. Presumably, Kuhse should be understood as toying here with different understandings of the metaphysicians' proposal that counterfactuals be understood as claims about what obtains in those possible worlds "closest" to the actual. If we imagine that the patient will not die, and we change everything causally connected to her death, either as cause or as effect, then what seems to follows is not that the medical equipment is "needed to keep the patient alive," but that she does not have a life-threatening illness. After all, the equipment is needed to keep her alive in the situation where she would die without it. If we suppose that she does not die when it is turned off, then it must be that it was not needed for life. Given that, I see no basis for Kuhse's insistence that the physician in the extraordinary means case would not "act the same way," that is, would not turn off the equipment.

15. Kuhse 134. She seems not to notice that my action can be one of turning off an iron lung, and thus in one respect acting the same way, whether or not my action is also one of therein causing (or, as some would describe it, allowing) someone to die. Whenever we vary the circumstances in which an agent acts, or the results or intentions with which she acts, we insure that in some respects she acts differently even if in other respects she acts the same way. That follows from the obvious fact that an action can have different descriptions, determined by different aspects. Kuhse talks as if it made sense to say that an agent, in two situations or possible worlds, did or did not act the same way *simpliciter* when in fact this is always a relativized concept. Two ways of acting can never be exactly the same, share *all* properties, for then they would not be two but one and the same. All the counterfactual test inquires about is whether the agent would perform relevantly similar physical movements with relevantly alike results.

16. Note that the test-question Kuhse discusses constitutes only a rough criterion for intention anyway, because a relevantly changed plan might involve the same action. If Crook pulls a human shield in front of her, Cop may not abandon her original plan to shoot Crook. But even if she does not, she must nonetheless alter her plan, for now Cop plans to shoot *through* the human shield. The external behavior is identical, but it is performed with different intentions, ones whose difference is quite important morally.

17. Kuhse 147.

18. See Bratman (cited in n.10); Gilbert Harman, *Change in View* (Cambridge: MIT Press, 1986); or G. E. M. Anscombe, *Intention* (Ithaca: Cornell Univ. Press, 1957) for some current views that support a moderate conception of the intended. Unlike Kuhse and me, several of these authors allow what the agent intentionally does to extend beyond what she intends to do. Thus, they may support a broad conception of the intentional, but not in a way that helps Kuhse's case against intention-sensitive ethics. What an attack on the latter requires is a broad view of the intended. The allies Kuhse needs, then, have to support not just a broad view of what the agent intentionally does but of what she actually intends. On this, all the thinkers cited reject her position.

19. Rachels 93, 94.

20. For additional arguments against intention-sensitivity, some of them similarly question-begging, see Judith J. Thomson, "Self-Defense" in *Philosophy and Public Affairs* 20 (1991) 283-310 and Holmes (cited in n. 8). For criticism of Thomson's reasoning, see J. L. A. Garcia, "Intention-Sensitive Ethics" in *Public Affairs Quarterly* 9 (1995) 201-13; of Holmes', see

J. L. A. Garcia, "Intentions and Wrongdoing" in *American Catholic Philosophical Quarterly* 69 (1995) 605-17.

21. I suspect that technical talk of "direct killing" and "direct abortion" entered ethical discussions because it is useful to have a term to pick out the types of killing that are always intentional. Notice that, unlike lying, rape, kidnapping, etc., killing need not be intentional. (See Kuhse's discussion of "direct" killing at Kuhse, sec. 3.3, especially pp. 103, 124.)

Incidentally, Kuhse is wrong if, as she there suggests, she thinks that traditional Christian medical ethics permits direct killing of innocents in tubal pregnancies or self-defense. I will not discuss self-defense here: the topic is not within the realm of medical ethics, and efforts to understand some medical quandaries as instances of self-defense (as in cases where pregnancy endangers the woman's life or health) have generated absurd, sophistical claims. (E. g., the fantasy that one might profitably think of a fetus as a kind of aggressor.) In ectopic pregnancies, suffice it to say that, in my limited understanding of the medicine, the mother's blood vessels are normally damaged, so the arteries leading to the tubes may properly be clamped to stop hemorrhaging there with no intent to deprive the fetus within of life. The diseased tube can likewise be licitly removed with the fetus inside in what clearly counts as an indirect abortion. (Kuhse 107ff.)

22. Williams' complaint is explicitly directed against what he calls the "Doctrine of Double Effect," but he is concerned only with that so-called "doctrine's" embrace of intention-sensitivity, not its other elements. So, like similar philosophical treatments of double effect reasoning, it is relevant for our discussion. (Glanville Williams, *The Sanctity of Life and the Criminal Law* [London: Faber and Faber, 1958] 286)

By the way, I should acknowledge that Tom Cavanaugh convinced me that, since double effect is too complicated to be considered a single principle, and seems never to have been explicitly taught in its entirety by highest religious authority, it is best conceived of a special form reasoning rather than as either a "principle" or "doctrine."

23. See Anscombe.

CONTRACEPTION AND ABORTION: FRUITS OF THE SAME TREE

Richard J. Fehring

IN HIS RECENT encyclical *Evangelium Vitae* ("The Gospel of Life") Pope John Paul II links abortion and contraception as life-issues with similar characteristics but of different moral magnitudes.[1] Conventional wisdom, however, rejects the contraception-abortion link and commonly encourages contraception as a means to decrease the incidence of abortion. Furthermore, the Catholic church is often criticized for outlawing contraception and is accused of actually increasing the incidence of abortion (instead of decreasing it) because of its rejection of contraception. The Pope in his encyclical says that this is a mistake and argues that a "contraceptive mentality" predisposes a person to accepting abortion.

Why contraception is linked to abortion both as an attitude and in regard to cause-and-effect is addressed in this paper by analyzing John Paul II's statements on contraception in his encyclical *Evangelium Vitae* and by analyzing how abortion and contraception violate basic assumptions of health, nursing and biological laws of nature. I also discuss Natural Family Planning (NFP) as a moral contrast to contraception and as a means to engender openness to life.

VIOLATIONS OF BASIC HEALTH-ASSUMPTIONS

The American Nurses Association's (ANA) Social Policy Statement is a major document on the basic philosophical stance that the profession of nursing holds on nursing and health-care.[2] The first health-assumption formulated by the ANA is that the human person manifests an integration (unity) of the mind, body and spirit. The ANA rejects the dualistic split of the mind and body and believes that if you manipulate the body, the mind and spirit will also be affected. Nursing encourages and works towards the integration of individuals, families and communities. Professional nurses, in caring for individuals, seek to engender wholeness (of body-mind-spirit) and avoid interventions that fail to aid in that integration.

Another value or assumption of professional nursing is that nurses should work with nature rather than against it. This assumption has its origins in the writings and work of Florence Nightingale.[3] In her "Notes on Nursing" Nightingale advocated that professional nurses place the patient in the best position to work with nature—not against it. She also concluded that there can be dire consequences when work is directed against nature. Nature, to her, was simply the manifestation of God.

A similar health-assumption or corollary to "working with nature" that is accepted by professional nursing and in particular by the American Academy of Nurse Midwifery is that health-care professionals should not treat normal body-systems or processes as a disease.[4] This principle is usually directed towards the process of child-birth but can be applied to other body-systems as well. There is no need to medicalize a normal process, and by doing so you not only interfere with the process but also can cause more problems. Using medicine to aid normal processes and to treat actual diseases, however, is advocated and supported.

Another strongly-held principle of nursing is that nurses should help persons to trust their own bodies.[5] The body has signs and symptoms to indicate when one is well or not. Likewise the body will provide us with warning signs of health-problems such as a headache when we are overstressed. Nursing advocates that people should listen to their bodies and trust the signs that it is giving.

CONTRACEPTION AND ABORTION CONTRADICTS HEALTH-ASSUMPTIONS

Contraception is a violation of the above health-assumptions and values. Contraception works against nature and treats fertility as a disease. The basic mechanisms and processes of artificial contraception are either using a powerful chemical to suppress fertility, a device to block or subvert fertility, some type of process to destroy fertility, or some type of mechanism that causes an early abortion. Blocking, suppressing, destroying or aborting new life is not integrating a bodily process. How can you have unity of mind, body, and spirit if you destroy, block or suppress a normal body-process? And if you do interfere with that body-process, will not the mind and spirit be affected also? An example of how far we have come in the United States to rejecting the integration of our fertility is the fact that the number one method of family planning (for women) is surgical sterilization, i.e., destroying one's fertility.[6] You cannot integrate something that you destroy.

In 1994 Dr. Warren Hern, the Chair of the Population, Family Planning and Reproductive Health Section of the American Public Health Association, addressed the International Conference on Population and Development sponsored by the United Nations in Cairo, Egypt. He stated that there were no social goals more important "than liberating women from the tyranny of their own biology."[7] What kind of message is Dr. Hern sending to women when he refers to women's biology (i.e., their fertility or reproductive capacity) as the biggest social tyranny in the world? You would think that the women attending that conference would have jeered at this notion. According to Hern, the cure for this tyranny is contraception and abortion. This thinking is representative (at an extreme) of the notion that a woman's fertility is a disease that needs to be altered, destroyed or suppressed. The use of contraception is one of the only uses of medicine (that I know of) where a normal (essential or important) biological system is treated like a disease and is suppressed or destroyed. The only other is abortion.

Although the moral magnitudes of abortion and contraception are quite different, the similarities and boundaries between abortion and contraception are often blurred. Many of the forms of so-called contraceptives are not contraceptive in function, in that either some of the time or all of the time they abort early human life.[8] It is obvious that the abortion pill RU-486 acts as an abortifacient, but not as obvious that some oral contraceptives (especially the mini-pill or the low-dose estrogenic pills and the progestin-only pills) and the IUD do so also.

A method of family planning that respects the integration of the whole person, that works with nature (not against it), that does not treat fertility as a disease, and that helps men and women to trust the signs of the body is Natural Family Planning. NFP is based on monitoring the body's signs of fertility; with that knowledge, one can determine whether one is fertile or not, and how one should act, whether one wants to achieve or avoid pregnancy. NFP respects (not rejects) the biological laws of nature.

With artificial contraception there is no monitoring the signs of the body to determine fertility (or infertility) and there is no fertility integration (physically, mentally, or spiritually). In fact the signs of fertility are destroyed or subverted. With contraception there is an overall mistrust of the body. With contraception you cannot achieve a pregnancy but only avoid or destroy it. With contraception there is no respecting the biological laws of nature. As Mary Joyce (a philosopher) has stated, contraception is an expression of the failure to integrate the functional and competent expression of a holistic human sexuality.[9]

Abortion is an extreme act of mistrust of the normal processes of pregnancy and birth. Abortion treats as undesirable not only the process of pregnancy and reproduction but also the product—the unborn child. Abortion, therefore, like contraception treats the normal process of reproduction as a disease and treats the unborn child in this way as well. Abortion is simply an extreme on the continuum with contraception in violating the unity of the mind-body-spirit. If individuals have not integrated their fertility (understanding it and accepting it), then how would you expect that person to accept the products of that process, i.e., pregnancy and the unborn child? Contraception is a violation of the integrity of the process, and abortion is the violation of the product. Both contraception and abortion violate basic health-assumptions and values. Abortion is certainly an extreme expression of these violations, but there is no doubt that they are connected.

POPE JOHN PAUL II AND THE CONTRACEPTIVE MENTALITY

In *Evangelium Vitae* Pope John Paul II recognizes that there is a continuum between contraception and abortion when he refers to them as the fruits of the same tree. In the encyclical the Pope calls attention to the functional link between contraception and abortion when he points out that many contraceptives function (always or some of the time) as abortifacients. The Pope also points out the psychological continuum between contraception and abortion in what he calls the "contraceptive mentality."[10] With this mentality abortion is a response to failed contraception. Women on contraception do so to avoid pregnancy. They also do so to feel responsible and to have control over their lives and goals. When contraception fails (and they become pregnant), procreation then becomes (as the Pope says) an obstacle to personal fulfillment and goals. Abortion is "needed" as a back-up because the pregnancy was not intended.

Research that I have conducted supports the notion that fertility and pregnancy are viewed by couples as a threat to personal goals.[11] My co-researchers and I have conducted in-depth interviews with couples on contraception. Consistent responses by these couples were that they were using contraceptive methods because they feared pregnancy and that they had goals to achieve (e.g., material or career goals) for themselves or their children. They also felt that they needed to be in control of their procreative powers and that contraceptives provided them with this control. The control, however, was external. There was no felt integration of their fertility. Rather, fertility was something to be avoided as an obstacle.

Another link between abortion and contraception that needs further research is the effects that contraception has on the marital bond. For years a variety of authors (including Pope Paul VI in the encyclical *Humanae Vitae*, Mahatma Ghandi in his writings, and modern authors such as Janet Smith, a Professor of Philosophy at University of Dallas, and John Kippley, author and founder of the Couple to Couple League) have speculated that contraception weakens the marital bond. With contraception the woman is more likely to be treated as an object of desire. So too, as Pope John Paul II has pointed out in *Evangelium Vitae* and other documents, contraception is an expression of a conditional type of love. It is a lie of the body that "contradicts the full truth of the sexual act as the proper expression of conjugal love."[12] The sexual act of intercourse is meant as a totality of giving. If a person (in effect) says "I love you but I am not willing to give you my fertility or to deal with yours," then love becomes conditional and the marital bond can be weakened. There are also many (physical and aesthetic) side-effects of the various forms of contraceptives that could interfere with the marital bond. For example, depression and bloating from being on oral contraceptives, the messiness of spermacides, and the disruption of the sexual act with the placement of condoms. The reason that this is important is because if the marital bond is weakened, then the acceptance of life between two individuals is less likely to be present. In fact, according to the Alan Guttmacher Institute, trouble with a relationship is one of the biggest reasons that women give for wanting to have an abortion.

EVIDENCE FOR THE LINK BETWEEN ABORTION AND THE

CONTRACEPTIVE MENTALITY

The empirical evidence of the contraception-abortion link is not clear from a cause-and-effect standpoint. There seems, however, to be some indirect evidence. There have been a number of articles that have demonstrated that as contraception is introduced into an area or country the incidence of abortion increases (as well as divorce and sexually transmitted diseases).[13] Likewise, as contraceptive-oriented awareness/education programs are promoted (especially among the adolescent populations) abortion also goes up.[14]

We also know from data supplied by the Alan Guttmacher Institute (the research-arm of Planned Parenthood) that about half of the pregnancies in the United States are unintended and that almost half of unintended pregnancies end in abortion.[15] Furthermore, "although almost all women at risk of unintended pregnancy use contraceptives... the small proportion who do not [use contraception] account for more than half (57%) of all unintended pregnancies."[16] These figures reflect either failed contraception, non-compliance with use or a failure to integrate and understand fertility. Unintended pregnancies are important because about half (47%) of unintended pregnancies end in abortion. If women and men could monitor their fertility, there would be less (unintended) pregnancies, i.e., people would know whether they are fertile or not on any given day.

What is also known is that only 9% of abortion-patients in the U.S. have never used contraception to avoid pregnancy.[17] Or, to express this in another way, 91% of women who have had an abortion have used some form of contraception in the past. Furthermore, approximately 43% of unintended pregnancies occur with women who were currently using some form of contraception.[18] So, to say that more contraception will decrease abortions does not fit the data. Nor does the common assertion that the Catholic Church's position against artificial contraception is actually promoting the incidence of abortion. As the Pope says in *Evangelium Vitae*, "when looked at carefully, this objection is clearly unfounded."[19]

But does the contraceptive mentality and the use of contraception actually strengthen the temptation to have an abortion when the pregnancy is unintended? According to the data from the Alan Guttmacher Institute, the main reasons that women have abortion are responsibilities (such as employment or school), economic circumstances, and unstable relationships.[20] The Pope recognizes this in *Evangelium Vitae* by saying that "it is true that in many cases contraception and even abortion are practiced under the pressure of real-life difficulties."[21] Still, he points out that many abortions result from being unwilling to accept responsibility in matters of human sexuality.

Part of this unwillingness is the refusal to see sexuality in its whole context. The "natural," inherent purpose of the conjugal act is for procreation and bonding, not just to fulfill the impulse of instinct and passion, what the Pope calls the trivilization of human sexuality.[22] Sexuality only becomes whole when it enriches the whole person and involves the total giving of two persons in love. When couples are able to control their sexual passions and respect the biological laws of nature, they will more likely maintain an attitude of openness and service to life even under difficult circumstances.[23]

EVIDENCE OF OPENNESS TO LIFE

A method of family planning that respects the laws of nature, helps couples to control sexual passions, and respects the integration of the conjugal act is NFP. If so, then NFP should also help to generate in couples an openness to life, and there should be some empirical evidence for this human response.

The Marquette University Natural Family Program, has been in existence since 1985. From 1985 to 1995 approximately 435 couples have sought NFP services. Each couple in the program attends an introductory session on NFP and individual follow-up sessions with an NFP practitioner. At the end of each follow-up session couples are asked (by the practitioner) to rate their receptivity to an unplanned pregnancy. The ratings are on a 1-5 scale: 1 = very unreceptive; 2 = unreceptive; 3 = not sure or undecided; 4 = receptive, and 5 = very receptive.

Of the 435 couples who have participated in the Marquette NFP program, there were 60 married couples who have attended at least 8 follow-up sessions in the first year. During that first year the intentions of these 60 married couples were either temporarily to avoid pregnancy (N = 49) or permanently to avoid pregnancy (N = 11). The remaining couples in the program were not yet married (engaged), were attempting to achieve pregnancy, switched their intentions in the first year of use from avoiding to achieving, were infertile, dropped out of the program before the first year, or did not attend a minimum of 6 follow-up sessions.

The 60 couples (120 individuals) analyzed for this paper had a mean age of 29.6 years, were married for an average of 4.5 years, had an average of 1.3 children, were mostly Roman Catholic, had at least a high school education, and (all but four) were White-Americans.

The mean receptivity to an unplanned pregnancy expressed by these 60 couples at the first follow-up session was 3.41, at the second follow-up 3.58, and the third 3.93 (See graph 1). There was a significant increase (using both parametric paired t-tests and non-parametric signed ranked statistical tests) from the first to third session and from the second to third.

Of the 120 individuals (i.e., 60 couples) analyzed for this paper, 49 individuals rated themselves either 3 (undecided) or less receptive to an unplanned pregnancy at the first follow-up session. These 49 individuals had a mean receptivity to an unplanned pregnancy of 2.27 at the first follow-up session, 2.79 at the second and 3.31 at the third. Like the total group these increases were statistically significant (See graph 2).

Although this data was not generated from a controlled- research focus, it does lend some evidence that following the biological laws of nature through NFP (and developing control over passions) can lead to being more open to life. It should be noted that this sample of couples was very selective and that virtually none would actually have had an abortion.

Data from the Alan Guttmacher Institute also seems to support the notion that as the method of family planning more closely follows biological laws there is more openness to life by the user.[24] Their data shows that of women who use either the pill or IUD and have an unwanted pregnancy, 58% will obtain an abortion and 30% will give birth. Among women who use barrier-methods and have an unwanted pregnancy, 29% will have an abortion and 56% will give birth, and among the users of periodic abstinence and withdrawal who have unwanted pregnancies, 20% will have an abortion and 65% will give birth. An argument could be made that this data reflects the effectiveness of the given method of family planning (rather than the naturalness) to avoid pregnancy, i.e., as the method becomes less effective there is less of a willingness to have an abortion as a result of an unwanted pregnancy. The data could also reflect the mentality that as individuals use the more effective method of family planning, then they are being more responsible, and if they do become pregnant while contracepting, then they do not feel responsible for the pregnancy and abort the pregnancy as a result.

MANIPULATORS (RATHER THAN LOVERS) OF LIFE

In many of his writings before *Evangelium Vitae*, John Paul II has explored the dynamics of contraception and human sexuality.[25] In *Familiaris Consortio* he called upon scientists to deliniate further the moral and anthropological differences between artificial contraception and recourse to the natural, i.e., natural family planning.[26] By exploring these differences a greater appreciation and understanding of the damage that contraception does to society and marital relationships can emerge; so too can the connections between contraception and abortion.

This author and others have found some evidence to support differences between contraception and NFP.[27] With NFP, couples are challenged to live with their fertility and to integrate it into their lives. There is a working with nature and a growing appreciation and understanding of the nuances and rhythms of their natural cycles of fertility and sterility. The control that NFP couples achieve through this understanding is an internal control. There is also a sense and vision of their fertility in cooperation with a generous and generative God—couples see themselves open to God's will and as co-creators with God.

As opposed to NFP, couples on contraception do not choose to integrate and live with their fertility. They wish to have control over it, usually out of feeling a need to be in control of their lives. Often that control is stimulated by career, educational goals, material wants and financial demands. Contraceptive couples do not see their fertility in relationship to God. As such, contraceptive couples at times reject God's gift of fertility and do not remain open to the possibility of new life.

It is obvious that there are many similarities in the dynamics of contraception and abortion—besides the obvious connection in that many types of contraception actually function by aborting newly developing life. Abortion and contraception are also similar in that they do not involve an integration of fertility or the products of that fertility. There is also a lack of trust of the body and the spirit.

There is no recognition of the sense that God is a co-creator of life. The fertile time with its potential for new life is not a holy time. Rather, fertility (and the product of fertility) is something to control and manipulate. In one sense, being on contraception and accepting abortion attempts to make the individual the author and manipulator of life rather than to see God as the author of life and to be open to His will—even under difficult circumstances.

If, as the Pope says in *Evangelium Vitae*, abortion and contraception are fruits of the same tree, then what is that tree? In the garden of Eden, there was a tree with forbidden fruit. It was called the tree of the knowledge of good and evil. Eating of the fruit would make man like God.[28] The tree of which abortion and contraception are fruits is by nature the same type of tree. When humans use contraception and abortion, they wish to be the controller of life and to be their own gods; they do not wish God to be in control. Abortion and contraception are both a turning away from and a rejection of God. Abortion is an extreme rejection but contraception is on the same continuum of rejection.

There are many similar characteristics between abortion and contraception that can be placed on a continuum. Figure One below illustrates and summarizes some of those characteristics as discussed in this paper. Figure One also provides some of the fruits discovered when couples use NFP. The model shows, however, that there is a continuum of use (or integration) of NFP and that even NFP can be used with a contraceptive mentality.[29] The opposite of this mentality is allowing God's will to be part of the procreative decision-making.

Couples who use NFP often see themselves as co-creators with God in the decision and in the act of generating new life. They are able to know the fertile time of a woman's cycle and realize that it is a holy time with the possibility of creating new sons or daughters, i.e., creating new images of God. As John Paul II stated in *Evangelium Vitae*, "thus a man and woman joined in matrimony become partners in a divine undertaking: through the act of procreation, God's gift is accepted and new life opens to the future."[30] Contraception and abortion are a rejection of God's gifts and a rejection of this divine undertaking.

FIGURE ONE:
CONTINUUM-MODEL OF ABORTION AND CONTRACEPTION

CONTRACEPTION_____ABORTION

Fertility not integrated	Baby not integrated
Fertility is a disease	Baby is a disease
Fertility is an obstacle	Baby is an obstacle
Closed to generating life	Closed to life
Control fertility	Control life
Destroy fertility	Destroy life
Reject God's gift	Reject Image of God

NFP

CONTRACEPTIVE_____OPEN TO
MINDSET   GOD'S WILL

Integration of fertility
Fertility Natural Process
Trust of the body
Self-control
Appreciation of fertility
Generous to life
Co-creators with God

Graph One:

Mean Receptivity to Pregnancy:
At 1st, 6th, and 12th Month (N = 120)

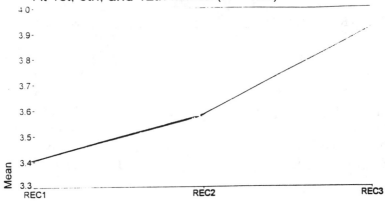

Graph Two:

Mean Receptivity to Pregnancy:
At 1st, 6th, and 12th Month (N = 49)

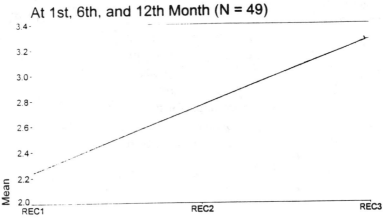

NOTES

1. Pope John Paul II, *The Encyclical "Evangelium Vitae" (The Gospel of Life)* in *Origins* 24/42 (April 6, 1995) 694-95.

2. *Nursing's Social Policy Statement* (Washington, D.C.: American Nurses Association, 1995) 1-22.

3. Janet Macrae, "Nightingale's Spiritual Philosophy" in *Image: Journal of Nursing Scholarship* 27/1 (1995) 8-10.

4. *Philosophy of the American College of Nurse-Midwives* (Washington, D.C.: The American College of Nurse-Midwives, 1989) 10. Cf. also Janet Scoggin, "How Nurse-Midwives Define Themselves in Relation to Nursing, Medicine, and Midwifery" in *Journal of Nurse-Midwifery* 41/1 (1996) 36-42.

5. *Today's Certified Nurse-Midwife* (Washington, D.C.: The American College of Nurse-Midwives, 1993).

6. "Still Fumbling in the Dark" in *Newsweek* (March 13, 1995) 61. Cf. also Cathleen A. Church and Judith S. Geller, "Voluntary Female Sterilization: Number One and Growing" in *Population Reports* (November 1990) 3.

7. Warren M. Hern, "The Role of Abortion in Women's Health and Population Growth," a paper presented at the *United Nations International Conference on Population and Development,* Cairo, Egypt (September 5-13, 1994).

8. Patrick McCrystal, "What Kind of Prescription? Do Contraceptive Drugs Prevent Life or Destroy It?" in *Celebrate Life* (May-June 1996) 23-25. Cf. also "Contraceptive Issues and Options for Young Women" in *Contemporary Studies in Women's Health* (an independent study, continuing education program from Wyeth-Ayerst Laboratories and the Association of Women's Health, Obstetric, and Neonatal Nurses, published by MPE Communications, Inc., at Fair Lawn, N.J., 1994) 1-32.

9. Mary Rosera Joyce, *Women and Choice: A New Beginning* (St. Cloud: Lifecom, 1986) 124-34.

10. *Evangelium Vitae* #13.

11. Richard J. Fehring and Donna M. Lawrence, "Spiritual Well-Being, Self-Esteem, and Intimacy Among Couples Using Natural Family Planning" in *Linacre Quarterly* 62/4 (1995) 22-28.

12. *Evangelium Vitae* 13.

13. William F. Colliton, Jr., "Contraception and Abortion: Is There a Connection?" in *Saint Louis University Public Law Review* 13/1 (1993) 315-26.

14. Stan E. Weed and Joseph A. Olsen, "Policy and Program Considerations for Teenage Pregnancy Prevention: A Summary for Policymakers" in *International Review* 13/3-4 (Fall/Winter 1989) 267-93.

15. Rachel B. Gold, *Abortion and Women's Health: A Turning Point for America?* (New York: The Alan Guttmacher Institute, 1990) 1-74. Cf. also Howard W. Ory, Jacqueline D. Forrest, and Richard Lincoln, *Making Choices: Evaluating the Health Risks and Benefits of Birth Control Methods* (New York: The Alan Guttmacher Institute, 1983) 1-72.

16. Ory *et al.* 13.

17. *Ibid.*

18. *Ibid.*

19. *Evangelium Vitae* #13.

20. Gold, 19-21.

21. *Evangelium Vitae* #13.

22. *Evangelium Vitae* #97.

23. *Ibid.*

24. Ory *et al.*

25. Pope John Paul II, *Love and Responsibility* (San Francisco: Ignatius Press, 1994). Cf. also Richard M. Hogan and John M. LeVoir, *Covenant of Love: Pope John Paul II on Sexuality, Marriage, and Family in the Modern World* (San Francisco: Ignatius Press, 1992).

26. Pope John Paul II, *The Role of the Christian Family in the Modern World* (Boston: Daughters of St. Paul, 1981) 52.

27. Fehring and Lawrence 22-28. Cf. also Richard J. Fehring, Donna M. Lawrence and Catherine Sauvage, "Self-Esteem, Spiritual Well-Being and Intimacy: A Comparison Among Couples Using NFP and Oral Contraceptives" in *International Review of Natural Family Planning* 13/3-4 (1989) 227-36. Cf. also Joseph Tortorici, "Conception Regulation, Self-Esteem, and Marital Satisfaction Among Catholic Couples: Michigan State University Study" in *International Review of Natural Family Planning* 3 (1979) 191-205.

28. Frank Sheed, *Theology and Sanity* (San Francisco: Ignatius Press, 1993) 191-207.

29. For a more in-depth description of the levels of integration of NFP, see Richard J. Fehring, "Toward a Model of Fertility Awareness" in *Life and Learning IV: Proceedings of the 4th Annual University Faculty for Life Conference* (Washington, D.C.: UFL, 1995) 216-29.

30. *Evangelium Vitae* #43.

THREE IN ONE FLESH

Mary A. Nicholas

A TOTAL OF 40,578 BIRTHS were reported[1] worldwide as a result of reproductive techniques in 1993.[2] The actual number is much greater, as there were 8,741 births resulting from assisted reproductive technologies in the U.S. and Canada alone, reported in 1995.[3] In addition, there were 6,869 frozen embryo transfer procedures reported in 1995, which represented 13.5% of total assisted reproductive treatments.[4]

This technology, which has a tremendous impact on our way of thinking and acting, represents a paradigm shift in all human relations, particularly the family, revealed in the telling statement by Edwards and Steptoe: "Indeed, several oocytes could be collected during the cycle...and stored as oocytes or embryos for successive transfers over a period of time, so that *a whole family* could be established by a single laparoscopy"[5] (emphasis added).

Human beings are now conceived of as by-products in the mechanization and industrialization of birth, reflected in common terminology such as "freeze-thaw" babies (babies born after initial incubation as an embryo in a freezer); "the quality of the embryos"; "weekend egg pick-ups"; and "vitrification" (the suspension of human embryos in solutions with a cryoprotectant followed by plunging them in liquid nitrogen).

Significantly, the change in terminology preceded the technology, as Cardinal Ratzinger noted: "Until the present moment the origin of the human being has come to be expressed through the concepts of 'generation' and of 'conception,' and the theology within which the process would be included, through the concept of 'human procreation.' Now it would seem that the word, 'reproduction,' is gradually describing the transmission of a human life with greater precision."[6]

This new reproductive terminology masks the fact of what is—in many cases—technological genocide of the youngest and most innocent members of the human species—embryos. A scientific ethos of reproduction has invented a new type of killing—which can be termed *embryocide*. (We need to retain the phrase "in many cases" because the late Dr. Jerome LeJeune was careful to distinguish between freezing embryos for preservation, even though there is an inherent risk of loss; and taking an "embryo which has been frozen" and putting him "briskly at normal temperature so that he will die," which is "killing the embryo."[7])

The germ of these ideas was planted with the preliminary steps of contraception and abortion. The first step, contraception, separated sexuality from procreation. At least one researcher has explicitly linked the right to this technology to contraception: "The couples retain control over their own embryos and have the right to keep them in storage, dispose of or donate them. These conditions are consistent with couples' rights to contraception...."[8] The second step, abortion, alienated the fetus from his own mother's womb. *In vitro* fertilization represents a further progression of the inner logic of these two ideas: the possibility of the death of one or more embryos is accepted as a new starting point for life.

Nature, though, known as mother, communicates in a language of her own which can be discerned by sensitive observation and respect. Can she be a guide for scientists, philosophers and physicians? (The etymological root of the word physician is *physis*, meaning nature.) What can be discerned about the process of Motherhood and Fatherhood on a biological level, since the natural and the supernatural are one package: "Their respective truths are mirror images of one another and are, in essence, one integral truth."[9]

Man, desiring to penetrate more deeply beneath the surface of nature's workings, is immediately confronted with the fact that his own eyes are insufficient—to penetrate he needs the light of the microscope, laparoscope, and embryoscope. With these magnifications, the first thing we notice about nature's care is that as a primary oocyte forms, connective tissue (we could say protective tissue) forms around it, surrounding it with an external layer of cells. In essence, during a woman's entire childhood, the oocyte lies *protected and hidden* from others. Its beginnings are wrapt in silence.

Photographs by Lennart Nilsson[10] have shown the magnificent silence of a woman's oocyte within the folds of the fallopian tubes, flesh within flesh, awaiting fertilization. Such a glimpse at nature elicits reverence, respect, and expectation. Contrast this with the laboratory reality of an oocyte immobilized by a metal instrument in preparation for injection of sperm. A petrie dish is not a *mother*.

Is the introduction of a technologist and manipulation by metal instruments consistent with the nature, i.e., the ontology of the conjugal act? Adjusting our view to the personal level, the conjugal act is *the most intimate physical act of man*, an act of exclusive communion between persons. The language of the body is clearly one of intimacy. Since the conjugal act takes place between persons, "it is inseparably corporeal and spiritual."[11] Consequently, the transmission of life is inseparably corporeal and spiritual.

By contrast, *in vitro* fertilization lacks intimacy, creates an artificial separation from another, and severs human relations. In the natural course of procreation, the oocyte within the fallopian tube is the woman's own and it awaits the possible fertilization from her husband. The "story," or history, includes both human flesh and human genealogy. For Christians, the gospels included both of these elements before telling of Christ's birth: they told the genealogy of Christ and the fact that He was conceived within the womb of His mother. This was important for His "story."

In contrast, with *in vitro* fertilization the oocyte is "captured" from the mother and awaits fertilization from the husband's sperm. In a further progression of this technology—gamete-donation—flesh is separated from flesh and the donor remains deliberately anonymous. A document submitted to the Warnock Committee of England specifically stated that the donor should be "absolutely anonymous, and the donor surrenders unconditionally all responsibilities for care and contact with the child."[12] Figure 1 (all figures are printed below, after all the notes) represents a typical advertisement for anonymous donors now found on U.S. hospital bulletin boards.

Returning to the microscopic level, a closer look at an oocyte shows us that it has several layers. From the exterior to the interior, it contains the corona radiata, the zona pellucida, the vitelline space, and a cell membrane. To enter the oocyte, the sperm must penetrate the very interior of the oocyte. Are these cellular actions symbolic of what occurs on a personal level? We can then follow the magnificent steps in the fusion of the two cells. First the sperm penetrates the layers of the oocyte (Figure 2). As indicated, the large circular area to the right is the female pronucleus. It is the norm of nature that from this point on no other sperm can penetrate the oocyte. The oocyte's boundaries become sealed. Figure 3 shows both male and female pronuclei. At this stage, the single-cell embryo has two genetic centers: the male and female pronuclei. The pronuclei work together in an integrative fashion for the good of the organism. Through regulatory genes and feed-back loops, "communications are established that allow genes to influence each other's state of activity. In short, the genes in an organism are not independent, isolated entities...."[13] They are not acting autonomously. The next event is the fusion of the male and female pronuclei (Figure 4). Figure 5 shows that the zygote has now formed. This process, the passage of the head of the sperm into the cytoplasm of the oocyte with subsequent fusion of the male and female pronuclei, is called syngamy.

The word "marriage" could be used to describe syngamy. It is not just a symbolic coming together, but a physical joining of two different cells. They become one, while retaining the individual genetic contributions from the sperm and oocyte. This process can have no other ontological meaning than unity—communion. It represents a *"primordial" biological event that demonstrates "the two shall become one flesh."*

St. John Chrysostom speaks of this "one flesh" as including the child as well. Referring to Christ's words, that the "two shall become one flesh," he says: "For he shews that a man leaving them that begat him, and from whom he was born, is knit to his wife; and that then the one flesh is, father, and mother, and the child, formed from the union of the two. For indeed by that union is the child produced, so that the three are one flesh."[14]

It is within the fallopian tube that an embryo first begins physically bonding with his or her mother, here where the sperm and oocyte joined. A new, entirely unique individual begins here. *The person comes into being within the person of another.* He is immediately related to that intimate other—the mother. *The family then, begins interiorly.* The three are one flesh. Cells, genes, and gametes show an activity and rhythm of communion which is intimate.

If a family, in all traditional cultures until recently, began this way, we must ask what effect *in vitro* fertilization will have on family solidarity, both the couple and the child. *In vitro* fertilization, when it severs the corporeal bond, simultaneously severs the spiritual bond, and annihilates the intimacy of the family. These consequences can be seen at several levels:

1. Alienation of the early human being from his/her mother if he/she is frozen. There are two types of alienation that can occur at this level. The first type of alienation possible is physical and hopefully temporary. If an embryo is consigned to a cryopreservation tank (LeJeune used the phrase "concentration can"), he is physically separated from his mother's womb. By contrast, in Japanese, uterus is written: *ski-kyu. Ski* means infant, and *kyu* is the word for palace. This language reveals a culture which understood a womb as an infant palace. A recent issue of *Scientific American* showed photographs of cryopreservation tanks.[15] A tank is not an infant palace.

While preparing slides for a presentation, an extremely nice gentleman from a photography firm placed the art work carefully in an envelope and then placed this in a plastic container. The top of the container had a sign which said: "ORIGINALS, DO NOT DESTROY." How careful, what personal attention he gave to the slides. Yet this is the sign that should be placed over cryopreservation tanks.

The second type of alienation of the early human being is permanent—death from freezing or thawing. Figures from the Society for Reproductive Technology give some indication of the loss involved in procedures with cryopreserved embryos. Of 9,100 reported procedures which yielded embryos for cryopreservation, only 984 resulted in pregnancies and of these only 791 resulted in a delivery.[16] Death can also result from cryopreservation when the embryo is deliberately discarded.

A recent study indicated that while donation of a "supernumerary" embryo is the most frequent choice of a couple "destruction is tolerated by almost all the couples(92%)."[17] Recent reports from England have confirmed that thousands of embryos were destroyed in British fertility clinics to comply with a law limiting storage to five years.[18]

2. A second consequence of in vitro fertilization is the later alienation of the child from his or her biological parent; and parent from child if he/she is the result of an anonymous donor. If the IVF child is the result of an anonymous donor, he or she is deprived of an essential aspect of his identity and self-understanding which is essential for his integration into the family. Suzanne Rubin, one of the first children born from artificial insemination by donor described her search to identify her genetic father: "It's an obsession. I must find my father even if it's only to discover what kind of man sells his sperm and ultimately his own flesh and blood for $25, then walks away without any thought of the life he may have created. How is a child supposed to feel about a father who sold the essence of his life so cheaply and is a total stranger."[19] This psychological syndrome has been termed the "genealogical bewilderment syndrome."[20]

Additionally, a father whose wife has received donor sperm will never be able to say with Adam: "flesh of my flesh."

3. The alienation of the child from God. A child's earliest knowledge and impressions about God the Father are influenced by the relationship he has with his own father. If the case is one of separation, this can be implanted into the child's first knowledge about God. This truth, that a child's ideas about God the Father are influenced and in some cases originate from his own father, has profound implications in the case of an embryo placed in the womb of a lesbian woman.

4. The alienation of the couple from each other. When one introduces an anonymous donor's gamete into the act of procreation, there is an *implicit* acknowledgment that a third party can be personally present in the act of begetting. While the sexual bond may remain unbreached by an alien personal presence, the donor is present in his genetic contribution, as a third party who will be the 'father' of the child.[21] The question then arises: "How can the third party be personally present in the act of begetting, without being intrusive"[22] into the married couple's relationship?

A study of IVF patients found that almost all the women felt less inclined to intimacy, as one woman expressed: "The whole area is so painful I want to deny it exists. The other night...I thought 'this isn't something special between the two of us, it is something which involves all these other people."[23]

Alienation between the couple also occurs during decision-making throughout the process of assisted reproduction. *In vitro* fertilization programs admit that the husband and wife often disagree about discarding an embryo. They also disagree on the number of embryos to transfer.[24]

5. The alienation of the couple from God. With *in vitro* fertilization, the act of procreation becomes a soliloquy, rather than a dialogue, with God. If a couple believes that they are merely making or producing children, "then they do not believe that they are operating in a way that intimately unites them to God. Thus they are alienated from God."[25]

In vitro fertilization is an implicit acknowledgment by the couple of an understanding of being independent from God. Yet, the human person's true understanding of his own being is as a "being-from" which admits to the existence of reality anterior to the self. "The absolutely primary status of our being, of our substantial *esse* itself, is receptivity: it is a gift received *from another*, i.e., from God our Creator."[26]

6. The alienation of the feminine from the experience of motherhood. In *vitro* fertilization reveals a masculine mechanical model of reproduction which attempts to separate the feminine from reproduction. Alice Rossi has said: "There are intimate connections between sexuality and maternalism in the female of the species that Western society has not reckoned with. Indeed, it could be argued that the full weight of Western history has inserted a wedge between sex and maternalism so successfully that women themselves and the scientists who have studied their bodies and social roles have seldom seen the intimate connections between them. Yet the evidence is there in female reproductive physiology, thinly covered by a masculine lens that projects male fantasy onto female functions."[27]

Fletcher has gone even further. His analysis shows that separation of the feminine from reproduction causes not only a definitive separation in this process but results in perversion: "Not only is laboratory reproduction acceptable, it is "radically human compared to conception by ordinary heterosexual intercourse. It is willed, chosen, purposed and controlled, and surely these are traits that distinguish *homo sapiens* from others in the animal genus, from the primates down. Coital reproduction is, therefore, less human than laboratory reproduction—more fun, to be sure, but with our separation of babymaking from lovemaking, both become more human because they are matters of choice, and not chance."[28]

Reproductive technologies disregard the unique nature of woman and attempt to substitute the experience of motherhood with a scientific experiment. In this process, these

techniques are creating for women the same kind of discontinuous reproductive experience men now have. 'That is one of the absolutely crucial things about them, the woman begins to feel that the baby is not hers.... The more complex the technologies become, the more a woman must use her intellect to figure out in what way she contributed to the child's birth. Through her egg? Through her womb? Through her labor? As paternity always has been, maternity is becoming an act of intellect—for example, making a causal connection between the extraction of an egg and the birth of a child to another woman nine months later.'[29]

The truth is that, while a male reproductive specialist may be less affected by such technologies, a woman *by nature*, is profoundly affected by them. As Edith Stein has observed, a distinct characteristic of woman's nature is to be *more* affected by what happens to her body:

Woman's soul is present and lives more intensely in all parts of the body, and it is inwardly affected by that which happens to the body,...,This is closely related to the vocation of motherhood. The task of assimilating in oneself a living being which is evolving and growing, of containing and nourishing it, signifies a definite end in itself. Moreover, the mysterious process of the formation of a new creature in the maternal organism represents such an intimate unity of the physical and spiritual that one is well able to understand that this unity imposes itself on the entire nature of woman.[30]

7. The possible alienation of the child from a normal marriage. If an embryo is placed in the womb of a lesbian, he or she will be separated from a heterosexual marriage, with exposure to both a father and a mother.[31] Again, following nature's example, we have seen that syngamy on a biological level requires distinct genetic contributions from both the sperm and oocyte.

8. Alienation of the child from his mother or parents if he/she is aborted. The possibility of abortion, if not explicitly discussed prior to the initiation of treatment, is implicit in the process of assisted reproduction. In order to increase the possibility of pregnancy, greater than one or two embryos are usually transferred. As a result, there are often multifetal pregnancies with associated complications. Many physicians "advise multifetal pregnancy reduction for women pregnant with four or more fetuses. Women pregnant with triplets are given the option of reduction.[32]

Figure 6 provides some statistics on induced abortions in women who have chosen assisted reproduction.

Conclusions. *In vitro* fertilization attempts to treat the relational aspect of personhood as accidental, rather than intrinsic. *It contradicts the biological reality of the person coming into being as essentially related bodily,* and disregards man's essential *dimension of intimacy.* Kenneth Schmitz has noted that:

intimacy is not grounded in the recognition of this or that characteristic a person has, but rather in the simple unqualified presence the person is.... Indeed, it seems to me that the presence in which intimacy is rooted is nothing short of the unique act of existing of each person. Presence is but another name for the being of something insofar as it is actual, and in intimacy we come upon and are received into the very act of existing of another. We are, then, at the heart, not only of another person, but at the heart of the texture of being itself.[33]

In vitro fertilization implies a radical change in the understanding of the person, and represents the reproduction of an autonomous individual from two separate individuals rather than an intimate third from the "two in one flesh." Each step is a word in the language of alienation—of man from himself and from others. *In vitro* fertilization demonstrates above all else a total loss of the sense of "incarnation," that "infinitely mysterious act by which an essence assumes a body, an act around which the meditation of a Plato crystallized, and to which modern philosophers only cease to give their attention in so far as they have lost the intelligence's essential gift, that is to say, the faculty of wonder."[34]

Nature, in cellular events, transmits not only genetic messages *for* the transmission of life, but speaks a language about *how* life is transmitted. It transmits a hermeneutics. Nature's language is an utterance about man himself. If the dignity of man is his personal bond with God, and the dignity of marriage is a personal bond with another, then the dignity of the bond between parent and child must also be founded on an intimate, bodily communion.

The embryo we have been considering in these techniques is small and does not yet resemble a person. Could a mother recognize it? Can nature tells us anything? Dr. LeJeune illustrated this precise point with the natural history of kangaroos:

After two months of development in an insufficient uterus, the kangaroo infant is aborted. About two centimeters long, one could say it is like a little sausage supplied with rudimentary members. It does not know where the maternal pouch is located and does not even know that it exists but it senses weight. As soon as it has left, it climbs vertically in the fur of its mother and, without fail, it reaches the pouch and falls inside. Comfortably installed, it firmly grasps a minuscule nipple and continues its growth for six or seven months. The remarkable fact is that the mother kangaroo lets it do this, while at the same time she will tolerate no other animal in her pouch.[35]

NOTES

1. Reporting is not mandatory.

2. Alan O. Trounson and Carl Wood, "IVF and Related Technology" in *Medical Journal of Australia* 158:12 (June 21, 1993) 854. These are the latest figures available for worldwide activities.

3. Society for Assisted Reproductive Technology, "Assisted Reproductive Technology in the United States and Canada: 1993 Results Generated from the Amer. Soc. for Reproductive Medicine/Society for Assisted Reproductive Technology Registry" in *Fertility and Sterility* 64:1 (July 1995) 13.

4. *Ibid.*

5. R.G. Edwards and P. C. Steptoe, "The Relevance of the Frozen Storage of Human Embryos" in the Ciba Foundation Symposium: *The Freezing of Mammalian Embryos* (Amsterdam: Elsevier, 1977) 235.

6. Joseph Cardinal Ratzinger, "A Theologic Glance on the Subject of Human Procreation" in *Avvenire* (May 14, 1988), translated by Robert Constable, quoted in Donald DeMarco, *Biotechnology and the Assault on Parenthood* (San Francisco: Ignatius Press, 1991) 35.

7. Jerome LeJeune, M.D., Ph.D., *The Concentration Can* (San Francisco: Ignatius Press, 1992) 78-9.

8. Trounson, *ibid.*, 855. (John Rock, who was responsible for the clinical trials of the contraceptive pill, worked from approximately 1938 to 1944 on *in vitro* fertilization.) See John Rock and Miriam F. Menkin, "*In Vitro*

Fertilization and Cleavage of Human Ovarian Eggs" in *Science* 100: 2588 (1944) 105-07.

9. Henri De Lubac, *The Mystery of the Supernatural* (New York: Herder & Herder, 1967), quoted in Herbert Ratner, M.D., "The Physician: A Normative Artist" in *Listening* 18:3 (1984) 183.

10. See: Lennart Nilsson, *A Child Is Born* (New York: Delacorte Press, 1977).

11. William E. May, "'Begotten Not Made': Catholic Teaching on the Laboratory Generation of Human Life" in *Marriage: The Rock on Which the Family Is Built* (San Francisco: Ignatius Press, 1995) 67.

12. Oliver O'Donovan, *Begotten or Made?* (Oxford: Clarendon Press, 1984) 41.

13. Rudolph B. Brun, "Principles of Morphogenesis in Embryonic Development, Music and Evolution" in *Communio* 22:3 (Fall, 1993) 530.

14. St. John Chrysostom, "Homilies on the Epistle to the Ephesians of St. John Chrysostom" in *A Library of Fathers of the Holy Catholic Church Vol. V* (Oxford: John Henry Parker, 1840) 320.

15. See Gina Maranto, "Embryo Overpopulation" in *Scientific American* 274:4 (April 1996) 16.

16. See endnote 2.

17. Chantal Laruelle, M.Sc. and Yvon Englert, Ph.D., "Psychological Study of *In Vitro* Fertilization-Embryo Transfer Participants' Attitudes toward the Destiny of Their Supernumerary Embryos" in *Fertility and Sterility* 63:5 (May 1995) 1047.

18. See "British Clinics, Obeying Law, Destroy Thousands of Embryos" in *The New York Times* (August 2, 1996), A3. This moral dilemma was fully anticipated as early as 1992. Howard W. Jones, Jr., M.D., noted that situations could arise in which the "original reproductive intent of the prospective parents could be thwarted," including "The cryopreserved material remains in storage beyond the reproductive limit of the prospective mother or beyond some other agreed-upon time limit...." See his "A Step Toward Solving Some of the Problems of Cryopreservation" in *Fertility and Sterility* 57:2 (February 1992) 278.

19. Anthony Fisher, *IVF The Critical Issues* (Melbourne: Colllins Dove, 1989) 73.

20. *Ibid.*

21. *Ibid.*, 95-96.

22. Fisher, *Ibid.*

23. *Ibid.*

24. James Goldfarb, M.D., "Attitudes of in Vitro Fertilization and Intrauterine Insemination Couples toward Multiple Gestation Pregnancy and Multifetal Pregnancy Reduction" in *Fertility and Sterility* 65:4 (April 1996)

819.

25. Donald De Marco, *Biotechnology and the Assault on Parenthood* (San Francisco: Ignatius Press, 1991) 39.

26. W. Norris Clarke, "Response to David Schindler's Comments" in *Communio* (Fall 1993) 595.

27. Alice Rossi, "A Biosocial Perspective on Parenting" in *Daedalus* (Spring 1977) 1-31, quoted in Ratner, *ibid.*, 207.

28. Joseph Fletcher, S.T.D., "Ethical Aspects of Genetic Control," in "Genetic Engineering of a Technological Issue" in *Report to the Subcommittee on Science, Research, and Development, of the Committee on Science and Astronautics U.S. House of Representatives* (Washington: U.S. Government Printing Office, 1972) 72.

Fletcher has also commented on the "unnatural" possibility of making men mothers. "Furthermore, transplant or replacement medicine foresees the day, after the automatic rejection of alien tissues is overcome, when a uterus can be implanted in a human male's body—his abdomen has spaces—and gestation started by artificial fertilization and egg transfer." By decreasing the activity of the testes, physicians could also "stimulate milk from the man's rudimentary breasts—men too have mammary glands. If surgery could not construct a cervical canal the delivery could be effected by a cesarean section and the male or transsexualized mother could nurse his own baby."

In this way, reproductive technologists, like the alchemists, would be conferring "the magic of maternity" on men...." Cf. Joseph Fletcher, *The Ethics of Genetic Control: Ending Reproductive Roulette* (Garden City: Anchor Press, 1974) quoted in Alpern, 226.

29. Gena Chorea, *The Mother Machine* (New York: Harper & Row, 1985) 283-317, quoted in Alpern.

30. Edith Stein, *Woman* in *The Collected Works of Edith Stein*, L. Gelber, ed., vol. II (Washington: ICS Publications, 1987) 95.

31. See: Daniel Wikler and Norma J. Wikler, "Turkey-baster Babies: The Demedicalization of Artificial Insemination" in *The Millbank Quarterly* 69:1 (1991) 5-40.

32. Goldfarb, *ibid.*, 816.

33. Kenneth Schmitz, "The Geography of the Human Person" in *Communio* 13 (Spring 1986) 45.

34. Jacques Maritain, *Science and Wisdom* (New York: Charles Scribners and Co., 1940) 27.

35. Jerome LeJeune, *The Concentration Can* (San Francisco: Ignatius Press, 1992) 114-15.

Figure 1

EGG DONORS WANTED

IVF PROGRAM IS URGENTLY
SEEKING YOUNG HEALTHY WOMEN
TO DONATE EGGS ANONYMOUSLY
TO A COUPLE WHO WOULD OTHERWISE
HAVE NO CHANCE OF ACHIEVING
A PREGNANCY

DONORS WILL BE COMPENSATED $3,000.

**FOR MORE INFORMATION
CONTACT:
EGG DONOR PROGRAM AT 697-8999**

CENTER FOR REPRODUCTIVE MEDICINE

(Approved by IRB)

Figure 6
Abortions in sub-populations of women undergoing assisted
reproductive technology for pregnancy

		Spontaneous Abortions	Induced Abortions	Total Abortions
A. Stimulated cycles	Women <40, no male factor	12.4%	6.1%	18.5%
	Women >40, no male factor	30.2%	4.2%	34.4%
B. GIFT	Women <40, male factor	15.2%	0	15.2%
	Women >40, male factor	25%	0	25%

Source: Society for Reproductive Technology[12]

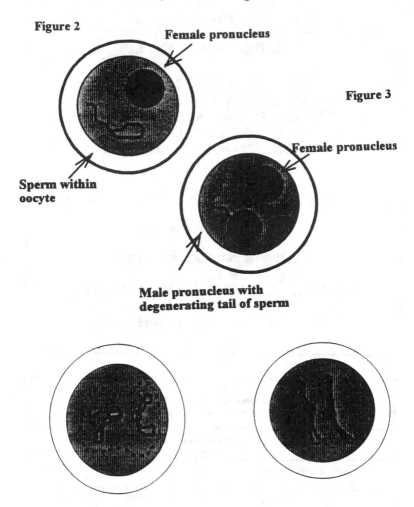

Figure 2

Female pronucleus

Figure 3

Female pronucleus

Sperm within
oocyte

Male pronucleus with
degenerating tail of sperm

Figure 4   Figure 5

SEXUALITY EDUCATION: DEVELOPING AND IMPLEMENTING A PEER PROGRAM IN COLLEGE RESIDENCE HALLS

Mary Lee O'Connell

THE CHALLENGE

Human immunodeficiency virus (HIV)/AIDS is the sixth leading cause of death among 15-24 year olds in the United States according to the Centers for Disease Control and Prevention (1995). One in five reported AIDS cases are diagnosed in the 20-29 year age group. Most of these cases are the result of an HIV infection acquired ten years before during the teen years. One in four sexually active teenagers becomes infected with a sexually transmitted disease each year (The Alan Guttmacher Institute, 1994). Many of these STDs act in synergy with HIV to enhance the transmission of both (Center for Disease Control and Prevention, 1992).

Women account for the largest increase in HIV infection through heterosexual contact (Guinan, 1992). Heterosexual exposure is responsible for 50% of the accumulated cases among women ages 13-19 years and 49% of the accumulated cases among women ages 20-24 years (Centers for Disease Control and Prevention, 1993). Many young women lack good communication skills in sexual matters placing them at additional risk for heterosexually transmitted HIV infection (Guinan, 1992).

In spite of massive international research efforts, education remains the only effective way to prevent the rising rates of STD/HIV infection. But information alone does not change behavior. According to the National Survey of Adolescent Males (1988), 73% of 15-19 year olds received formal instruction about AIDS, 79% about birth control and 58% about the skills needed to resist sexual activity. The skills needed to resist sexual activity had a stronger independent influence on reducing sexual activity than the instruction about AIDS or birth control. The authors concluded that the skills needed to resist sexual activity should coexist with education about contraception and condom use (Ku, Sonenstein & Pleck, 1992). The Centers for Disease Control and Prevention (1988) also recommends a combined education approach.

Although abstinence is the only method to provide 100% protection from pregnancy and STD/HIV infection, many "safe sex" programs present statistics that are confusing and misleading. No highly effective method exists to protect a sexually active woman against pregnancy and infection (Cates & Stone, 1992a). The effectiveness rates of birth control methods reflect only pregnancy prevention, not the prevention of STD/HIV infection (O'Connell, 1996). A woman can only get pregnant during a part of her cycle, but the risk of infection exists throughout her cycle. This is not reflected in the theoretical effectiveness rates of birth control methods that are presented in most "safe sex" programs.

Health educators have the opportunity and responsibility to develop programs that do more than present information on AIDS and birth control. These programs can present opportunities for students to develop their communication skills and identify their feelings and values about sexuality. Students cannot make an informed choice on whether to become sexually active without first understanding the separate risks of pregnancy and STD/HIV infection.

A SOLUTION

Sexuality, Personhood & Relationships © (SPR) is an education program developed at Catholic University of America and sponsored by the Student Health Advisory Council (SHAC). SPR's goal is to assist peer educators in identifying their personal values and feelings about sexuality. The program, developed by Mary Lee O'Connell, RN, MSN, assists students to identify the physical, psychological and spiritual components of sexuality and to become more effective communicators. SPR integrates the positive values of the Catholic Church's teachings on human sexuality as it prepares students to take an active role in the development and implementation of residence hall sexuality programs.

PEER EDUCATION

Peer education provides a low cost opportunity to reach many at-risk students and at the same time provide benefits for the peer educators. Peer educators learn current health information, presentation skills, active listening, role playing and value clarification. Effective peer educators integrate what they have learned, interpret for fellow students, and synthesize information into meaningful presentations. They are also likely to incorporate their knowledge of health promotion and risk reduction into their own lives. The goal of a peer health education is to help students make healthier choices and to develop a campus community to support and assist them in maintaining these choices (Fabiano, 1994).

Students who might be lost to professionals' education outreach share a common language and culture with peer educators. These educators live in the same environment, have unlimited access and have a better opportunity to confront risky behavior and intervene at the "teachable moment." They can share health information, encourage behavior change, and serve as role models (Gould & Lomax, 1994).

DEVELOPMENT OF THE PROGRAM

The SPR programs evolved from student teaching projects at the School of Nursing in N525 Contemporary Women's Health and N531 Human Sexuality in Health and Illness. Both courses were open to nursing and non-nursing students and encouraged students to develop and evaluate peer education programs in the residence halls. The programs provided an opportunity to pilot different content, experiment with different formats and identify a combination that met the needs of the undergraduate students.

The residence hall programs included nutrition, exercise, stress management, skin cancer, breast cancer, sexually transmitted diseases, and natural family planning. Although attendance ranged between three to eight students, the programs received excellent evaluations and repeated requests for more information on women's health and sexuality. Peer educators suggested the development of a specific program to address students' sexuality questions with the general and non threatening title, "Know Your Body Class."

PEER EDUCATION'S GOALS

The following semester a new group of students collaborated to develop and present a "Know Your Body Class for Women" in the residence halls. The peer educators' goal was not to teach everything that a woman needed to know but to help students realize that they needed more information about their bodies. Peer educators wanted to assist each woman to know more about her body, recognize normal changes, and know when to seek professional care. Peer educators attended the Archdiocese of Washington's Natural Family Planning classes to increase awareness and appreciation of their own fertility and the Catholic Church's teachings on sexuality.

EVALUATION

In evaluating the "Know Your Body" classes, peer educators stated that they were well prepared and confident in presenting the class content. Resident Assistants (RAs) concluded that the peer educators were both knowledgeable and professional in presenting the class material and answering students' questions. Peer educators and RAs concluded that the "Know Your Body Class" for women worked best when held in the RA's room with a maximum of ten women. The private setting and small room encouraged students to ask personal questions. Students commented that this format was "not too big so one felt crowded and not too small that one felt uncomfortable." They stated that the program "cleared many questions and concerns we've had but would never attempt to explore with friends over dinner table conversation." One RA commented, "This was my best program all year."

During the evaluations the peer educators consistently expressed concern about the content of the students' questions and the small numbers of students attending the programs. The questions that college freshmen typically asked were basic anatomy questions covering information that should have been learned in grade school. Peer educators commented that the number of basic questions confirmed the need for the programs. Although the programs received excellent evaluations from those attending, getting the students to attend was a consistent problem despite extensive advertising. Students questioned whether an informal, group participation format would encourage more students to attend.

INCREASING STUDENT PARTICIPATION

In an attempt to increase student participation, a game show format was developed to incorporate the health promotion content of the nutrition class. "Nutrition Jeopardy" was developed and eighteen students attended the first program. The following semester "Sexual

Jeopardy" was offered and twenty-five students attended. The goal was to use the game show format to awaken student interest and to follow this program with a "Know Your Body Class" for women and a separate class for men.

The "Know Your Body Class" and "Sexual Jeopardy" program evolved over the semesters. The name of the "Sexual Jeopardy" program was changed to "Sexual Trivia" by the new peer educators from the SPR program. Presenting teams now consist of at least one male and one female peer educator. New student volunteers join the current peer educators in determining the categories and questions as well as choosing the questions that they will personally ask. Mary Lee O'Connell, RN, MSN attends the first two programs that each peer educator presents. She serves as a resource for one or two questions, but the peer educators soon find they are well prepared and can anticipate the group's questions. During a program, if peer educators do not know the answer to a question, they can send the students the information through a follow-up note to the R.A.

Peer educators experimented with different game show formats such as "Jeopardy" and "Hollywood Squares," as well as female students against male students, or one residence hall against another. Evaluations indicated that large teams did not give enough opportunity for individual participation. It was decided that the most successful format was teams of four. Each team was given a color and the RAs kept score on large posters. The team captain was given a packet of cards marked A, B, C, D or True, False to raise up and indicate the group's answer. Small teams gave all students the opportunity to contribute to the discussion and help decide the group's answer. After the correct answer was given, the peer educators gave an explanation and answered any questions. RAs provided refreshments and prizes for the winning team.

EVALUATIONS

Students evaluating the programs stated that the content was "not the same old stuff." That it was "informative and the questions were interesting," the "competition made tough issues cool to handle," and the atmosphere was friendly. Students also asked for more written information and more information on sexually transmitted disease. The "12 Secrets of Sexual Health" for men and women, handouts reflecting a holistic approach to health, were developed (See Appendix 2 & 3).

These handouts are given out at the end of the program when the educators encourage students to come to a "Know Your Body Class." Peer educators also use the this time as an opportunity to explain the services that are available at the campus student health center and emphasize that strict confidentiality is maintained.

The peer educators evaluation indicated that no one had difficulty with the subject matter but numerous suggestions were offered to improve the wording of the questions. More categories and additional questions were developed as a result of the evaluations. There are currently nine categories (See Figure 1) and one hundred and fifteen questions.

Although the programs were well received, there were not enough peer educators to meet the requests for the residence hall programs. Students who taught the classes were seniors who developed the programs as part of the women's health or human sexuality classes. Once their courses were completed, students graduated and were no longer available to present the programs. Additional students were needed to fulfill the requests for residence hall programs. "Sexuality, Personhood & Relationships" (SPR) was developed to meet this need.

DEVELOPING AND IMPLEMENTING A PROGRAM

SPR began as the result of a meeting with Fr. Michael Mannion, The Catholic University of America's Chaplain and Director of Campus Ministry. Fr. Mannion brought together members of Campus Ministry, Housing and Residential Services, Student Health, the School of Nursing, the Archdiocese of Washington's Office of Natural Family Planning and student representatives to assess the needs of the university community. The need to continue and expand residence hall programs was recognized, as well as the need to develop an ongoing program to prepare peer educators. SPR was developed to meet this need. The broad-based sponsorship and Fr. Mannion's active recruitment of the students contributed to the success of the program.

Initially the SPR program was held in the Campus Ministry offices. But because student evaluations indicated that the high profile of Campus Ministry may intimidate some students, the program was presented in one of the residence halls. The sponsorship of the SPR programs also changed. A Student Health Advisory Committee (SHAC) was established to address the health needs of the campus community and the SPR programs became a part of SHAC. Donna Gray, the moderator of SHAC, Terry Brady Novak, Director of Student Health Services, and Fr. Mannion reviewed and edited all of the residence hall programs. Fr. Mannion named the program, "Sexuality, Personhood & Relationships."

The peer educators' program is based on the content of N525 Contemporary Women's Health and N531 Human Sexuality in Health and Illness. Four sophomore students, two men and two women, are asked to serve as peer facilitators for the SPR program. These students receive four hours of preparation that includes the content and philosophy of the program as well as the opportunity to become more effective communicators in discussing sexuality issues. The six one-and-a-half hour evening programs are divided so that each male-female team is responsible for three programs. Peer facilitators lead the small group discussions that begin each evening's program, introduce faculty and guest speakers, and contribute to the ongoing evaluation of the program. They become more comfortable with and effective in communicating about sexual concerns and are recognized by other students as an integral part of the SPR program.

The SPR program is presented during the third week of the spring semester. This allows time to recruit students during the fall and early spring semester and to be completed before the spring break. There is no requirement to serve as a peer educator after the completion of the program. All students are welcome but sophomore students are more actively recruited as they are available as peer educators during their junior and senior years.

Advertised across the campus, the program receives high marks for its student-friendly timing with a commitment to begin and end on time, e.g., "Thursday—8:30-10:00PM—After 'Friends' and before 'ER'." Thursday evenings are chosen by the peer educators as a time when busy students begin to wind down from the week's academic demands and have more time to participate in a volunteer program.

SEXUALITY, PERSONHOOD & RELATIONSHIPS ©

Although the SPR program is developed by the author, other members of the faculty and community also serve as presenters. This approach enriches the program and shares the demands of this all volunteer program. SPR consists of six evenings:

1. The History of Sexuality—Cultural and Religious Influences—Mary Lee O'Connell, RN, MSN

>   What messages are given by society?
>   What attitudes and beliefs are promoted in the '90s?
>   What does it mean to be a man and woman in the '90s?
>>   Small group activity: The "Slang Game"
>>   Homework activity: Male and Female Anatomy Quiz

2. God's Plan for Sexuality—Anne Lanctot, Director of Natural Family Planning, Archdiocese of Washington

>   What is the Bible's message on sexuality?
>   What are the Catholic Church's teachings on Sexuality?
>   How does Natural Family Planning fulfill God's design?
>>   Small group activity: "Adolescent Memories"
>>   Homework activity: "Marriage Contract"

3. Relationships—Integrating the Physical, Psychological and Spiritual Person—Mary Lee O'Connell, RN, MSN

>   How does the male and female body function?
>   What makes an intimate loving relationship?
>   How do you develop trust in a relationship?
>>   Small group activity: "Marriage Contract"

4. Homosexuality—Answering Concerns and Questions—Fr. Bob Keffer, University of Maryland, Campus Ministry

>   What are the cultural, historic and religious influences?
>   What is/are the cause/causes of homosexuality?
>   Homosexuality in the 90s—the individual and the family.
>>   Small group activity: Role Playing Exercise
>>   Homework: "How much does the man in your life know?"

5. The Full Picture—Birth Control Methods and STD/HIV Risk—Mary Lee O'Connell, RN, MSN

>   What are a man and woman's risk of STD/HIV infection?
>   Why isn't "safe sex" safe?
>   "The Full Picture": the effects of birth control methods on pregnancy prevention and STD/HIV risk.
>>   Small group activity: "A Sexual Act Should Be..."

6. Taking Care of the Gift of Your Fertility
   —Female— Dr. Benita Walton-Moss, CUA School of Nursing
   —Male—Terry Brady Novak, Director, CUA Health Services

>   Listen to your body, recognize early signs of illness.
>   Health habits that can hurt you, healthy steps to take
>   Health Tests and Screenings: what do they mean?
>   Student Health Service, working with you to promote your health.
>>   Small group activity: Looking at Memories and
>>>   Planning the Future

CONCLUSION

SPR assists students to identify the physical, psychological, cultural, and religious factors that affect sexual choices. During group activities students clarify their feelings and beliefs and become more aware of the opinions of others. SPR provides the knowledge and skills which peer educators need to encourage others to make healthy choices (See Appendix 1, SPR Evaluation). In day-to-day interactions in the residence halls, peer educators have the opportunity to correct misinformation and stimulate an environment to support healthy sexual choices.

SHAC wants to reach more students by recruiting more peer educators for the SPR program. These peer educators can serve as role models using teachable moments in the residence halls to encourage healthy behaviors and life style changes. Since the Resident Assistants (RAs) provide daily advice and guidance in the resident halls, the SPR program content may be used as part of their orientation or continuing education program. Future plans also include outreach to area high schools. The "Know Your Body Class for Women" has already been piloted with high school freshmen. Their teacher commented that the peer educators were well prepared and were well received by the students. The SPR program was also well received when the author and peer educators presented it to high school seniors in a local parish.

The author and the peer educators are committed to help others develop and implement sexuality education programs. Students and faculty from other universities have been welcome to attend the programs and the SPR content and handouts are willingly shared.

Address for correspondence:
Mary Lee O'Connell, RN, MSN, FACCE,
4524 Cheltenham Drive, Bethesda, Maryland 20814
e-mail: mloconne@erols.com

FIGURE 1 - SEXUAL TRIVIA CATEGORIES

Sexual Statistics
Differences Between Men and Women
Sexual Identity and Homosexuality
Know Your Body for Men
Know Your Body for Women

Relationships
Sex and Drugs
Love Bugs
Sex and Violence

APPENDIX 1 — SPR EVALUATION *

1) How do you rate SPR?

not helpful at all	0%	somewhat helpful	8%
extremely helpful	25%	not very helpful	0%
very helpful	67%		

2) SPR has given you a greater understanding and control over your emotions.

no difference	9%
somewhat greater understanding and control	64%
much greater understanding and control	27%

3) SPR has given you a greater understanding and empathy for the moods and emotions of others.

no difference	9%
somewhat greater understanding and control	73%
much greater understanding and control	18%

4) Have you and your friends talked about things you learned or discussed in SPR?

many times	27%	once or twice	27%
several times	36%	never	9%

5) How does your knowledge and understanding of fertility and procreative capacity influence your current sexual behavior?

It makes me determined not to have sex as an unmarried person	100%
It makes me less likely to have sex as an unmarried person	0%

6) Number of SPR students who volunteered to help with residence hall programs.   More than 50%

*Evaluation adapted from "Holistic Sexuality 1994-1995" Survey
    Property of NFP Center, Washington, DC

APPENDIX 2 — 12 SECRETS OF MALE SEXUAL HEALTH ©

1. RESPECT YOUR BODY AND YOUR MIND—Communicate honestly with one another to protect both of you and avoid dangerous situations.
2. EAT MORE FIBER—fruits, vegetables, whole grains, and beans. Lack of fiber was associated with decreased sexuality. Fiber helps remove estrogen from the male intestines.
3. LIMIT FAT INTAKE—No more than 30% of daily caloric intake from fat. This lowers the risk of high blood pressure and diabetes; both conditions impair the ability to have an erection.
4. LIMIT ALCOHOL INTAKE—Shakespeare's Macbeth was right, alcohol "provokes the desire, but...takes away the performance." Alcohol decreases testosterone and the hormone balance required to make an erection.
5. DON'T SMOKE—Impotence is more prevalent among heavy smokers. Testosterone levels return to near normal a week after quitting.
6. PROTECT YOUR TESTICLES WHEN EXERCISING—If you are uncomfortable wearing a jock, snug support brief underwear provide the support that you need.
7. EXAMINE YOUR TESTICLES ONCE A MONTH to feel for any abnormal lumps, cysts, or swelling. If you detect anything abnormal, consult your doctor.
8. EXERCISE, BUT DON'T OVERDO. At least 20 minutes of aerobic exercise two/three times a week improved men's sex lives. Always warm-up and cool down.
9. REPORT ANY BLISTER-LIKE LESIONS in the genital area. If you are sexually active, this may be a herpes infection. This can occur 2 to 30 days after exposure. Infection may have no obvious symptoms.
10. REPORT ANY PAINFUL, BURNING URINATION AND PUS-LIKE DISCHARGE from the penis. If you are sexually active, this may be a warning that you have gonorrhea or chlamydia. These are sexually transmitted diseases (STDs) that can be cured by antibiotics. Even if *the symptoms disappear, you can still be infected.*
11. TREATMENT—All sexually active men with burning on urination and their partners should be treated with antibiotics even if their cultures are negative. Men who have chlamydia often have negative cultures but if untreated they can become infertile
12. EDUCATE YOURSELF ABOUT YOUR BODY AND YOUR HEALTH. Knowledge is the best defense in disease prevention. If you are diagnosed with any STD, consult your physician about additional sources of information as well as support groups.

APPENDIX 3 — 12 SECRETS OF FEMALE SEXUAL HEALTH ©

1. RESPECT YOUR BODY AND YOUR MIND—Communicate honestly with one another to protect both of you and avoid dangerous situations.
2. LIMIT FAT INTAKE—Goal no more than 30% of daily caloric intake from fat. High fat diets are associated with increased estrogen-receptor positive breast cancer.
3. MAINTAIN A "HEALTHY" WEIGHT—A body fat content greater than 22% is needed for estrogen production. 10-15% below normal weight can cause irregular cycles and interfere with fertility and calcium absorption.
4. LIMIT ALCOHOL INTAKE—Women have lower tolerance than men and the effects of alcohol are more intense before a woman has her period. 76% of convicted date rapists used alcohol to seduce their dates. Women who have two drinks a day increase their risk of breast cancer by 40-100%.
5. DON'T SMOKE—Toxic chemicals from cigarette smoke were found in cervical fluid and cells. Smoking increases the risk of infection with human papilloma virus (HPV) that causes genital warts. Some of these can cause cervical cancer especially during puberty when cells are rapidly changing.
6. EXERCISE, BUT DON'T OVERDO—Women who do not exercise 2-3 hours a week double their risk of breast cancer. Always warm-up and cool down.
7. EXAMINATIONS—Do self breast exam each month 4-5 days after your period. If you are 18 years old or sexually active, get a pelvic exam each year. 50 to 80% of chlamydia and gonorrhea may have no symptoms but can cause infertility.
8. CLOTHING CONCERNS—Avoid tight jeans, nylon underwear, wet bathing suits, and damp exercise clothing. All increase the dampness of your vagina and provide a place for harmful germs to grow.
9. CHEMICAL CONCERNS—Avoid feminine hygiene sprays, and deodorant or scented tampons, pads, and panty liners. These can change the natural chemistry that protects you and increase your risk of irritation or infection. They may also mask unpleasant odors that alert you to a vaginal infection.
10. DOUCHING—Don't unless told to by your health practitioner. The chemicals may irritate you, wash away your normal protection and lubrication, or spread a vaginal infection into your uterus. This increases your risk of pelvic inflammatory disease.
11. TAMPONS CAN INCREASE INFECTION—only use on heavy flow days. On light flow days tampons can dry out the vagina and scratch it, increasing the risk of infection. Change tampons every 3-4 hours so harmful germs do not have time to collect and grow.
12. WIPE FROM FRONT TO BACK when going to the bathroom to avoid transferring germs from the bowel movement to the vagina.

REFERENCES

Alan Guttmacher Institute (1994). Sex and American Teenagers . New York: Author.

Centers for Disease Control and Prevention (1995, December). Facts about adolescents and HIV/AIDS. *CDC HIV/AIDS Prevention.* Atlanta: CDC.

Center for Disease Control and Prevention (1993). HIV/AIDS surveillance report, 5(1) 1-10.

Center for Disease Control and Prevention (1992, July). *Sexually Transmitted Disease Surveillance, 1991, U.S. Department of Health and Human Services, Public Health Service.* Atlanta: Centers of Disease Control.

Center for Disease Control and Prevention. (1988). Guidelines for effective school health education to prevent the spread of AIDS. *Morbidity and Mortality Weekly Report,* 37 (Suppl. 2).

Fabiano, P. M. (1994). From personal health into community action: Another step forward in peer health education. *Journal of American College Health,* 43, 115-121.

Gould, J., & Lomax, A. (1994, January). More schools starting peer education programs to change student behavior. *Student Insurance Division Health News,* 2(1), 1-2.

Guinan, M. E. (1992). HIV, heterosexual transmission, and women. *Journal of the American Medical Association,* 268, 520-521.

Ku, L. C., Sonenstein, F. L. & Pleck, J. (1992). The association of AIDS education and sex education with sexual behavior and condom use among teenage men. *Family Planning Perspectives,* 24, 100-106.

O'Connell, M. L. (1996). The effects of birth control methods on STD/HIV risk. *Journal of Obstetric, Gynecologic, and Neonatal Nursing,* 25, 476-480.

INDUCED ABORTION AS A VIOLATION OF CONSCIENCE OF THE WOMAN

Thomas W. Strahan

WHY SHOULD WE CONCERN ourselves as to whether or not a woman's conscience is violated when she obtains an abortion? What difference does it make? Is it important? Whether conscience is followed, or whether it is violated, is of considerable importance. This is particularly the case in the faith-communities in which many of us are affiliated. If one does not follow one's conscience, it is a sin. There is guilt. A violation of conscience alienates a person from God. Confession and repentance are necessary to restore that relationship. That is very important. The eternal destiny of the individual may depend on it.

In its 1965 Declaration on Religious Freedom, Vatican Council II said: "On his part, man perceives and acknowledges the imperatives of the divine law through the mediation of conscience.... In all his activity a man is bound to follow his conscience in order that he may come to God, the end and purpose of life. It follows that he is not to be forced to act in a manner contrary to his conscience.... Nor, on the other hand, is he to be restrained from acting in accordance with his conscience, especially in matters religious."[1] In this statement the conscience of the individual is very important. But God is the sovereign, not only with respect to divine revelation, but also in order that a person may come to know and have a relationship with Him.

Consider also the statement of a major Protestant denomination regarding abortion. It declared that the right to have an abortion is a necessary prerequisite to the exercise of conscience, and it urges its congregations and individual members to "affirm women's ability to make responsible decisions, whether the choice be to abort or to carry to term."[2] In this statement it is the woman's conscience which is autonomous. All that is required is that the decision be "responsible" in the eyes of the woman. Whatever the decision, the other members and congregations are admonished to affirm it. Under this abortion-doctrine there is no higher authority than a "responsible decision," no requirement of the imperatives of divine law, no Biblical authority, and (not incidentally) no acknowledgement of the beliefs of the founder of the denomination, who condemned abortion as a monstrous crime and killing.[3] There is a particular irony in all of this because this denomination is the very one that was known to stress the sovereignty of God. Now, instead of God as sovereign, it is Eve, the one who ate of the tree of the knowledge of good and evil in the Garden of Eden. This is not merely a debate within a single denomination but has a close parallel in the legal arena as well.

Conscience also has legal significance. For example, the Minnesota State Constitution says: "the right of every man to worship God according to the dictates of his own conscience shall never be infringed"—that is, beliefs are absolute. "Nor shall any control of or interference with the rights of conscience be permitted... but the liberty of conscience hereby secured shall not be so construed as to excuse acts of licentiousness or justify practices inconsistent with the peace or safety of the state."[4] Other states have similar provisions, e.g., "actions based on conscience are not absolute."[5] The distinction between beliefs being absolute and actions or practices based upon those beliefs as subject to regulation or prohibition is an important one to remember, although it appears to have been forgotten by the U.S. Supreme Court in its abortion-decisions.

The most significant legal connection between conscience and abortion is found in *Planned Parenthood v. Casey* (1992), which re-affirmed *Roe v. Wade*. In *Casey* the Court attempted to establish abortion as a liberty protected by the Constitution by an appeal to conscience. The Court stated: "The abortion decision may originate within the *zone of conscience* or belief.... The destiny of the woman must be shaped to a large extent by her own conception of her *spiritual imperatives* and her place in society" (emphasis added).[6] Is the decision to have an abortion an exercise of conscience, and does it, as the decision of the Supreme Court indicates, represent a "spiritual imperative"? The Court, although it made such a suggestion, offered no evidence or support for these statements that abortion is a matter of conscience or spiritual imperative.

In regard to abortion, conscience has important social and political aspects. For example, in an interview while considering becoming a candidate for the U. S. Presidency, Colin Powell addressed the situation of a woman considering abortion: "If it is her choice to abort, it's a matter between her, her doctor, her family, *her conscience and her God.*"[7] Similarly, President Bill Clinton in a letter to Senator Orrin Hatch about the proposed ban on partial-birth abortions, said: "I have always believed that the decision to have an abortion should be between *a woman, her conscience, her doctor, and her God.*"[8] Some have speculated that the reference to abortion as a matter of conscience is part of a new strategy of those who support legalized abortion in order to replace the previous "I'm personally opposed, but..." rhetoric. Some observers believe that this new strategy arises out of a *Newsweek* poll which asked about support for abortion using the phrase "It's a matter between a woman, her doctor, her family, her conscience, and her God." Reportedly, when asked in that form, 72% of those responding called it "about right." This represents a gain of thirty points over the abortion-rights support registered in the latest Gallup poll, which asked about abortion without using the words *God* or *conscience.*[9]

But do those who use the word *conscience* understand its meaning? Do they understand what happens to the conscience of women before abortion, at the time of abortion, and in the days, months, and years that follow? A careful analysis of the meaning of the word *conscience* and an understanding of how the decision to have an abortion is made make clear that having an abortion violates the conscience of at least most women.

DEFINING THE MEANING OF *CONSCIENCE*

In order to demonstrate that having an abortion generally violates the conscience of women, it is first necessary to determine what the word *conscience* means. It has had different meanings over the years. Older decisions tend to view conscience in a Judeo-Christian perspective, which recognized the sovereignty of God. For example, in a conscientious objector case decided by a Federal Court of Appeals in 1943, the court stated, "Religious belief arises from a sense of the inadequacy of reason as a means of relating the individual to his fellow men and to his universe.... It is belief finding expression in a conscience which categorically requires the believer to disregard elementary self-interest and to accept martyrdom in preference to transgressing its tenets.... It may be justly regarded as a response of the individual to an inward mentor, call it conscience or God, that is for many persons at the present time the equivalent of what has always been thought a religious impulse.[10] At least as late as 1952 the U.S. Supreme Court declared in a case upholding release-time education that "we are a religious people and our institutions presuppose the existence of a Supreme Being."[11] And in 1954, in response to the perceived threat of "atheistic communism," the words *under God* were placed into the Pledge of Allegiance: "one nation under God." But this declaration was short-lived as a matter of public-policy.

In *U.S. v. Seeger*, a 1965 case involving a conscientious objector, the Supreme Court defined "religion" as "a given belief that is sincere and meaningful that occupies a place in the life of its possessor parallel to the belief in another orthodox belief in God."[12] In the case of *U.S. v. Nordolf* (1972), a draft-board attempted to order a person who claimed to be a conscientious objector to report for induction into military service without considering the claims of conscience of the draftee. In this case the court defined conscience as "a knowledge or feeling of right and wrong, with a compulsion to do right; moral judgment that prohibits or opposes the violation of a previously recognized ethical principle."[13]

In a 1971 conscientious objector case decided by the Supreme Court, Justice Douglas stated (in dissent) that "conscience and belief are the main ingredients of First Amendment rights.... Conscience is often an echo of religious faith. But... it may also be the product of travail, meditation, or sudden revelation related to a moral comprehension of the dimension of a problem, not to a religion in the ordinary sense."[14] An example of conscience not based upon religious belief was recognized by the U.S. Supreme Court in the case of *U.S. v. Welsh*, a case in which the Court granted a conscientious objector an exemption from military service on the basis of conscience. The essence of Welsh's conscientious objector beliefs were quoted in the opinion thus: "I believe that human life is valuable in and of itself; in its living, therefore, I will not injure or kill another human being. This belief (and the 'duty' to abstain from violence toward another person)... is essential to every human relation."[15]

The beliefs of Welsh were praised by Justice Douglas as representing the essence of religion. In fact, his beliefs appear remarkably close to the statements of Jewish theologian Martin Buber as to what represents the obligations of conscience. This case, although favorable to protecting human beings, had no precedental value in *Roe v. Wade*, decided only a few years later. There the court permitted violence and destruction of human life in the womb, based upon the "choice" made by a woman and her doctor. In *Roe v. Wade* human life was no longer considered valuable in and of itself, but only if someone else placed value on it. In order to do so, it said that life in the womb was only "a theory of life" and created the fiction of "potential life"—in fact, there is actual life in the womb with potential, not potential life. Thus in *Roe v. Wade* a medical model replaced a moral model. No longer was there a duty to abstain from violence, and the value of life became relative, not valuable in and of itself.

Eminent authorities in other fields have also attempted to define the meaning of *conscience*. Origen, a theologian of the early Christian church, defined "conscience" as a correcting and guiding spirit accompanying the soul, by which it is led away from evil and made to cling to good.[16] German philosopher George Friedrich Hegel stated that "true conscience" is the disposition to will what is absolutely good.[17] Philosopher Immanuel Kant observed that when a moral issue presents itself and demands action, then "conscience speaks involuntarily and inevitably."[18] Martin Buber defined conscience as "the capacity and tendency of man to distinguish between those of his past and future actions which should be approved and which should be disapproved. Conscience only rarely fully coincides with a standard derived from the society or community."[19] The Catholic theologian Thomas Aquinas observed that "conscience implies the relation of knowledge to something applied to an individual case.... Conscience is said to witness, to bind, to stir up, and also to accuse, torment, or rebuke."[20]

A violated conscience is recognized by disapproval, accusation, torment or rebuke. Those who express personal guilt, remorse, regret, or other self-reproach can be said to feel that they have violated their conscience. Perhaps the most important single aspect of a violated conscience is guilt. However, influential elements of modern society believe that guilt should be trivialized, relativized, or eliminated entirely. In his book *Without Guilt and Justice* Walter Kaufman stated that "Guilt feelings are a contagious disease that harms those who harbor them and endangers those who live close to them. The liberation of guilt spells the dawn of autonomy."[21] Swiss psychiatrist Paul Tournier has lamented the modern loss of conscience. In a book entitled *The Whole Person in a Broken World* he writes: "Modern man thinks he has eliminated the world of values, the world of poetry, the world of moral consciousness; but he has only repressed it and is suffering from it.... Our materialistic and amoral civilization no longer answers the deepest needs of the soul.... Modern man suffers from a repression of conscience."[22]

THE INFLUENCE OF THE THERAPEUTIC MODEL

A very important influence on the loss of significance of conscience and the attempt to eliminate guilt and remorse is the modern rise of the therapeutic model. Sociologist Christopher Lasch has written, "The contemporary climate is therapeutic, not religious. People today hunger not for personal salvation... but for the feeling, the momentary illusion of personal well-being, health, and psychic security."[23] Another observer has written, "Morality is no longer a prominent feature of civil society. In the 80s politicians abandoned it, Wall Street discarded it, televangelists defiled it... but as virtue drained out of our public lives, it reappeared in our cereal bowls... and our exercise regimens... and our militant responses to cigarette smoke, strong drink and greasy food. We redefined virtue as health."[24]

Sociologist Philip Rieff says that the therapeutic model follows the model of psychological man, whom he describes as "a child not of nature but of technology—not committed to the public life and most unlike religious man. Psychological man is anti-heroic, shrewd, carefully counting his satisfactions and dissatisfactions, studying unprofitable commitments as the sins most to be avoided."[25] Thus terms such as *free will, guilt, good* or *evil* have no place in the therapeutic model.[26] The therapeutic tolerates no revealed, eternal, and commanding truths. Instead, it represents an assault, more and more successful, upon all sacred barriers, according to Rieff.[27] The therapeutic model is far removed from the person who disregards elementary self-interest and accepts martyrdom in preference to transgressing conscientiously-held beliefs.

But these modern elements fail to recognize that guilt as a result of the violation of conscience has an intrinsic aspect not derived from external influences. Nor can it be eliminated by science or technology or by a perfection of the technique of abortion. Nor can conscience be reduced to a calculation of the various risks and potential benefits from taking a certain course of action. Neither can it be trivialized because the consequences of violating one's conscience can have a profound influence on subsequent behavior and also may result in influencing or determining one's eternal destiny.

Influential elements in modern society have also attempted to claim that guilt or its absence is merely a matter of social conditioning, and some have claimed that it is the pro-life opposition to abortion that causes the woman to feel guilt about abortion. But Buber points out that guilt is not simply acquired from transgressing ancient taboos or social customs or laws or parental values. In a 1948 presentation made to an international conference on medical psychotherapy he stated, "there exists real guilt, fundamentally different from all the anxiety-induced bugbears that are generated in the cavern of the unconscious. Personal guilt, whose reality some schools of psychoanalysis contest, and others ignore, does not permit itself to be reduced to the trespass against a powerful taboo. Each person stands in an objective relationship to others.... It is that person's share in the human order of being, the share for which that person bears responsibility. This responsibility or share in the human order is the action demanded by conscience."

ABORTION COUNSELING PRACTICES

With this as background, let us examine contemporary abortion-counseling practices. An examination of the literature on abortion-counseling as well as various forms used to provide information and consent by the woman at the time of the abortion, reveals that there is no discussion of (or even information about) the morality of abortion. Abortion-counseling does not use concepts of right or wrong. There is no effort made whatsoever to encourage a woman to examine her conscience. In abortion-counseling the woman is autonomous and the presence of another being in the womb is down-played or eliminated entirely. In abortion-counseling there is no human order of being. No reference to even a possible or potential relation to another is mentioned.

When abortion-techniques are described to women *via* film or models, the womb is empty. The impression is left that there is nothing being aborted. Personnel in the abortion-facility use terms such as *tissue* or *products of conception* and never *baby* or even *fetus*. These dehumanizing terms are also used in consent-forms and in other information provided to the woman at the time of the abortion. The failure accurately to describe exactly what is being removed has been criticized as a deprivation of informed consent and a moral decision by the doctor on behalf of the woman.[28] The woman is also autonomous. The role of the male is marginalized or non-existent, at least in the legal context, and at the abortion-clinic as well. The U.S. Supreme Court has guaranteed this by its 1992 ruling in *Casey* that a husband is not even entitled to notice before his wife obtains an abortion.

While abortion-counseling, in theory, is supposed to be non-directive, in actual practice it is contrived and manipulative. It makes "therapeutic" exceptions instead of providing full and complete information. In abortion-counseling the emphasis is placed on effective contraceptive usage, but there is no attempt to encourage abstinence from sexual intercourse out of wedlock. (The vast majority of women who obtain abortions are unmarried.[29]) These counseling techniques rely on a risk-benefit analysis with a pronounced bias in favor of the benefits of abortion and the detriments of childbirth. Abortion-counseling claims to be in response to the "choice" of the woman but does not protect the woman's conscience.

The risks and benefits which are discussed omit any reference to moral or religious considerations. Instead they concentrate on bodily and reproductive concerns. If the church with which the woman may be affiliated has taken a position in opposition to abortion, it is not respected. The sole authority is the autonomous self. This is the hallmark of abortion-counseling. This sole appeal to the autonomous self has been criticized by psychologist Paul Vitz as "almost guaranteeing the breakdown of higher ideals into a rationalization of selfishness permeated with narcissism."[30]

Abortionists may also manipulate the women into obtaining an abortion by appealing to her fears. This is done by identifying a predominant fear and then using that fear to gain compliance and "sell" another abortion. Examples may include a fear that parents or a husband will find out that she is pregnant, fear of interruption of school- or career-plans, or fear of death. Those who work in abortion-facilities may themselves have had an abortion. If so, these counselors may actively encourage a woman to obtain an abortion in order that the counselor may feel a little better about having had an abortion herself. Other counselors may include radical feminists, who as an exercise in power and control encourage abortion.

Abortion-clinics may also prominently display pro-abortion slogans on their walls in the waiting room and provide literature from such groups as Catholics for Free Choice in a deliberate attempt to erode and undermine any existing religious precepts or idealistic values which may be different from a decision for abortion. In one particular abortion-malpractice case, a woman had an abortion at age 16. Afterwards, she promised God that she would never have another abortion. In later years she got married and had three children. Marriage-problems ensued and her husband left when she was pregnant. She had severe economic difficulties. Despite her vow to God that she would never have another abortion, she found herself at an abortion-clinic. At the clinic she was very ambivalent. Despite her financial difficulties, the abortion-counselor told her not to take money from the pro-lifers protesting outside. And instead of respecting the woman's Catholic beliefs, she gave the woman literature from Catholics for Free Choice and urged her to obtain an abortion.

Possible psychological problems following abortion, including guilt, regret, and remorse, receive little attention in abortion-counseling, and when they are discussed the presentations tend to be misleading and inaccurate. For example, in a handout at a Planned Parenthood affiliate on "Facts about Early Abortion," the information is primarily limited to a brief description of how the abortion is done, with foreseeable problems limited to possible bodily injury or future reproductive problems. Under a section entitled "Emotional Problems" it states that "emotional problems after abortion are uncommon, and when they happen they usually go away quickly. Most women report a sense of relief, although some experience depression or guilt. Serious psychiatric disturbances (such as a psychosis or serious depression) after abortion appear to be less frequent than after childbirth." Although guilt is acknowledged as a possibility, it is trivialized and the emotional problems are greatly understated.

Another informational handout used by an abortion-facility entitled "Voluntary Interruption of Pregnancy Aftercare" includes a section on "Feelings after the Abortion." It states: "What's important for us to realize is that positive, negative, ambivalent feelings are natural after an abortion. Any of the negative or confused feelings tend to pass away with time. We need to accept them as part of us and not put ourselves down for having them.... It is possible, though rare, to have a few days of depression. This may be due to hormonal changes that take place in our body when a pregnancy ends, whether by abortion, miscarriage, or full-term delivery." This informational handout makes no reference at all to guilt, only to possible "negative feelings." It attempts to place induced abortion in the same category as miscarriage or childbirth by reference to "hormonal changes." Again, the range of psychological and emotional problems following abortion is considerably understated. Still another abortion-facility which is part of a chain of abortion-clinics in several states has no discussion at all relative to emotional or psychological problems following abortion in any of its forms or the handouts provided to women.

The frequent experience of guilt by women following abortion exists even in the absence of legal prohibitions against abortion. Nor is the personal guilt eliminated by counselors or others attempting to be "non-judgmental." Abortion-counseling makes the assumption of modern liberalism, which believes that every individual is a person of many parts who assembles him or herself. Every person can be a self-constituting creature, manufacturing oneself by choosing purposes and values by whatever principle he or she wishes from the universe of possibilities. In this view freedom is defined as a hostility toward conventions.[31] The possibility that there is an objective reality of general application is never considered. Thus, counseling at abortion-clinics is at least indifferent to the conscience of the woman, and at worst actively exploits and manipulates her into a decision for abortion that violates her conscience.

Instead of better health for the woman, her health is now worsened, despite the claims of the proponents of abortion to the contrary. Childbirth is protective against breast-cancer; induced abortion is not. Women who have abortions are much more likely to be found in a psychiatric hospital than child-bearing women. Induced abortion leads to more destructive and impaired relationships than other pregnancy-outcomes. The evidence of physical, psychological, and social deterioration following repeated abortion is particularly persuasive. This is most important, because about 60% of U.S. women age 30 and over have repeated abortions.[32] At least 32 areas of health and well-being have been identified where this deterioration takes place. These include increased isolation, lower self-esteem, distress and anxiety, less stable relationships, increased psychiatric hospital admissions, suicide attempts, more depression, increased smoking, drug and alcohol use, more grief, communication-breakdowns, increased risk of ectopic preg-nancy, miscarriage and infertility.[33] Dietrich Bonhoeffer once said, "whoever does injury or violence to the natural will suffer for it.... The natural is the true means of protection of the preserved life.... The natural is the safeguarding of life against the unnatural.... This is what underlies the maintenance and recovery of physical and mental health."[34] The myriad number of medical, psychological, and social problems tell us that abortion is unnatural—it destroys life, not only of the life in the womb, but of individuals and societies.

THE DENIAL OF CONSCIENCE AT THE TIME OF ABORTION

Perhaps the most important evidence that making the decision for abortion does not fall within the legally protected zone of conscience or spiritual imperatives is found in a comprehensive articled entitled "Abortion Counselling" written by Uta Landy, then Executive Director of the National Abortion Federation (NAF). The NAF is one of the foremost advocates of abortion and has about 400 abortion-clinics as members of the organization. It has established standards for the practice of abortion. A review of this article leads to the inescapable conclusion that women who decide to have an abortion most often are in the midst of a major personal crisis in the face of an unplanned pregnancy and deny their conscience in the process. The article examines the various behavioral patterns of women who seek abortion. Ambivalence, guilt, anger, and deep confusion are identified as "major themes" that consistently arise in the decision-making that leads to abortion. These themes are a strong indication that, for most women, the decision to abort most likely represents a violation of conscience or ideals.

Landy identifies four types of reaction by women in a crisis-situation. These include the "spontaneous approach" in which the woman makes the decision quickly without thinking too long about it. Landy warns that, while this approach produces a quick resolution, the decision and its consequences might result in regret later. A second type of reaction to a crisis is the "rational-analytical" type in which the woman weighs her options carefully. But this type of woman is so pre-occupied with being rational that she fails to take her emotions into account.

A third type is the woman who takes the "denying-procrastinating" approach in which she initially denies she is pregnant and has many reasons why she cannot make a decision. Fourth, there is the "no-decision-making" approach, in which case the woman refuses to make a decision herself and instead allows others, such as her husband, boyfriend, parents, doctor, or counselor, to make the decision for her. She consequently refuses to take responsibility for the decision and is prone to blame others for having the abortion.[35] Based upon the findings of this article, it is reasonable to conclude that women who make decisions to abort without adequate reflection, or are overly rational, or who engage in procrastination and denial, or who let others decide, are very likely to leave their moral or religious values behind in the process.

The findings and conclusions in Landy's article are not unique. Several other studies have also shown that the abortion-decision may be severely conflicted, as indicated by high levels of pre-abortion stress, as well as by guilt or anger, self-reproach, anticipatory grief, or high levels of anxiety. Those who have observed women prior to their induced abortion have noticed pronounced personality-changes. For example, a psychiatric counselor has said, "the 24-hour period prior to the woman obtaining an abortion is a period of intense anxiety and ambivalence."[36] Researchers at Duke University who studied women upon their arrival at a Raleigh abortion-clinic also found a generalized stress-response syn-drome. Four distinct coping styles were identified. Women tended to be either "approachers" or "avoiders" and marked by anxiety, depression, denial and intrusion. These researchers found similar responses between the women who sought abortion and bereaved populations.[37]

Similarly, an intense grief-response was found in a 1982 study of 80 women at Midtown Hospital (Atlanta GA) at a pre-abortion counseling-session. Pre-abortion grief was found to be higher than grief-responses six weeks later. The authors concluded that the decision to abort may initiate the grief-reaction.[38] A 1981 study of 55 British women who requested abortion for mental health reasons used a hostility-questionnaire which measured the urge to act out hostility, to criticize others, and to project delusional (paranoid) hostility, self-criticism, and guilt. Prior to their abortion, the mean hostility-score was about two standard deviations above the normal mean. The hostility-scores were similar to those of psychiatric populations. The predominant direction of hostility was toward self-criticism and guilt.[39] All of these studies tend to demonstrate that the woman is in a crisis at the time of her abortion and is attempting to cope with guilt, grief and remorse.

In Carol Gilligan's frequently cited book *In a Different Voice*, Kohlberg's theory of justice was contrasted with the values considered by women, both before and after abortion.[40] She found that nihilism was an important aspect of the thinking process as revealed in their personal stories. She observed that women frequently seemed to want separation but also attachment. They tended to recast the moral judgment from a consideration of the good to a choice between two evils. Moral dilemmas were seen in terms of conflicting responsibilities. The women asked themselves, "Why care?" in a world where the strong end relationships. The author concluded that the abortion-decision centers on the self. The woman focuses on taking care of herself because she feels that she is all alone.

The patterns of thought described in Gilligan's book contrast sharply with Buber's idealistic views. He says, "Each person stands in an objective relationship to others.... It is that person's share in the human order of being, the share for which that person bears responsibility. This responsibility or share in the human order is the action demanded by conscience."[41] Not only is it the woman obtaining the abortion, but those who may have encouraged her to do so, or otherwise participated, also bear their share of responsibility for the abortion.

CRISIS-BEHAVIOR AS A REASON FOR VIOLATION OF CONSCIENCE

Isolation of the woman by treating abortion as her personal and private choice also fails to take adequate account of the crisis-situation in which women involved in decisions regarding abortion often find themselves. The types of coping methods described by Landy provide ample evidence that the woman is frequently in a crisis. According to those who have studied crisis-theory and crisis-situations, one of the worst things a person can do is to become isolated. Isolation often leads to bouts of depression and self-pity and to loss of self-control. It may result in primitive methods of coping behavior in an attempt to resolve the crisis. Persons in crisis are also very susceptible to the influence of others who may try to aid in resolving the crisis. Thus, with a minimum effort on the part of the counselor, mental health professional, or family-member, a maximum amount of leverage may be exerted upon the individual.

Various studies have demonstrated that the influence of others is frequently a significant factor in the decision to have an abortion or to bring a child to term. In one study by the Alan Guttmacher Institute during 1987-88 of 1900 women obtaining abortions at various facilities throughout the U.S., it was found that 23% stated as a reason that their husband or partner wanted them to have an abortion and 7% stated that their parents wanted them to do so.[42] Other studies have found even higher figures. A study of post-abortion women in 1993-94 recruited from local post-abortion counseling services found that 58% of the women had abortions because of pressure from a husband, boyfriend, or parents.[43] However, if women in a crisis-situation are pressured to have an abortion, or take that action to please others, it is likely that the values of these others will be dominant in the process.

WOMEN AS MORAL AGENTS

Other research has also identified various coping strategies used by women who obtained abortions. In one of the studies, all of the coping strategies appeared to be based on abortion as a moral problem. In a 1978 doctoral dissertation by Janice Muhr, a model of abortion decision-making was developed which weighted three kinds of issues: volitional, practical, and moral.[44] In-depth interviews revealed that women tended to generate rationales which excluded or minimized conflictual levels of meaning and came to view their decisions as relatively free or forced. Four post-abortion adjustment styles were identified, with each characterized by cognitive and behavioral coping strategies: *status quo*, maturation, victim, and victim-persecutor. It was hypothesized that all adjustment-styles were organized around concern for abortion as a moral problem, even for women who did not raise personal moral concerns. For women who experienced abortion as a loss, mourning-processes were blocked because of the moral and volitional nature of the decision. An affective cycle of guilt and loss was identified in some women which did not resolve itself over time.

Maturation as a possible response following abortion might be categorized as a "wake-up" call. For example, one woman who had an abortion at age 16 later related that it made her realize that she was a sinner. She made the important step of taking responsibility for her actions. In later years she committed her life to Jesus Christ. Another "wake-up" call type of response might be to obtain a tubal ligation to prevent further pregnancies, or to decide to abstain from sexual intercourse in the future. Women who view themselves as victims are those who will join organizations such as Victims of Choice, American Victims of Abortion, or Women Exploited by Abortion (WEBA). Those who see themselves as victims are conflicted by the fact that they saw themselves as victims if they bore a child but also as aggressors by their involvement in the death of their unborn child.[45]

TYPICAL THOUGHT-PATTERNS APPEAR TO EXCLUDE CONSCIENCE AS THE BASIS OF ABORTION DECISION-MAKING

There is other evidence, based upon the typical thought-processes of women who obtain abortions, that conscience and moral or spiritual imperatives are not controlling the decision. For example, in a study of women who had abortions in a Baltimore area clinic in 1983-85, it was found that 2 out of 3 exhibited a histrionic personality, 1 out of 3 was narcissistic, and nearly 1 out of 4 had an anti-social personality. Histrionic individuals are prone to denial, may display rapidly shifting and shallow emotions, and will likely over-react to situations when they arise. Usually they tend to show little interest in careful, analytic thinking and tend to be easily influenced by others or by fads. The narcissistic personality is characterized by extreme self-centeredness or self-absorption. The emotional reactions of narcissistic individuals are frequently dominated by rage or shame. Thus they may not express guilt-feelings, at least until they have matured at some time in the future. Anti-social personalities frequently engage in unlawful acts, are irritable and aggressive, often fail to plan ahead or are impulsive. They also tend to lack regard for the truth and are reckless regarding their own or others' personal safety. The author concluded that the clinical picture of personality-disorders exhibited by these women suggests that "it is one of somebody who has been wounded early in life, has difficulty in relationships, and has tremendous difficulty with intimacy."[46]

PRAGMATISM PREVAILS OVER PRINCIPLE

The reasons given by women for having abortions indicate that the basis for decision-making is pragmatic and not based on conscience. The 1987-88 Guttmacher survey found that the most important reasons for obtaining an abortion were: (1) the woman is concerned that having a baby would change her life, (2) the woman can't afford a baby now, (3) the woman has problems with a relationship or wants to avoid single parenthood, (4) the woman is unready for responsibility, (5) the woman is not mature enough or is too young to have a child.[47] All of the reasons given in the survey were pragmatic in nature, and none referred to religious or spiritual reasons. All reasons involved the avoidance or dissolution of human relationships, whether existing or potential. The reasons appear to be far removed from God or a religious impulse. Instead, they appear to be motivated by abandonment, self-interest, weakness, or the influence of others.

THE INFLUENCE OF LEGALIZED ABORTION

The fact that induced abortion is legal also appears to be an important influence on the decision to have an abortion. In a study of 252 women-members of WEBA, 70% said the law had played a major role in their moral perception of abortion, only 6% said it played a moderate role, and 13% said it played little or no role.[48] When these same women were asked whether or not they would have sought an illegal abortion if a legal abortion had not been available, 75% said they definitely would not have sought an illegal abortion. One woman was quoted as saying, "If it's legal, it must be all right." Similarly, in a study of 344 post-abortion women who were receiving a variety of services at Akron Pregnancy Services in Akron, Ohio from 1988-93, 91% reported legal abortions and only 5% reported illegal abortions.[49] When asked if they would have illegal abortions, only 12% said yes, 58% said no, and 30% had no response. Thus, according to the self-assessment of the women, they were far less likely to have an illegal abortion compared to a legal abortion.

The fact that abortion is legal also appears to influence women before they even become pregnant. Recent studies have reported that many women will decide to obtain an abortion even before they become pregnant.[50] However, even if these women obtain an abortion after becoming pregnant, stress-reactions indicating internal conflict are still reported among them in the time-period shortly before their abortion. Again, the influence of legalized abortion on decision-making is apparent.

LONG-TERM GUILT OR REGRET OR OTHER ADVERSE REACTIONS

An investigation of the medical, psychological, and social literature following legal abortion reveals that women may experience depression on the perceived date of the aborted child's birth, anger at not receiving accurate information from abortion-counselors prior to the abortion, resentment at the manipulation by others, or increased sexual activity in an attempt to atone for the destruction of the aborted child by having another replacement-child. Women may contemplate or attempt suicide after abortion. A significant number will initiate or expand their use of alcohol or drugs following abortion. Any of these symptoms represent evidence that women have violated their own standards when they obtain abortions. Specific examples include a 1989 study of 232 post-abortion women seen at crisis-pregnancy centers across the U.S. approximately ten to eleven years post-abortion and who indicated some evidence of post-abortion syndrome. Virtually all expressed guilt from their abortion and 36% said that they had suicidal thoughts following their abortion. Most of these women (76%) were Protestants.[51] A study conducted by Open Arms, a religiously oriented post-abortion support ministry, of 828 post-abortion women an average of 8 years thereafter, among centers with which they are associated throughout the U.S., found that 81% expressed guilt from their abortion.[52]

Severely adverse reactions following abortion are not limited to Christian or religious women. In a 1965 study of Japanese women (a society not known for being particularly religious) conducted by a Japanese newspaper-chain, only 18% of those polled said that they had no guilt-feelings at all, while more than 60% admitted to some degree of regret or remorse.[53] In a small study published by Anne Speckhard of 30 post-abortion women who were stressed by their abortion-experience, all expressed feelings of grief, sadness, regret and loss, 92 % expressed guilt, 60% increased drug or alcohol use, 31%

made suicide-attempts, and 65% had suicidal thoughts following their abortion, among their negative reactions. In this sample 72% said that they had no identifiable religious beliefs at the time of their abortion.[54] In a sample of 80 women who had abortions at a Baltimore area clinic during 1984-86, intrusive or avoidance behavior was present in two-thirds of the women, even three to five years after their abortions. Some 67.5% of these Baltimore women reported that religious worship was not important in their lives at the time of their abortion.[55]

In David Reardon's 1987 study of 252 women about ten years following their abortion and who were members of WEBA, 94% had negative psychological reactions which they attributed to their abortion-experience. In a further study of a sub-group of 100 WEBA women from the original sample of 252, 91% said that they experienced feelings of guilt and sorrow after their abortion. When asked about their choice for abortion, 54% said it was inconsistent with their prior beliefs and a betrayal of their own ideals, 14% were uncertain, and 28% said it was consistent with their prior beliefs. When asked if they were religious persons prior to their abortion, 38% agreed or strongly agreed, while 47% disagreed or strongly disagreed, with 29% uncertain.[56] The fact that many women (47%) who said they were not religious when they obtained their abortion and yet still subsequently had severely negative psychological reactions is evidence that there is "a law written on the heart" and that obtaining an abortion violates that law.

Random studies on U.S. women who have been asked about their emotional reaction to abortion are very few. In March 1989 a random telephone-interview study of 2533 women aged 18 or older was conducted by the *Los Angeles Times*. Among these women 8% admitted to having had at least one abortion. Of those admitting abortion, 56% expressed a sense of guilt about having had an abortion, and 26% of the women said they "mostly regretted" the abortion.[57] The elapsed length of time since their abortion would have varied widely. The percentage reporting guilt in the *Los Angeles Times* study is higher than guilt-feelings expressed by women in a number of other studies where women were questioned shortly after their abortion. This suggests that guilt as a reaction to abortion may increase over time.

The percentage of women reporting abortion was lower than the actual percentage of U.S. women who would have actually obtained abortions because, at the time of the study, about 13% should have reported one or more previous legal abortions. Based on previous studies comparing women who participated in post-abortion studies with those who dropped out or refused to participate, the women dropping out or not participating were likely to have had more emotional difficulties, be more likely to be repeating abortions, and less likely to want the abortion than the women who participated.[58]

Non-randomized long-term studies of women stressed or traumatized by abortion have found very high percentages of women expressing guilt-feelings. In the Akron study of 344 post-abortion women receiving services at Akron Pregnancy Services from 1988-93, 66% expressed guilt and 54% expressed regret or remorse from their abortion approximately six years afterward. The average age of these women at the time of their abortion was about 18 years.[59] In Reardon's 1987 study, 91% expressed guilt when interviewed about eleven years later. A 1990 study by a Minneapolis-based post-abortion support-group among religiously oriented women ten to fifteen years after their abortions found that 90% expressed guilt from their abortion.[60] And a 1989 study of 232 women seen at various crisis-pregnancy center in 39 states who exhibited evidence of some post-abortion stress found that virtually all had guilt-feelings from abortion.[61]

Some short-term studies on special populations have also shown high levels of moral conflict and resulting guilt following abortion. A San Diego study published in 1973 of unmarried women aged 14-20 who had structured, in-depth interviews found that 90% had moral conflicts over the decision, 61.5% expressed strong guilt, and 38.5% expressed minimal guilt, while 42% thought abortion was murder. The average length of time since their abortions was about six months.[62] In a North Carolina study adolescents seeking abortion were asked their beliefs about abortion. The study found that 34% opposed abortion on request, 20% thought abortion was justified only on medical recommendation, and yet all of the adolescents had abortions without giving any of those reasons for doing so. It was concluded that many had rationalized their guilt by considering themselves "exceptions to the rule."[63] A British study which personally interviewed women two to three months post-abortion found that 55% of the women reported guilt from their abortion.[64]

In one of the leading, early U.S. studies on post-abortion psychological reactions, 24% of New York women reported much guilt or moderate guilt when interviewed about one month post-abortion.[65] Other reviewers have reported short-term guilt reactions ranging from 10 to 36% in five other studies published in 1972-73.[66] Because of these and other studies, some observers have concluded that existing beliefs about abortion may be inadequate guides for decision-making in the face of an abortion-dilemma. In order to overcome this disequilibrium, the woman develops new cognitive constructions of the situation.[67]

GUILT AS THE GUARDIAN OF OUR GOODNESS

The encouragement of behavior that does not result in guilt is most important in a social context. Dr. Willard Gaylin, a psychotherapist and author of *Feelings: Our Vital Signs*, has stated in an article that "contrary to the tenets of pop psychology, guilt is hardly a useless emotion.... Guilt..., the sense of anguish that we have fallen short of our own standards, is the guardian of our goodness. It is necessary to the development of conscience in our children and to the avoidance of anti-social behavior. The failure to feel guilt is the basic flaw of the psychopath, who is capable of committing crimes of the vilest sort without remorse or contrition.... Guilt results when we betray an internalized model of behavior."[68] Many women betray that internalized standard of behavior when they obtain an abortion.

A VIOLATION OF A BASIC HUMAN RIGHT

The violation of conscience of these women is a violation of a basic human right. Virtually all of the state constitutions in the U.S. protect the rights of conscience from interference by others. The Universal Declaration of Human Rights adopted in 1948 by the United Nations also recognizes that the right of conscience is part of the dignity of the individual. Thus, a violation of conscience violates the basic rights and dignity of the woman. Those who claim that abortion represents a decision based upon conscience simply do not know the facts.

NOTES

1. *Declaration on Religious Freedom*, Vatican Council II (December 1965) as quoted in *Religious Liberty and Conscience*, ed. Milton R. Konvitz (1968) 23.

2. Covenant and Creation: Theological Reflections on Contraception and Abortion. Policy Statement of the 195th General Assembly of the Presbyterian Church (USA), 1983, p. 60.

3. Harold O. J. Brown, *Death Before Birth* (Grand Rapids: Eerdmans, 1977) 126, citing John Calvin's *Commentaries on the Last Four Books of Moses*, trans. Charles W. Bingham, 3: 41-42.

4. *Minnesota State Constitution* of 1857, Article 1, 16.

5. Virtually all state constitutions protect liberty of conscience, usually by absolutely protecting the right of religious worship, but they make a distinction between liberty and license relative to acts or practices.

6. *Planned Parenthood v. Casey* 112 S. Ct. 2791 (1992).

7. *National Right to Life News* (Oct. 11, 1995) p. 2, quoting the Colin Powell interview with Barbara Walters of Sept. 15, 1995 on the *20/20* program.

8. *National Right to Life News* (March 15, 1996), p.7, quoting a letter dated Febr. 28, 1996.

9. Naomi Wolf, "Our Bodies, Our Souls" in *The New Republic* (Oct. 16, 1995) 33.

10. *U. S. v. Kauten*, 133 F. 2d 703, 708 (2nd Cir 1943).

11. *Zorach v. Clauson*, 343 U.S. 306, 313 (1952).

12. *U.S. v. Seeger* 380 U.S. 163, 170-71 (1965).

13. *U.S. v. Nordolf* 440 F. 2d 840, 843-44 (C.A. III 1971).

14. *U.S. v. Gillette* 401 U.S. 437, 465 (1971), J. Douglas dissenting.

15. *U.S. v. Welsh* 398 U.S. 333, 343 (1970).

16. Origen, *Commentary on Romans* 2:15 (PG 14: 892) as quoted in *Thomas Aquinas: Summa Theologica*, vol. 1 of the edition within *Great Books of the Western World*, ed. Robert M. Hutchins (Encyclopedia Brittanica, 1952) 426.

17. Georg Friedrich Hegel, *The Philosophy of Right* in the edition reprinted in *Great Books of the Western World* (Encyclopedia Britannica, 19523) 48.

18. Immanuel Kant, *Critique of Practical Reason*, ed. Longmans (1954) 311-12.

19. Martin Buber, "Guilt and Guilt Feelings" in *Proceedings of the International Conference on Medical Psychotherapy*, vol. 3: International Conference on Mental Health, London 1948 (New York: Columbia Univ. Press, 1948).

20. Thomas Aquinas, *Summa Theologica*, vol. 1 of the edition within *Great Books of the Western World*, ed. Robert M. Hutchins (Encyclopedia Brittanica, 1952) 426.

21. Walter Kaufman, *Without Guilt and Justice* (1973) 114.

22. Paul Tournier, *The Whole Person in a Broken World* (1964) 11.

23. Christopher Lasch, *The Culture of Narcissism* (1979) 33.

24. Barbara Ehrenreich in *Lear Magazine*, as quoted in *Minneapolis Star-Tribune* (August 30, 1990).

25. Philip Rieff, *Freud: The Mind of the Moralist* (Chicago: Univ. of Chicago Press, 1961) 327, 391.

26. Nicholas Kittrie, *The Right to Be Different: Deviance and Enforced Therapy* (Baltimore: The Johns Hopkins Univ. Press, 1971) 39.

27. Philip Rieff, *The Triumph of the Therapeutic: The Uses of Faith after Freud* (New York: Harper and Row, 1987) x, xii.

28. "Regulating Abortion Services," letter by Virginia P. Riggs, M.D., in *New England Journal of Medicine* (Feb. 7, 1980) 350.

29. Abortion Surveillance: Preliminary Data, United States, 1992, MMWR 43/5 (Dec. 23, 1994) 930.

30. Paul Vitz, *Psychology as a Religion: The Cult of Self-Worship* (Grand Rapids: Eerdmans, 1977) 101.

31. George Will, *Statecraft as Soulcraft: What Your Government Does* (1983) 60.

32. S. K. Henshaw, K. Kost, "Abortion Patients in 1994-95: Characteristics and Contraceptive Use" in *Family Planning Perspectives* 28 (1996) 140.

33. T. Strahan, "Women's Health and Abortion. I. Deterioration of Health among Women Repeating Induced Abortion" in *Association for Interdisciplinary Research Newsletter* 5/1 (1993) 1-8.

34. Dietrich Bonhoeffer, *Ethics*, trans. Neville Horton Smith (New York: Macmillan, 1955) 105.

35. Uta Landy, "Abortion Counselling: A New Component of Medical Care" in *Clinics in Obstetrics and Gynecology* 13/1 (1986) 33.

36. Joyce Dunlop, "Counselling of Patients Requesting an Abortion" in *The Practitioner* 220 (1978) 847.

37. L. Cohen and S. Roth, "Coping with Abortion" in *Journal of Human Stress* (Fall 1984) 140-45.

38. Larry Peppers, "Grief and Elective Abortions: Breaking the Emotional Bond?" in *Omega* 18/1 (1987-88) 1-12.

39. R. Schmidt and R. G. Priest, "The Effects of Termination of Pregnancy: A Follow-up Study of Psychiatric Referrals" in *British Journal of Medical Psychology* 54 (1981) 267.

40. Carol Gilligan, *In a Different Voice: Psychological Theory and Women's Development* (Cambridge: Harvard Univ. Press, 1982) 75, 101, 124.

41. Buber.

42. A. Torres, J. D. Forrest, "Why Do Women Have Abortions?" in *Family Planning Perspectives* 20/4 (1988) 169.

43. Frederica Matthewes-Green, "Listening Groups, Summary" in *Real Choices, Offering Practical Life-Affirming Alternatives to Abortion* (1994) 247-48.

44. Janice Muhr, *Psychological Responses to First-Trimester Abortion*, Dissertation Abstracts International (1979) 4045-B.

45. Robert C. Erikson, "Abortion Trauma: Application of a Conflict Model" in *Pre- and Perinatal Psychology Journal* 8/1 (1933) 33.

46. Catherine A. Barnard, "Stress Reactions in Women Related to Induced Abortion" in *Association for Interdisciplinary Research in Values and Social Change Newsletter* 3/4 (1991) 3.

47. Torres, Forrest (cited in n.42 above) 169.

48. Reported by David Reardon, *Aborted Women: Silent No More* (1987) 336.

49. Lee E. H. Gsellman, "Physical and Psychological Injury in Women Following Abortion: Akron Pregnancy Service Survey" in *Association for Interdisciplinary Research in Values and Social Change* 15/4 (1993) 5.

50. K. Holmgren, "Time of Decision to Undergo a Legal Abortion" in *Gynecol. Obstet. Invest.* 26 (1988) 289-95.

51. Helen P. Vaughan, "Canonical Variates of Postabortion Syndrome" (Portsmouth, NH: Institute for Pregnancy Loss, 1990) 32-33, 21.

52. Abortion Information Sheet Project, Open Arms, P. O. Box 1056, Columbia MO 65205 (March 1993).

53. Minoru Muramatsu, ed., *Japan's Experience in Family Planning—Past and Present* (Tokyo: Family Planning Federation of Japan, 1967) 78, as cited in Daniel Callahan, *Abortion: Law Choice, and Morality* (New York: Macmillan, 1970) 70.

54. Anne Speckhard, *The Psycho-Social Aspects of Stress Following Abortion* (Kansas City: Sheed and Ward, 1987).

55. Catherine Barnard, "The Long Term Psychological Effects of Abortion" (Portsmouth, NH: Institute for Pregnancy Loss, 1990).

56. Reardon (1987) 334; see also David Reardon, *A Survey of Postabortion Reactions* (Springfield: Elliot Institute, 1987).

57. George Skelton, "Many in Survey Who Had Abortion Cite Guilt Feelings" in *Los Angeles Times* (March 19, 1989) 28.

58. E. W. Freeman, "Influence of Personality Attributes on Abortion Experience" in *American Journal of Orthopsychiatry* 47/3 (1977) 503; N. E. Adler, "Sample Attrition in Studies of Psychosocial Sequelae of Abortion: How Great a Problem?" in *Journal of Applied Social Psychology* 6/3 (1976)

240.

59. Lee Gsellman, "Physical and Psychological Injury in Women Following Abortion: Akron Pregnancy Services Survey" in *Association for Interdisciplinary Research Newsletter* 5/4 (1993) 1-8.

60. Jeanette Vought, *Post Abortion Trauma: 9 Steps to Recovery* (Grand Rapids: Zondervan, 1991) 97.

61. Vaughan.

62. Cynthia Martin, "Psychological Problems of Abortion for the Unmarried Teenage Girl" in *Genetic Psychology Monographs* 88 (1973) 32.

63. M. Perez-Reyes, R. Falk, "Follow-up after Therapeutic Abortion in Early Adolescence" in *Archives of General Psychiatry* 28 (1973) 120.

64. J. R. Ashton, "The Psychosocial Outcome of Induced Abortion" in *British Journal of Obstetrics and Gynaecology* 87 (1980) 1115.

65. J. D. Osofsky, H. J. Osofsky, "The Psychological Reaction of Patients to Legalized Abortion" in *American Journal of Orthopsychiatry* 42/1 (1972) 48.

66. Paul Dagg, "The Psychological Sequelae of Therapeutic Abortion—Denied and Completed" in American Journal of Psychiatry 148 (1991) 578.

67. M. L. Friedlander, T. J. Kaul, C. A. Stimel, "Abortion: Predicting the Complexity of the Decision-Making Process" in *Women and Health* 9/1 (1984) 43.

68. Willard Gaylin, *Feelings: Our Vital Signs.*

BREAKING THE LINGUISTIC PERMAFROST OF CURRENT AMERICAN ANTI-LIFE FICTION: A GUIDE FOR STUDENTS OF LITERATURE

Jeff Koloze

RECENTLY I PRESENTED A PAPER at a medieval conference at McMaster University wherein I noted that many women in Thomas Malory's tales of King Arthur's Knights of the Round Table are often not the sweet virginal creatures denoted by the term "damsels." I noted further that, since the term is popularly joined to the prepositional phrase "in distress," the combination phrase ("damsels in distress") was an example of how some words have become frozen in a "linguistic permafrost."

Contemporary American fiction, shackled by a corrupted, anti-life, feminist literary theory and by the oppression of nine-month legalized abortion, presents few works of fiction where women characters can be in any way denoted as "damsels in distress." As I pronounced those words to my audience then, I had two thoughts. First, what a, as our students would say, "cool" idea to enunciate. Secondly, I thought that, regarding the presentation of the right-to-life issues of abortion, infanticide, and euthanasia in contemporary American fiction, there is a similar linguistic permafrost perpetually freezing terms such as "abortion," "choice," and "rights" in anti-life writing.

There is a summer, however, even in Siberia. I believe that the linguistic permafrost which has enveloped contemporary fiction will eventually shatter, for there are fissures in the surface of the ice now. You can hear the subterranean rumbling. It will be my task here to present evidence of the breaking of the linguistic permafrost so that it will be obvious not only to ourselves but also to our students that the literature of the United States—even now, as it is being churned out in these nightmare decades of legal killing of the unborn child, the handicapped newborn, and the elderly—even now, our literature supports life-affirming principles.

The first half of this paper will focus on current fiction-titles which primarily present an anti-life theme.[1] What are some defining features of current anti-life fiction? Faulty characterization of pro-lifers tops the list of attributes of anti-life fiction, followed closely by a corollary point, a blindness to the pro-life viewpoint. On a secondary level, anti-life fiction frequently suffers from poor diction and historical inaccuracy. Finally, in at least one noticeable case, spelling, grammatical, and even typographical errors abound in one work of anti-life fiction. I will focus on Sue Robinson's *The Amendment*,[2] Walter Kirn's *She Needed Me*,[3] and Mary Logue's *Still Explosion*.[4]

The plot of Sue Robinson's *The Amendment* is unique in its boldness to "solve" what the author presents as a future "problem": how to bypass a constitutional amendment which restores the first civil right to life. Once the Human Life Amendment has been ratified, Robinson's characters engage in guerrilla-warfare tactics to enable mothers to have abortions. Underground abortion-clinics spring up around the country to do their killing work. Frances Foster is an elderly woman who lost not only her grandchild but also her daughter in a botched abortion in one of these illegal underground abortion-clinics. She is resolved to guarantee that mothers continue to have the right to kill their unborn children. She suggests to her accomplices that they can frustrate the protection of the Human Life Amendment by kidnapping the head of the pro-life movement, First Lady Mary Morgan. Unlike our unfortunate real First Lady, Mary Morgan is the force behind the national pro-life organization which brought about ratification of the Human Life Amendment, the Rights for the Unborn League. This kidnapping is a plausible feature of the plot because Foster has documentary evidence that it was Frances Foster's secret-abortionist father who aborted the future First Lady's child.

In Robinson's fictive world, the strategy works; a blow is struck against the protection of the Human Life Amendment. The First Lady and pro-life groups are forced to deposit $100 million into a Swiss bank account so that Frances Foster and her pro-abortion gang can open an abortion-clinic in Sweden which would cater to the killing needs of the mothers who come to them.

The plot of the novel can be torn apart with one stroke of deconstruction. One statement by a minor character can be deconstructed enormously. At the University Faculty for Life conference last year, I suggested that, as current literary theories have been used to distort and contort texts into versions foreign to the author's intention, or at least what has been considered the canonical reading for decades or centuries, these same literary theories can be used to valorize pro-life readings of texts. While many academics may argue over the profound philosophical assault which decon-struction makes on substantive readings, the theory can be used in the case of this novel to unravel its anti-life rhetoric.

Just before she is abducted, the First Lady's hairdresser exclaims, "I want to live" (188). Note that the character does not say merely "Oh" or "What's happening?" This spontaneous life-affirming exclamation is an odd statement to admit into a novel ostensibly concerned with declaring the acceptability of killing. The statement should immediately enable students to polarize themselves around two camps: those for the right to life and those against it. Here is a character, blacking out from the application of chloroform, whose last thought before losing consciousness is life-affirming. Immediately, the case can be made that any human being automatically responds to the threat of death by declaring the opposite, perhaps because this automatic response is that innate right to life with which we are endowed by the Creator. Since J. Hillis Miller asserts that deconstruction is not nihilistic, once the polarities of life and death are established, students can deconstruct the anti-life intent of the novel and replace it with a life-affirming criticism.[5]

Moreover, pro-life academics and students will be struck by the vengeance dominating the anti-life characters in the book. Note that, instead of working legislatively to overturn the constitutional amendment restoring the first civil right to life, Frances Foster and her pro-abortion gang resort to illegal activities: kidnapping, threatening government-officials, and deliberately breaking a national constitutional law. What is the paramount emotion directing Frances' and other characters' behavior? Hatred of the First Lady, who is reduced either to a "little bitch" (162) or a "pricey little bitch" (205). Hatred of the pro-life movement, which is described by one anti-life character as "an organization she detested with a pure hot loathing that made her tremble with fury" (93). Hatred of individual pro-lifers; the same anti-life character trembles with hatred again as she dehumanizes a pro-life character by calling him "the loathsome creature from the Rights for the Unborn League" (93). Frances Foster similarly voices her violent thoughts. At one point, looking at another pro-life character, Thomas B. Tuttle, she feels the urge "to grab Mr. Thomas B. Tuttle by his skinny neck and wring it until he was dead" (141). She reduces his humanity to a synecdoche; he is part of a larger "monster," the Rights for the Unborn League (141). Specifically, Frances Foster reduces the pro-life man to being only "a curling fingernail, a piece of dirt under its claw" (141).

Of course, such dehumanization should be typical. If anti-lifers do not respect human life in the flesh, why should they respect fictional human life on the printed page?

Walter Kirn's *She Needed Me* is another boiler-plate, anti-life novel. The main characters are the descriptively-named Weaver Walquist, pro-life activist, and Kim Lindgren, with whom he has a sexual relationship.[6] There is also a pro-lifer named Lucas Boone, who is the leader of the Conscience Squad, an Operation Rescue-type activist organization.

Walter's bossy mother eventually helps Kim obtain an abortion. Using a cultural-criticism approach, pro-life academics and students are able to note the absences of pro-life educational groups and positive pregnancy-support centers in the novel.

The trio of Weaver, Kim, and her brother Ricky (perhaps even Lucas in substitution for Ricky) is reminiscent of the characters in Richard Brautigan's *The Abortion: An Historical Romance 1966* (the Librarian, Vida, and Foster), all of whom collaborate in securing the killing of Vida's unborn child.[7]

As is typical with anti-life fiction, Kirn's novel contains some faulty legal citation. A reference to state law is questionable: "*If all Kim does for the next four weeks is watch TV and eat, she'll have to keep the baby. At the end of the first trimester, state law will tie her hands*" (88, all italics in original to show that this is what Weaver is thinking). Perhaps it would be too shocking for Kirn to acknowledge that in the reader's real world abortion is legal throughout the nine months of pregnancy and that, even if a state were to outlaw abortions, federal law in its abortion-distortion dominates the will of the people at the state-level.

Again, as is typical of most anti-life novels I have read, the baby, unfortunately, is aborted at the end of the novel. The reader is left with the distinct impression at closure, however, that Weaver's and Kim's romantic/sexual relationship has ended. Moreover, Kim, the aborted mother, hints at what pro-life academics and students would recognize as Post Abortion Syndrome. Weaver relates that "Kim said it sometimes after sex, in the dark: 'I can still be a mother someday'" (227).

In any respect, Kirn's book is tame contrasted with the more invidious *Still Explosion* by Mary Logue. The cover of *Still Explosion* has the following quote from Nancy Pickard: "The best I've read in a long time." Apparently, Pickard hasn't been reading very much lately. Critical reviews of the novel have been equally faulty.[8]

The plot is stereotypically anti-life. An abortion clinic is bombed; pro-lifers are "obviously" suspect. Anti-life journalist Laura Malloy solves the crime with little police help. All is saved so that the abortion-clinic can continue to kill unborn babies, harm their mothers, and estrange the fathers of aborted children from their former lovers. In essence, *Still Explosion* has such a predictable plot that anybody could write it.

The characters are not only typically rendered by someone who probably is an anti-lifer; they are stereotypically rendered. Pro-life activists are described either as devout Roman Catholics or fundamentalist Christians. Furthermore, pro-life people are portrayed as chauvinists. The leading pro-life activist, Tom Chasen, treats his wife as an inferior. Another pro-life character, Paul Jameson, is portrayed not only as one who suffers from the abortion of his own child, but also as someone who resents women.

Another character, who "got pregnant when she was in high school" and decided to give birth to her unborn child, is described gratuitously as a young woman who "said there was no way she could have had an abortion. Catholic and all" (136).

Pro-lifers know that many talented people contribute to this, our civil rights movement of the 1990s. Pro-lifers are liberal and conservative, religious and atheist, Christian and Jewish, Democrat and Republican. There is even, reportedly, a pro-life homosexual group. The diversity of the pro-life movement is something which certain anti-life writers cannot understand.

By novel's end, the major pro-life characters are taken away (as in "by the police") or blown away (as in "by a bomb"). Perhaps this is Logue's subliminal desire to "solve" the "problem" of pro-lifers.[9]

In fact, the most engaging "character" in the novel is Fabiola, Laura Malloy's pet ferret. (Gee, I wonder if, unlike her owner, Fabiola is pro-life? Maybe that's why the heroine keeps poor Fabiola in a closet.)

Immediately, the pro-life reader is hit with one of the favorite assumptions proclaimed by anti-lifers. Malloy wonders about the mothers going for abortions and wants to "find out what had brought them to this point in their lives and how they would feel if this right were taken away from them" (3). What "right"? Abortion is a wrong, not a right.

The moral blindness on abortion from which all anti-lifers suffer is evident in several passages. One in particular is quintessential anti-life rhetoric. Malloy enumerates the following as sufferings in the world which greatly disturb her:

AIDS killing babies and otters caught in oil spills. The otters always got to me, I could picture them so clearly just swimming along like they had done all their lives and then this black, smelly, gluey stuff would get in their eyes and noses, cover their bodies and they would drown. (27)

Pro-lifers immediately would query how someone could be more sensitive to the needs of the world's seals than to the needs of the unborn. In fact, we who are pro-life academics can use the above passage as an assignment for either an old-fashioned in-class writing exercise or a new-fashioned reader-response revision by having our students "translate" the passage into "pro-life":

Abortionists killing babies in saline abortions. The babies always got to me. I could picture them so clearly just swimming along like they had done all their unborn lives and then this burning, saline solution would get in their eyes and noses, and burn their lungs and the skin of their unborn bodies and they would drown in a saline ocean.[10]

Again, Malloy must be either ignorant of fetology or unwilling to accept the truth enunciated by the pro-life movement when she states to pro-lifer Tom Chasen, "Well, for one thing, it isn't a child. And for another when a couple decide to use birth control, they are making a decision together about whether they want her to get pregnant" (125). First, if the unborn child is not a child, what is he or she? A rock? A clump of cells from the mother's body which magically—poof!—becomes a unique human being? A car? Second, birth-control is either contraception or other non-artificial means of reproductive control. What does that have to do with the fact that after fertilization a human life exists?

Quick: a test. Take out your pens and put all books under your desk. Circle whatever might be incorrect with this next passage while I hum to myself the tune played during the final Jeopardy question:

I remembered when some members of a militant pro-life organization called Pro-Life Action Ministries raided a dumpster behind a family planning clinic in Robinsdale and found twelve "aborted babies." ...The legislature had passed a "fetal disposal law" and even though Planned Parenthood sought an injunction on the grounds that it was unconstitutional, the law was finally made official. It asked that the "human remains of an aborted or miscarried fetus be disposed of in a dignified manner, either burial or cremation." (149)

What's wrong with the above passage? Right, Alex! When not quoting someone or introducing a word used in a different and unique manner, the use of quotation-marks around certain terms diminishes the importance of those terms. It is as though the "being" of the term or phrase is lessened. Why are there quotes around "aborted babies"? Either the pro-life activists (note that they are gratuitously called followers of a "militant" pro-life group) actually did find babies who were aborted or they found objects which they purported to be babies which (not "who", since that pronoun denotes humanity) were aborted. Which one is it? Of course, an anti-life author would not want her readers to sympathize with pro-lifers in this matter. Finding bodies of aborted babies in a dumpster is gruesome and could sway some people who are undecided on abortion closer to the pro-life side.[11] Why, too, is it necessary to use quotes around "fetal disposal law"? The same line of reasoning can assert that the words are used correctly and need not be called into question with quotation-marks.

Malloy speaks a fundamental dishonesty about the theological issue

of when the soul enters the human body when she states "that was
the crux of all the controversy. When did the soul come into the
body? At conception, at quickening, at birth?" (185). Today's anti-
lifers can be respected for at least one thing: when they advocate the
killing of an unborn child, they do not consider this theological
argument. Permit me to make more sweeping generalizations. Anti-
lifers do not care about the theology of abortion. They demand
taxpayer funding of abortions. They demand censorship of pro-lifers.
They know human life begins at fertilization, but so what? Women
must be able to kill their unborn children if they so desire. An anti-
life author shows great disrespect for the intellectual underpinnings
of the abortion wrongs movement, and lowers his or her own
credibility within that community, when he or she classifies abortion
as a theological issue.

When "pro-life" Paul Jameson recounts his girlfriend's abortion to
Laura Malloy, he states, "OK, I know it's not a baby, it's a fetus, but
in my mind it was a baby" (224). Logue reduces with one
prepositional phrase the entire war between pro-lifers and anti-lifers
as a version of the phenomenalistic argument: it's all in your mind.
If you think it's a baby, then it's a baby; if you think it's only a
choice, then it's a choice.

Similarly, when another mother describes her abortion to Malloy,
she states that the abortionist told her

the fetus was too little to see, but I didn't believe him. Not that I wanted
to see it (*sic*). I think about it (*sic*) a lot. It (*sic*) would've been a baby.
Right before the abortion, I tried to tell it (*sic*) it was nothing personal.
That at another time I would have felt different. (112)

Note the extensive use of the impersonal pronoun for a child who
was either a "he" or a "she." The use of the impersonal pronoun
presents another problem to readers who support the first civil right:
the necessary correction which such readers must make (as evidenced
by the numerous "*sic*"s which I introduced into the passage quoted)
impedes the progression of the text. Thus, the comprehension of the
anti-life intent of the passage is severely hampered.

As the opening pages of the novel hits pro-lifers with an assault of
anti-life rhetoric, so does the last page, which attempts to summarize
the functions of the characters and to bring closure to the book:

Christine's reasons for having an abortion, Tom Chasen's fears of women using it as a means of birth control, Sandy Chasen's religious fervor, Donna Asman's [the abortion-clinic director] commitment to providing women of all income brackets with a choice, Meg Jameson's Catholic views, and Sheila Langstrom's desire to have a baby, coloring her attitude on abortion, and Paul's question of where do men fit into the decision. (234)

Note that in the above litany, the anti-life characters are described positively. It is a definite good being communicated to the reader that Donna Asman, responsible for the deaths of thousands of unborn children, has her career of violation of the first civil right to life as a "commitment"—itself a powerfully positive word—"providing women of all income brackets with a choice." This positive description of Asman's abortorium-work needs to be translated by pro-lifers into something more accurate, such as:

Donna Asman's obsession with lowering the population, especially of poor minority women, and making sure that they understand that killing their unborn children is their only choice and that they owe it to society not to bring more of their kind—African American, Hispanic, Vietnamese—into the world.

Logue's diction makes the main character obviously anti-life, a fatal flaw for a newspaperwoman who admits her bias to the reader. Bemoaning the fact that she "had to cross the street and brave the cluster of protestors who were handing out pamphlets," the seasoned pro-lifer will halt at Laura Malloy's scorchingly negative continuation, "harassing the women who entered the clinic" (1). This first-page example of slapping pro-lifers continues throughout the book.

Prepositions show relationships between nouns and pronouns (a very positive and pro-life thing for a part of speech to do). An overuse of prepositions, however, can considerably slow down the reading and comprehension of a passage:

After I had been parked *in* front *of* the bondmen's offices *across* the street *from* the station *for* five minutes, I saw Tennison walk *in* the main doors *of* the station. I sat *in* my car *for* a few minutes to give him some time alone, then walked past the bronze Father *of* the Waters *in* the foyer *of* the building and down a long narrow hallway *to* his office. (21, emphasis added)

Despite the use of "for" in adverbial phrases, all of the above italicized words "read" to the eye (as does the "to" in the verb infinitive "to give") as prepositions and can distract the reader from the more important work of deciphering what the author tries to convey. The same can be said for the use of "down," although this is a truncation of the parallelism in the verb forms "walked past" and "walked down."

On several occasions Laura Malloy's comments read more as intrusions than as reminiscences or clarifying thoughts. Speaking about a fountain of which she is particularly fond, Malloy describes how she

went and stood by the fountain and watched the water squirt out of the fishes' mouths in a ring around the nymphet. Over the years, she had turned a light blue streaked-bronze color and seemed happy. It was nice to see women's art celebrating women in a public place. (172)

Malloy's comment about women's art being celebrated in public does nothing more to enhance her character; the reader is quite aware that Malloy is an anti-life feminist. It does, however, intrude a feminist political position unnecessarily.

Of lesser importance, yet annoying, are the numerous grammatical, historical, and typographical errors in the novel. Usually, readers are tolerant of such mistakes. Sometimes, however, when a novel contains numerous errors, the quality of the work as a whole suffers.

Two instances of grammatical errors cannot be attributed to the poor linguistic skills of the characters. It is Laura Malloy, supposedly a professional newspaperwoman, who states "the business and editorial office of the *Twin Cities Times* were on University Avenue, quite close to the dividing point between Minneapolis and St. Paul" (54). The principle of subject-verb agreement dictates that the sentence should either be "business and editorial offices ... were" or "office ... is on University Avenue." The other grammatical error is contained in a statement by the leading pro-life activist in the book, Tom Chasen: "One thing that is sacred to my wife and I is our time alone together" (67). We ain't got no ambiguity here. The sentence should read "sacred to my wife and me."

Is "analyzation" a word, as used in "Well, if I may do a little Malloy analyzation here, you don't give yourself a break" (136) or does Logue mean to say "analysis"?

An example of an historical error in the book is Saint Thomas Aquinas' statement, oft-repeated by anti-lifers, about when the soul enters the human body, which is mistakenly attributed to Saint Augustine: "But the quote that affected me the most ... was by St. Augustine from 1140: 'He is not a murderer who brings about abortion before the soul is in the body'" (185). Saint Augustine died in the year 430 A.D. Perhaps Malloy got confused; after all, anti-lifers are very confused people. "Augustine" sounds a lot like "Aquinas"—as much as "abortion" sounds like "reproductive choice."

Another historical inaccuracy occurs in Malloy's brief history of abortion (cited by Kuda in her review):

In 1812, the first abortion case in the United States was heard and the Supreme Court ruled that abortion was legal with the woman's consent if it was done before quickening, which is when the woman feels the fetus move within her, usually near the mid-point of gestation.... At this time abortion was often called "menstrual regulation." (185)

I will stand—and even sit—corrected on this if need be, but a search of legal databases using the terms "abortion" or "menstrual regulation" shows no such case decided by the United States Supreme Court in 1812.

Finally, the abortion-clinic has a variety of names. This can confuse the reader into thinking that there are several abortion-clinics involved in bombings. The abortorium is named the "Lakewood Family Planning Clinic" on page 1, "Family Planning Clinic" (capital letters) on page 206, and "family planning clinic" (lower case letters) elsewhere. Finally, on page 234 it is called "Lakeview Clinic." Which one is it?

Is dwelling on such minor points justifiable? Isn't this merely an *ad hominem* attack on an anti-life character, or, at the least, evidence that the author exercised her freedom of choice by choosing a poor printer? No. When the quality of an anti-life work suffers in so many areas, maybe this is evidence that the writer, having no respect for the unborn child, has subconsciously demonstrated her lack of respect for the born reader.

But wait, the book is so bad ... maybe Laura Malloy is, like her pet ferret Fabiola, a closet pro-lifer? Maybe this book is written so poorly from an anti-life perspective that people will see through the anti-life rhetoric and become pro-lifers?

The three novels which I have highlighted all have a dominant anti-life them. I will now consider how certain novels which present a pro-life viewpoint contrast with these anti-life novels. These are novels which are forcing cracks in the linguistic permafrost of anti-life writing. I will change my presentation order, starting with Lois Lowry's 1993 book *The Giver*[12] and then proceed to Carlos Fuentes' *Christopher Unborn*, which was published in 1989.

There are few recent novels which primarily present a pro-life theme on infanticide and euthanasia.[13] Lois Lowry's *The Giver* is one novel which incorporates infanticide and euthanasia themes and combines the two issues from a thematically pro-life perspective.

In writing *The Giver*, Lowry has written a testament for respect for human life and thus qualifies as a hallmark of pro-life fiction. It is a vision of the future, a utopia which is frighteningly possible.

By definition utopian literature has the capability not only of depicting a futuristic society, but also of commenting on contemporary society. Utopian literature may also serve to warn contemporary society of what frightening changes may occur in the future. Consider this book a masterpiece along with B.F. Skinner's *Walden II*—another American novel of a utopia gone wrong. *The Giver* presents us with the utopia of American society gone wrong, where quality of life becomes the overriding concern versus the fact that human life, in whatever imperfect state it exists, is worth protecting.

Set in a time when it will have been possible to eradicate emotions, Jonas, the twelve-year-old hero of the story, is selected by the "Community" in which he lives to be the "Receiver" of memories. A corresponding character, the "Giver," is an older man who imparts to the boy all his memories. These memories include life as it once existed before the Community adopted stringent controls; they also include memories of emotions, especially the most powerful emotion—love.

Pro-lifers immediately know to be alert to certain words. When a novelist mentions the word "release," pro-lifers think immediately that the book they are reading will concern itself with euthanasia.

In Lowry's dystopia, however, the one term "release" applies not only to the killing of defective newborns, but also to the elderly, who have only a set number of years to be alive in the Community.

One infanticide-scene in *The Giver* is especially graphic. In the following scene, Jonas' father, whose job in the Community is that of "Nurturer," decides to release a newborn baby, called a "newchild," who has not met the Community's standards regarding birth-weight. Jonas is watching this on videotape:

> [Jonas'] father began very carefully to direct the needle into the top of newchild's forehead, puncturing the place where the fragile skin pulsed. The newborn squirmed, and wailed faintly. His father was saying, "I know, I know. It hurts, little guy. But I have to use a vein, and the veins in your arms are still too teeny-weeny." He pushed the plunger very slowly, injecting the liquid into the scalp vein until the syringe was empty. *Now* he cleans him up and makes him comfy, Jonas said to himself.... The newchild, no longer crying, moved his arms and legs in a jerking motion. Then he went limp. He (*sic*) head fell to one side, his eyes half open. Then he was still. *He killed it! My father killed it!* Jonas said to himself, stunned at what he was realizing. (149-150)

No doubt, anti-lifers will want to ban the book from high school libraries. Cuyahoga County Public Library, which serves the metropolitan Cleveland area, rightfully catalogs this title as a work of juvenile fiction—rightfully, because it is appropriate that our young people should come to realize how close to practicing euthanasia our nation has come.

Where Lowry's *The Giver* is bold enough to tackle infanticide and euthanasia, Carlos Fuentes' *Christopher Unborn*[14] directly assaults the anti-life distortion of abortion. *Christopher Unborn* may not qualify for inclusion in this study since it is, first, not an "American" (that is, North American) work of fiction. If it is necessary to affix any label to it, then it is a Latin American work, a work of fiction by a Mexican author.[15] Fortunately for me, Fuentes' novel has been translated into English and has made a stunning impact on critics in the United States.[16]

Fuentes himself is enigmatic; his political positions can only be expressed in a series of complex sentences. Fuentes, who is called a leftist, supported the Sandinistas in Nicaragua, yet he thinks that Cuba needs more democracy. Although his novels are replete with the Roman Catholic fascinations of politics, sex, and religion, he has ridiculed what he has called the Catholic Church's "repression" of sex. Finally, although he states that he has found "stability" after being married and having children with his wife Sylvia, feminist critics think that Fuentes has a fear of women.[17]

Given these skeletal biographical facts, how could such a person write *Christopher Unborn*, which has such a profoundly dominant pro-life theme? While he may have been thinking immediately of the holocausts which are universally known, Fuentes once declared that "Everybody is capable of violence in the twentieth century" (*Crossing Borders*). Thus, pro-life academics and students can demonstrate successfully that even a so-called leftist author like Carlos Fuentes acknowledges that not even the womb is as safe as it once was.

The plot of the novel is ultimately simple. Christopher, an unborn child, recounts in vivid, omniscient-narrator mode the circumstances of his conception, his fertilization, and the nine months of his gestation in his mother's womb. Christopher realizes that he has been conceived mainly because his parents want to win the Christopher Contest, sponsored by the government of Mexico in celebration of the founding of the New World by Columbus. This is the ostensible reason for the child's existence.

Fuentes has done in fiction what *The Silent Scream*[18] does in video educational efforts: the unborn child is given a voice. It is difficult to ignore a narrator as he describes how half of him was shot out of his father during his fertilization.[19] It is difficult to ignore a narrator who engages in frequent fetological descriptions according to the stages of his gestation, such as "I, Christopher, was a cluster of well-organized cells, with defined functions, learning the classic lesson, innocent that I was, about the unity of my person" (220).

Later, Christopher enumerates a wide variety of activities which he calls "essential":

My hands, for example, have grown more rapidly than the arms they're attached to, they first appear with the fingers looking like buds; the last phalanx has emerged from the palms of my hands, my fingertips have formed, little tiny nails have appeared on all my fingers and toes, and the transparent and cartilaginous skeleton I had in my first four months is now bone and I move my arms and legs energetically; I have little accidents, I scratch my face with my nails unintentionally; I have pleasures: I suck my thumb incessantly; I make discoveries: I can touch my face. (408)

It is difficult to ignore a narrator who describes how his life seems threatened by other characters in the novel who may want him dead. It is difficult to ignore a narrator who depicts from the unique perspective of one who resides in what should be a safe womb how assaulted he felt when his mother was violently raped. Moreover, it is difficult not to personalize a narrator, an unborn child, who, in the reverse of apostrophe, directly addresses an absent character who becomes a character by virtue of his willing it so: the "Reader."[20]

Finally, with the exception of the other thematically pro-life work I have discussed (Lowry's *The Giver*), *Christopher Unborn* can give to the reader for his or her patient efforts to plow through 531 pages of sometimes incomprehensible word-play a satisfaction which is absent at the conclusion of the other thematically anti-life novels. It is like the joy of being at a birth. Does anybody not at least have a tear in his or her eye when a baby is born? Or, considering the polar opposite, does anybody cry for joy as the parts of an unborn child are dragged piecemeal from the mother's womb, sucked through the vacuum-aspiration tube? Can anyone imagine future fiction where characters proclaim with rapture, "Oh look, there's the left arm! Why, look at those pieces there! That's the head! That's the head of the fetus we're aborting!" Of course not. While abortion may be sanitized as an abstract right in anti-life fiction, the birth of an unborn child still engenders happiness.

In fact, what happens to Baby Ba is an added treat for the patient reader. More importantly, the epiphany of Baby Ba is truly a surprise. Do you want to know what happens to Baby Ba? Do you want to know who Baby Ba is?

I won't tell you. You'll have to read the book.

Listen. Listen carefully. Let us tell our students also to listen, to listen carefully, to the cracking of the ice, the fissures in the permafrost.

Let us tell our students to listen for the voices of unborn children and comatose persons in our literature. They are there, trapped beneath the massive weight of a decades-long linguistic permafrost.

Fortunately, the love we show the unborn and others who have been marginalized in American fiction may warm the surface of the frozen ground and may melt just enough of the ice so that these nightmare decades of living without our first civil right to life may soon come to a close.

NOTES

1. Thus, while numerous other novels may contain characters who have had abortions, they will not be considered here since these novels are usually only tangentially concerned with the first right-to-life issue.

2. Sue Robinson, *The Amendment: A Novel* (New York: Birch Lane Press, 1990).

3. Walter Kirn, *She Needed Me* (New York: Pocket Books, 1992).

4. Mary Logue, *Still Explosion* (Seattle: Seal Press, 1993).

5. J. Hillis Miller, *The Ethics of Reading: Kant deMan, Eliot, Trollope, James, and Benjamin* (New York: Columbia Univ. Press, 1987) 9.

6. It is significant that the main character in this Minnesota-locale novel is not named a strongly-masculine "Mitch Viking" or "Todd Icelander." The name "Weaver Walquist" is particularly descriptive since it combines several items from the popular culture. "Weaver" resonates with the associations "wimp" and one who is uncertain about where he or she is to go, someone who literally "weaves" from one position to another. "Walquist" similarly resonates with at least one association, "quisling." In Kirn's prose, Weaver can indeed be a traitor not only to his girlfriend but also to his purported pro-life views.

7. Richard Brautigan, *The Abortion: An Historical Romance 1966* (New York: Simon and Schuster, 1971).

8. Not many reviewers have the conciseness of Rex E. Klett, a reviewer for *Library Journal* [118 (April 1, 1993) 135]. Designed with the needs of the librarian working in a public library in mind, Klett's review can be condensed to an abstract of a simple sentence: "A workable prose, plot, and issue make this appropriate for larger collections."

At the other extreme, consider Marie Kuda's abstracted review in *Booklist* [39 (April 1, 1993) 1415]: "As (Laura Malloy, the main character in the novel) goes after both the bombing and the abortion story that led her to it, Logue develops both major sides of the abortion issue and includes a capsule history of abortion. Then, what appears to be a bloody fetus is left on the doorstep of Bobby's grieving girlfriend, and the pace accelerates to an explosive ending."

Then, there is the ridiculously-biased and intellectually dishonest abstracted review by Gillian Gill which appeared in the *Women's Review of Books* [10 (July 1993) 40]: "Malloy is a sympathetic and persuasive detective, cast in many ways in the mold of the old detective hero as eulogized by Raymond Chandler—a tall loner (Malloy is five-ten) who searches for social justice in the city streets.... From the first tragic explosion that destroys a beautiful young man, Logue holds our attention and gives us the kind of excitement we expect from detective-thrillers. The violence is never gratuitous, however, as Logue wants not merely to entertain but to make some statement about abortion.... The pro-choice politics are upfront, expressed even more forcefully by the plot line and the characterization than in the journalistic conclusions written up by the fictional detective."

9. Perhaps, too, it was a Loguesque person who tried to kill one of the nation's most effective lobbyists for the pro-life movement. Ms. Jan Folger, Legislative Director for the Ohio Right to Life Society, recently had her car bombed. Presumably perpetrated by anti-lifers, the car bombing is a compliment to Ms. Folger's effectiveness with Ohio's representatives, senators, and governor. Whether the anti-life person responsible for the bombing thought of the idea on his or her own or was inspired to it by reading Logue's novel is an intriguing question, but one which I cannot answer at this time.

10. Of course, the revision would be purely to allow students to understand the contrast between an anti-life character and a pro-life one; we would never use the revision-process to proselytize as anti-life feminist literary critics have done.

11. Readers interested in one of the more well-known cases of unborn children's bodies found in a dumpster may wish to read S. Rickly Christian's account in *The Woodland Hills Tragedy* (Westchester, Ill.: Crossway Books, 1985).

12. Lois Lowry, *The Giver* (Boston: Houghton Mifflin, 1993).

13. We who study literature are, of course, all engaged in an archaeological effort: digging beneath accretions of anti-life criticism to get at the intent of a work which is essentially life-affirming. Instances of pro-life literature abound; stories which are thematically pro-life are being "discovered" continuously. For example, a literature-discussion in one of my research-paper classes excavated a thematic function behind Graham Greene's short story "The Destructors." I must thank a student in the course, Rob Poelking, for first pointing out what should have been obvious: the story can be interpreted in pro-life terms to be a story of euthanasia. In Greene's story, a centuries-old house in London, a house which survived natural catastrophes as well as the human-made holocaust of World War II, is destroyed from within by a gang of British youths who seem to have nothing better to do than to destroy artifacts of their society. My student's insight, that the story could have euthanasia overtones, was, I think, strikingly brilliant. The centuries-old house could be compared to an elderly

person of today: both are unwanted by some in society who see no value in either. The societal solution to the problem of old folks (and old buildings) which go nowhere and do nothing and do not contribute to the cash flow of the society is obvious: get rid of them both.

14. Carlos Fuentes, *Cristobal Nonato* (Mexico: Fondo de Cultura Economica, 1987), translated by Alfred MacAdam and the author as *Christopher Unborn* (New York: Farrar-Straus-Giroux, 1989).

15. There is another reason to justify the inclusion of this novel in the study. Now that we are more aware than ever of the "inclusion" principle which is working to expand the canon, especially to include those works from non-Western writers, it is only appropriate that we acknowledge the importance of such a cosmopolitan author like Carlos Fuentes.

Another conference-participant informed me that a Czech novelist, Jiri Grusa, included in his novel *The Questionnaire: or, Prayer for a Town and a Friend* (New York: Farrar, Straus & Giroux, 1982) a passage written from the perspective of the unborn child also. In the light of Ms. Mercedes Wilson's remarks about the oppression of the Third World by the anti-life First World nations, it is interesting and noteworthy that Second and Third World writers like Grusa and Fuentes are writing for the First World novels which are thematically pro-life.

16. Some reviewers, however, seem to have missed the pro-life point of the novel completely, arguing that it is more concerned with criticizing the Reagan years in the United States than it is with criticizing certain U.S. social policies and the deleterious effects of those policies on a nation such as Mexico. One reviewer's abstract reaches the generic conclusion that "Five hundred years after the discovery and conquest of Latin America, the utopia has become dystopia.... Only caustic, corrosive humour, it seems... can release new energies from the dead hand of history and state power...." John King in *Times Literary Supplement* (Dec. 15, 1989) 1386.

Another reviewer's abstract reads more as prophecy than literature review: "(Fuentes) has given an unborn babe the power of speech in order to bring the "odious eighties" to account.... Until American novelists take it upon themselves to muckrake the Reagan years with equal vigor, Carlos Fuentes, with this book, must rank as our leading North American political satirist." Suzanne Ruta in *The New York Times Book Review* (Aug. 20, 1989) 1.

17. See *Crossing Borders: the Journey of Carlos Fuentes*, written by Stephen Talbot, readings by Carlos Fuentes, directed and edited by Joan Saffa, a videocassette produced by Novel Productions in association with KQED, Inc. (n.p.: Novel Productions, 1989).

18. Donald S. Smith, *The Silent Scream: the Complete Text of the Documentary Film with an Authoritative Response to the Critics* (Anaheim: American Portrait Film Books, 1985).

19. Another tangential thought about *Christopher Unborn*. If the theme of the novel does not attract attention, then the playful and sometimes raunchy sexual scenes should.

20. In several instances Christopher addresses the reader as though he or she is a judge, but of what judicial authority is uncertain. The questions can then be begged of Christopher: are you on trial? what for? why are you on trial and not your parents? what will happen to you if you are found guilty? The reader of the novel is addressed as "your honor" (178), "your worship the reader" (210), or "your worships" (249). Does the Reader have the power merely to stop reading the book or does the Reader, especially by doing so, have the power to end Christopher's life? In several instances, Christopher engages in word-play with the quasi-judicial Reader, begging "mercy" from the Readers as though they were judges.

PRO-LIFE DIRECT ACTION CAMPAIGNS: A SURVEY OF SCHOLARLY AND MEDIA INTERPRETATIONS

Keith Cassidy

THE PRO-LIFE MOVEMENT is arguably one of the greatest grass-roots movements in American history, with millions of supporters and a crucial role in politics from the early 1970s to the present. A small but important segment of the movement went beyond pro-life voting and letter writing to a more direct role: picketing, sidewalk counselling and in some cases sit-ins and blockades of abortion clinic entrances. These and other examples of "direct action" were aimed both at stopping abortions and at dramatizing the abortion issue. Whatever else they achieved, they certainly succeeded in the latter objective.

A history of the pro-life movement must incorporate an understanding of its "direct action" wing. What do we need to know? Obvious questions include the following:

1) Its range—that is, how do you define "direct action"? This would entail a careful and exhaustive list of the actions lumped under the heading. In general it can be said that "direct activism" differs from "activism" in general in that it operates at the site of the abortion—it seeks to deter or block the action.
2) Its evolution over time—when do various forms of action appear, are there shifts in patterns, numbers involved, etc.
3) Its membership—who took part? how did they differ from other pro-lifers on various attitudinal and demographic variables? how many took part?
4) The effects of direct action on participants.
5) The effects of direct action on the pro-life movement and on the public perception of the pro-life movement.
6) The effects of direct action on the incidence of abortion
7) The public perception of direct action
8) The ideologies of direct action—why did people take part? What

did they think they were accomplishing? How did they deal
with issues of respect for law?

9) What opposition to direct action existed within the movement,
from individuals and organizations?

10) Inevitably—the question of violence. How much? by whom?
for what purposes? to what effect? how related to the
larger movement? how treated by the media? how did it
impact on public opinion? Of course, the whole issue of
violence *against* pro-lifers needs to be examined as well.

11) Parallels with other direct action movements.

This is hardly an exhaustive list of questions and lines of inquiry,
but it is a start. What help in answering them is given by looking
at the existing literature, both scholarly and journalistic? It would
be reasonable to assume that given the prominence and salience of
the topic a large literature should exist on it.

In fact, the paucity of material, and its generally low quality, is
striking. Searches of such databases as Social Science Citation Index,
Dissertation Abstracts and Sociofile reveal thousands of items under
the heading of "abortion": while some deal with "activism," far
fewer examine direct activism. As will be clear after review, the
literature is not only limited in quantity, but also limited by the
methodologies of the authors and frequently informed by their
palpable biases.

A three-stage approach to the literature seems appropriate: to
review first the scholarly literature of the topic, then media treatment
of it, and finally the movement's own accounts of what it was doing.

To begin a review of the scholarly literature at the most general
level, there is a good deal of writing on movement "activism," that
is, any activity on behalf of the cause. One approach relies on
survey research to discover the ways in which activists in this
movement differ from the population as a whole and from their
opponents in the pro-choice movement. The most significant of
these studies was carried out some years ago by Donald Granberg
who published the results in a number of papers on the attitudinal
and demographic characteristics of activists.[1] A different approach is
taken in one of the most famous of all studies of the abortion
controversy, Kristin Luker's *Abortion and the Politics of Motherhood*,
which declared that the abortion debate was primarily about the role

and importance attached to motherhood. In Luker's view pro-life activists were more attached to traditional female roles and saw in their opposition to abortion the opportunity to defend those roles. This thesis has been very influential but is certainly open to criticism.[2] Luker relied on interviews with a number of activists in California rather than on the survey approach employed by Granberg. While illuminating, this literature tells us very little about *direct* activism.

Studies of those who could more properly be called "direct activists" include Michael Cuneo's 1989 book *Catholics Against The Church*, which remains the best work yet.[3] Based on extensive observation and interviews, he suggests that there is a three-fold split in the activists who picket: civil rights activists, family heritage activists and revivalistic Catholic activists. This book is extraordinarily informative, but it is about the Canadian movement, and as Cuneo notes, there are significant differences between Canada and the U.S. The mainstream of the Canadian pro-life movement proved more openly supportive of direct action than its counterpart in the United States in part, it may be suggested, because the Canadian movement is more politically marginal than the American, with no major political party endorsing its objectives.

Another study of direct activists, also from 1989, is Faye Ginsburg's *Contested Lives*, which accepts the Luker thesis that pro- and anti-abortionists were fundamentally divided by their attitudes to motherhood. Ginsburg's work is an intensive study of one location, Fargo, North Dakota, and has the strengths and weaknesses of such a focus.

These studies were done before the rise of Operation Rescue thrust the issue of direct action very dramatically into the center of the public arena. That organization provoked study, as did the issue of violence directed at abortion clinics. Several scholarly studies of these topics appeared in the 1990s.

One is "Saving America's Souls: Operation Rescue's Crusade Against Abortion," also written by Faye Ginsburg. The thesis of this study is signalled by the fact that it appears in Volume Three of a series of studies published by the "Fundamentalism Project." Placed among studies of Hezbollah and Sikh militants, it is not surprising that she concludes that "Operation Rescue is the latest incarnation of the fundamentalist impulse to impose its religious culture on others."[4]   Unlike her study of North Dakota, Ginsburg did no field research for this essay and focused on two leaders, Joe Scheidler and Randall Terry.   She traces the rise of pro-life direct action to frustration felt by pro-lifers by the mid 1980s with the political and legal process.

Her discussion of the meaning direct action is interesting: "By the mid 1980s, groups that advocated direct action bordering on violence and terror—harassing patients, holding sit-ins, intimidating abortion providers—emerged with new confidence."[5] That a sit-in "borders" on violence and terror may surprise those who see it as a classic technique of peaceful civil disobedience.   She acknowledges the existence of an earlier tradition of pro-life civil disobedience—that begun by John Cavanaugh O'Keefe—but focuses on Terry.   She does discuss the tensions within the pro-life ranks over direct action. While the focus on fundamentalism as an explanatory theme is understandable in the case of Randall Terry, it is too limiting as a key to the ideology of the whole movement.

In a very similar vein is the work by Dallas Blanchard and Terry Prewitt: *Religious Violence and Abortion: The Gideon Project*. Focusing on clinic bombings in Pensacola, Florida in 1984, the authors trace the trials of the accused and then move to the larger of violence across the nation against abortion facilities.   They do not examine "direct action" as such, but focus instead on violence and like Ginsburg see it in the context of fundamentalism.

Their conscious linkage of direct action, and indeed of all anti-abortion activity, to violence is apparent in a chart in their book illustrating the "Levels of Involvement in the Anti-Abortion Movement"[6] which goes from an outer circle of "public opinion" through "education," "lobbying," "picketing," "mild violence," "moderate violence," to "radical violence."   The assumption is, of course, that anti-abortion activity reaches its logical culmination in extreme violence.   Since it could more reasonably be assumed that the highest level of involvement might be a total rejection of all violence (the "seamless garment" approach), it is hard to see how the authors reached their conclusion.   While they concede that the bombers are marginal to the movement, they nonetheless try to tie them to it.[7]

Similar themes appear in Blanchard's 1994 book, *The Anti-Abortion Movement and the Rise of the Religious Right: From Polite to Fiery*

Protest.[8] After such a title a review of the book's thesis may appear superfluous. Although the book is marred by numerous and serious errors, the author has been frequently interviewed as an expert. While conceding that people enter the movement for a variety of motives he asserts that "At this point in the history of the anti-abortion movement, the dominant motivation, particularly in the more activist organizations such as Operation Rescue, appears to be cultural fundamentalism. Closely informing cultural fundamentalism are the tenets of religious fundamentalism, usually associated with certain Protestant denominations but also evident in the Catholic and Mormon faiths."[9]

One study which does provide some insight into pro-life direct action is Carol Maxwell's "Where's the Land of Happy: Individual Meaning and Collective Antiabortion Activism" in Jelen and Chandlers's 1994 book, *Abortion Politics in the United States and Canada.*[10] This study arose from the research for her 1994 Ph.D. thesis, "Meaning and Motivation in Pro-Life Direct Action" and is one of a number of other papers derived from it.[11] While focusing on sit-in participants alone, she still adds to our knowledge by exploring a critical issue: why do some people become activists while others do not? Why are some active at certain times in their lives, but not others?

According to Maxwell the individual personal meanings of abortion change over time and so also do levels of involvement:

I argue that while prolife rhetoric expounded a perspective rescuers shared, it was not necessarily relevant to the factors actually impelling their activism.... The decision to rescue depended upon particular issues intimately entwined with the self identity and previously established ethics of individual listeners. However, both would be recruits' and practising activists' self-identities and ethics were influenced by factors that varied over time. Through the narratives of three direct activists, I will explore shifts in the balance of influence accorded by activists to their own emotional needs, ideology, and the practical constraints on their activism. The interplay of these factors created distinct understandings and motivations that frustrated the efforts of rescue organizers, whose rhetoric addressed the common concerns of an audience the organizers apparently conceived of as a collective.[12]

As she puts it later, "While rhetoric played a key role in many individuals' decisions to rescue, it did so as part of a complex process that was contingent on many aspects of the individuals' life circumstances and self-identities."[13]

Another study from the Jelen and Chandler book is by James Guth *et al.*, "Cut From the Whole Cloth: Antiabortion Mobilization among Religious Activists."[14] This study attempts to find out why some pro-lifers are attracted to Operation Rescue and others to non-direct action groups. It is based on a survey of nearly 5000 members of eight different groups, from across the ideological spectrum. Respondents were asked how close they felt to the National Right to Life Committee and to Operation Rescue. There were four groupings: those who opposed both, were neutral on both, supported only the NRLC or supported both. The conclusions are too complex for rapid summary, but one does stand out:

The findings are quite straightforward: one discriminant function accounts for the overwhelming amount of variance (91 percent), with a canonical correlation of .76, signifying excellent discriminating power. This function consists primarily of the moral traditionalism, religious fundamentalism, Christian militancy, and political conservatism variables...As the discriminant function shows, this is almost linear....The second function might be labelled activism, with strong correlations for disruptive politics, political interest, approval of conservative pulpit politics, and campaign involvement.[15]

There are some other studies of pro-life activism. One attempts to measure the effect of Operation Rescue's work in Buffalo, N.Y., on public support, and concludes that it caused a drop in support.[16] Another attempts to measure the relationship between religion and support for direct activism.[17] Yet another argues that pro-life activism is not really comparable to the non-violent protest of the civil rights movement.[18] While some of these works are useful and suggestive, the scholarly literature on direct action pro-lifers is generally weak and limited. With the exception of Cuneo's fine study it does not answer a number of the questions posed above. Moreover it often uses a single interpretive line: generally "fundamentalism" or else "motherhood." Hidden in the interpretive line is the usually not very subtle suggestion that what is being studied is a deviant and marginal phenomenon, with pathological characteristics. It often focuses obsessively on the subject of violence, most notably in

Blanchard's work and does not explore the real links to the civil rights movement. Another weakness is the use of either intensive interviews with a limited number of activists or else reliance on mass-media accounts. Nothing approaching an overview history of the topic, involving the use of a braod range of primary sources has been attempted.

What is particularly striking is the limited research: the same articles from *Time* and a few others are endlessly recycled. Blanchard did do research, but only on the most violent examples of direct action.

While relatively little scholarly work has been done on the topic, there is a large volume of journalistic writing on it. The activities of Operation Rescue were of course of huge interest, but even before some notice had been taken of sit-ins, but even more of Joe Scheidler's tactics and of clinic bombings.

A frequent theme is the use of the word "zealot" in connection with pro-life activists.[19] The word "crusade" was also widely used.[20] This religious imagery reinforces the image: these are not civil rights protestors, these are religious fanatics. Thus *Newsweek* spoke of "true believers" at the annual January 22 march in Washington.[21] Sometimes the parallels to the civil rights movement are allowed but are often discounted.[22] Book length studies have appeared as well, such as Marian Faux's *Crusaders: Voices From the Abortion Front*, which paints a very unflattering picture of Randall Terry.[23] The same pro-choice perspective is found in Sue Hertz's *Caught in the Crossfire: a Year on Abortion's Front Line*.[24]

Overlooked as a resource are the books by pro-life direct actionists themselves, such as the very important work by Joan Andrews, *I Will Never Forget You: The Rescue Movement in the Life of Joan Andrews* (which Blanchard does not include in his bibliography).[25] Also of interest is her earlier book, *You Reject Them, You Reject Me: The Prison Letters of Joan Andrews*.[26] Even Joe Scheidler's *Closed: 99 Ways to Stop Abortion*, while mentioned is not examined by Blanchard.[27]

Books by Randall Terry are also crucial to an understanding of the movement: his 1988 *Operation Rescue* and *Accessory To Murder* published two years later are essential reading.[28] Also of interest is his 1993 work, *Why Does A Nice Guy Like Me Keep Getting Thrown in Jail?*[29] In addition, a large literature sprang up discussing and defending pro-life direct action.   Titles include Paul Lindstrom's *4 Days in May: Storming the Gates of Hell*,[30] Philip Lawler's *Operation Rescue: A Challenge to the Nation's Conscience*,[31] Paul deParrie's *The Rescuers*[32] and Mark Belz's *Suffer the Little Children: Christians, Abortion and Civil Disobedience*.[33]

A true account of pro-life direct activism needs to be written, one which will set it in the frame of a long tradition of such activism rather than in one which treats it as aberrant.   Certainly the sources are there, in the activists themselves, their opponents and in the large written record.   When it written it will form another chapter in the history of American democracy.

NOTES

1. See for example Donald Granberg "The Abortion Activists" in   *Family Planning Perspectives* 3/4 (July/Aug 1981) 162; Donald Granberg, "Pro-Life or Reflection of Conservative Ideology? An Analysis of Opposition To Legalized Abortion" in *Sociology and Social Research: An International Journal* 62/3 (April 1978) 414-29; Donald Granberg and Donald Denney, "The Coathanger and the Rose" in *Society* (May/June 1982) 40. Also representative of this approach is Jacqueline Scott and Howard Schuman, "Attitude Strength and Social Action in the Abortion Dispute" in *American Sociological Review* 53/5 (1988) 785-93; J. C. Soper, "Political Structures and Interest Group Activism - A Comparison of the British and American Prolife Movements" in *Social Science Journal* 31/3 (1994) 319-34.

2. Kristin Luker, *Abortion and the Politics of Motherhood* (Berkeley: Univ. of California Press, 1984). For a critique see Michael Cuneo, *Catholics Against the Church: Anti-Abortion Protest in Toronto, 1969-1985* (Toronto: Univ. of Toronto Press, 1989) 82.

3. See n. 2 above.

4. Faye Ginsburg, "Saving America's Souls: Operation Rescue's Crusade Against Abortion" in Martin E. Marty and R. Scott Appleby, eds., *Fundamentalisms and the State: Remaking Polities, Economies and Militance* (Chicago: Univ. of Chicago Press, 1993) 557-88 at 579.

5. Ginsburg, "Saving America's Souls" 563.

6. Dallas Blanchard and Terry J. Prewitt, *Religious Violence and Abortion: The Gideon Project* (Gainesville: Univ. Press of Florida, 1993) 255. Other works on violence and abortion clinics include the following: David C. Nice, "Abortion Clinic Bombings as Political Violence" in *American Journal of Political Science* 32 (February 1988) 178-95 and Michele Wilson and John Lynxwiler, "Abortion Clinic Violence as Terrorism" in *Terrorism* 11/4 (1988)

263-273.

7. Blanchard and Prewitt, *Religious Violence* 215, 257.

8. Dallas Blanchard, *The Anti-Abortion Movement and the Rise of the Religious Right: From Polite to Fiery Protest* (New York: Twayne Publishers, 1994).

9. Blanchard, *Anti-Abortion Movement* 41.

10. Ted G. Jelen and Marthe A. Chandler, *Abortion Politics in the United States and Canada: Studies in Public Opinion* (Westport: Praeger, 1994) 89-106.

11. Carol J. C. Maxwell: "Meaning and Motivation in Pro-Life Direct Action," Ph.D. thesis, Washington University, 1994; "Coping With Bereavement Through Activism - Real Grief, Imagined Death, and Pseudo-Mourning Among Prolife Direct Activists" in *Ethos* 23/4 (1995) 437-52; "Commandos for Christ: Narratives of Male Pro-Life Activists" in *Review of Religious Research* 37/2 (Dec. 1995) 117-31; "Abortion, Salvation and Direct Activism" in *Social Justice Research* 7/4 (1994) 401-13.

12. Maxwell, "Where's the Land of Happy?" 90.

13. Maxwell, "Where's the Land of Happy" 106.

14. James L. Guth, Lyman A. Kellstedt, Corwin E. Smidt, and John C. Green, "Cut From the Whole Cloth: Antiabortion Mobilization among Religious Activists" in Jelen and Chandler, *Abortion Politics* 107-29.

15. Guth, *et al.* 26.

16. Catherine G. Ansuini, Julianna Fiddler-Woite and Robert S. Woitaszek, "The Effects of Operation Rescue on Pro-Life Support" in *College Student Journal* 28/4 (Dec. 1994) 441-45. While Operation Rescue's activities led to increased support at the time, their survey of over three hundred Buffalo residents found that it led to a long term decline in support.

17. Paul Raymond and Barbara Norrander, "Religion and Attitudes toward Anti-Abortion Protest" in *Review of Religious Research* 32/2 (Dec. 1990) 151-56.

18. Jay R. Howard, "A Comparative Analysis of the Civil Disobedience of Operation Rescue and Martin Luther King's Civil Rights Organization" in *Free Inquiry in Creative Sociology* 21/2 (Nov. 1993) 177-87.

19. *Newsweek* (Aug. 19, 1991) 18; *Time* (Feb. 12, 1990) 29, (July 19, 1993) 29.

20. *Newsweek* (Mar. 3, 1975) 22.

21. *Newsweek* (Feb. 4, 1985) 22.

22. *Newsweek* (Sept. 12, 1988) 25.

23. Marian Faux, *Crusaders: Voices From the Abortion Front* (New York:

Birch Lane Press, 1990).

24. Sue Hertz, *Caught in the Crossfire: A Year on Abortion's Front Line* (New York: Prentice Hall, 1991).

25. Joan Andrews, with John Cavanaugh O'Keefe, *I Will Never Forget You: The Rescue Movement in the Life of Joan Andrews* (San Francisco: Ignatius Press, 1989).

26. Richard Cowden Guido, ed., *You Reject Them, You Reject Me: The Prison Letters of Joan Andrews* (Manassasa: Trinity Communications, 1988).

27. Joseph M. Scheidler, *Closed: 99 Ways to Stop Abortion* (Toronto: Life Cycle Books, 1985).

28. Randall Terry, *Operation Rescue* (Springdale: Whitaker House, 1988); *Accessory To Murder: The Enemies, Allies, and Accomplices To The Culture of Death* (Brentwood: Wolgemuth and Hyatt, 1990).

29. Randall Terry, *Why Does A Nice Guy Lie Me Keep Getting Thrown in Jail?* (Lafayette: Huntington House Press, 1993).

30. Paul D. Lindstrom, *4 Days in May: Storming the Gates of Hell* (Arlington Heights: Christian Liberty Press, 1988).

31. Philip F. Lawler, *Operation Rescue: A Challenge to the Nation's Conscience* (Huntington: Our Sunday Visitor, 1992).

32. Paul deParrie, *The Rescuers* (Brentwood: Wolgemuth and Hyatt, 1989).

33. Mark Belz, *Suffer The Little Children: Christians, Abortion and Civil Disobedience* (Westchester: Crossway Books, 1989).

THE POLITICS OF A CULTURE OF LIFE

Kevin E. Miller

BY VIRTUE OF THE MANNER in which Pope John Paul II's 1995 encyclical letter *Evangelium Vitae* ("The Gospel of Life") provides an account and defense of "the value and inviolability of human life," it could be said to constitute the second volume of a two-volume work. The first volume of this work was *Veritatis Splendor* ("The Splendor of Truth," 1993). In that encyclical John Paul clarified, against certain tendencies in moral philosophy and theology today, that there exist exceptionless moral norms and that these express the meaning of the human person as this meaning can be discerned both from nature and, more fully, from the Gospel. *Evangelium Vitae* takes up this theme explicitly and develops it with respect to a set of concrete issues whose great importance owes both to their gravity and to their contemporary relevance, namely, those issues revolving around human life.[1]

A brief account of the argument is as follows: Human persons are created by God; they are destined for the fullness of communion with God; God's gracious granting to us of that communion is an act of mercy that cost the life of the Son of God in the flesh, because of human sin. This establishes the value of human life. In view of this value, directly to take an innocent human life is contrary to justice. Justice, furthermore, is but the beginning of love, and the dignity that is ours by God's grace makes us worthy of a love that transcends the minimal requirements of justice. These principles underlie unconditional opposition to such actions as abortion and euthanasia.

But the issues that John Paul addresses have a political dimension. The raging controversies concerning these issues are in part controversies about how they should be addressed legislatively, that is, by the political community as such. John Paul does not prescind from this dimension, since he calls for legal protection of all human life, especially the lives of those most vulnerable today, the unborn and the sick and elderly.[2] He even addresses a "life issue" that is by definition a political or legal issue, namely, that of capital punishment. Abortion and euthanasia are generally done by individuals, so that the political question concerning these issues (chiefly, when and whether the civil law should regulate individuals' choices) is not identical with the moral question (the rectitude of those choices). Capital punishment, by contrast, is an act of the political community. The moral question concerning capital punishment is therefore a question about the role of that community.

Fully to understand "the Gospel of life," then, requires that we grasp the vision of politics that John Paul wishes to communicate. His call for political protection of the vulnerable reflects not only the gravity of life issues but also a choice of one of several possible, competing accounts of the meaning or purpose of politics. In fact, not all such accounts are compatible with "the Gospel of life." This expression means not only "the Good News *concerning* life" but also "the Good News *represented by* life" in view of its value or dignity. Not all accounts of politics rejoice in life as "Good News."

It is my intention in this paper to clarify this connection by examining the basis in justice and love of the "culture of life" of which John Paul speaks and the political implications of such a culture. The true dignity of human life is recognized only when fundamental "rights" such as the "right to life" are seen as matters of an order of justice (and love) constituting a genuinely common good, so that it is essentially good for me to respect your life (and vice-versa). Such a recognition is necessary for life to be secure. If my respect for your life issues from a mere compromise designed to secure the individualistic good of my life at the price of my own dignity, your right to life will be ungrounded in principle and your life insecure.

A political community will therefore secure the right to life only if it is constituted with the end or goal of a common good of justice, of which absolute "rights" are an essential part.[3] A political community founded upon the principles of classical liberalism presupposes subjectivistic, individualistic rights-claims and a natural war of all against all over these claims, and makes justice an artifact of a merely contractarian politics that promotes peace for the sake of individuals' desires. Such a political community will not secure the right to life, because it will be opposed in principle to respect for life.

THE FAILURE OF CLASSICAL LIBERALISM

Politics based upon a common good identical with a real order of morality or justice does not take on every moral issue, prescribing every virtue and proscribing every vice. No one moral issue wholly encompasses the common good of the political community. Some matters, like life-issues, are so fundamental that no competing good takes precedence over legislation designed to bring about justice in their regard (*Evangelium Vitae* #71). In other cases, concern for such values as respect for the law or the integrity of a certain sphere of privacy for oneself or one's family, values that are also dimensions of the common good, may make "legislating morality" imprudent. This is most often the case when the "morality" at issue is that of actions that have little or no direct effect upon others without their consent.[4] However, it must be emphasized that the judgments needed in such cases are prudential and that prudence sometimes might require legislation touching consensual matters. Even actions in this category, and the absence of laws proscribing such actions when the actions are immoral, can easily affect the ethos of the community and therefore the common good.

The classical liberal understanding of politics, originated by Thomas Hobbes, stands in contrast. Classical liberalism founds politics only upon each citizen's subjective desire not to be injured or restrained, and upon his or her consent to a contract to minimize injury and restraint.[5] That is, its foundational concern is to maximize each citizen's sphere of autonomy. It therefore provides little or no basis for legislation proscribing "consensual" actions, no matter how immoral we might judge them to be. Classical liberals maintain as a matter of principle that the law may intervene only when an action would affect another without his or her consent.

Classical liberalism is attractive because it seems at first glance an excellent foundation for protection of human rights, including the right to life of the vulnerable, from violations by either individuals or a tyrannical state. In fact, a significant portion of the energy of the right-to-life movement has been expended upon elaborating precisely a classical liberal justification for laws against such actions as abortion.[6] Laws protecting the lives of the unborn are not, it is said in response to the objections of "pro-choice" opponents, mere instances of "legislating morality," for the unborn child is another human being, a person or at least destined for personhood. It is essential to the social contract (this classical expression may or may not be used, but it probably corresponds to the concept frequently in mind) whereby all of our lives are protected that we not begin to exclude classes of human beings from the protection of the law. Otherwise we run the risk of sliding down a "slippery slope," endangering our own lives as well.

The first thing that should be said about this classical liberal appeal to enlightened self-interest is that it has not worked. To speak only of abortion: A majority of Americans are not persuaded that the law should protect the lives of the unborn. A significant minority would allow few or no restrictions upon the practice of abortion. Many more would allow some restrictions, even significant ones, but they continue to deny, however uneasily, the proposition that it would ultimately be best to protect unborn life without compromise. And 23 years after *Roe v. Wade*, there have been few successful efforts to enact even such "moderate" restrictions upon abortion as the Supreme Court seems willing to deem constitutional.

A likely part of the problem is that people do not in fact see their own lives as imperiled. Compromise is necessary only if I am not strong enough to get what I want without the cost that compromise imposes. Conceivably, most Americans imagine they have the political strength to ensure that the social contract will continue to protect their lives for as long as they wish. And for the most part, for the foreseeable future, these people may be correct. Another possibly significant factor is that many people's conception of the good or worthy life includes such autonomy as would outweigh some attendant risk to themselves.

THE CULTURE OF DEATH

In view of these reflections upon our situation, I turn to some reflections upon *Evangelium Vitae* in the form of exegesis and commentary, in order to clarify why classical liberalism has not secured the right to life, and then to illumine the alternative. John Paul begins his encyclical by offering a diagnosis of our situation. He wishes to take up especially the problem of attacks against life "in its earliest and in its final stages" (#11). To understand the context of these attacks, John Paul says, we must consider a "reality, which can be described as a veritable *structure of sin*" (#12). Now, the pope is no more a cultural determinist than an economic determinist.

Significantly, he believes that nothing can wholly suppress our consciences (#24). But the way we see reality is conditioned, if not determined, by such lenses as that of our culture, and this will have implications when we make choices. And to the extent that our culture teaches us to see reality in a distorted way—to the extent, that is, that it leads us away from the truth—and to the extent that it thereby teaches us to sin in action, so that we are alienated, intellect and will, from God and from the reality of creation: to that extent, it is meaningful to speak of a "structure of sin."[7]

To explain the nature of this structure of sin, John Paul indicates that our culture denies solidarity and adds that it is excessively concerned with efficiency (#12). It is necessary to explicate the relationship between these characteristics. Denial of solidarity is denial that our flourishing is caught up with that of others by the nature of things, not only by the requirements of a compromise. Theologically, denial of solidarity goes so far as to deny the bond of love established among all human beings by the salvific actions of Christ, the universal Redeemer.[8]

But another way of expressing this is to say that denying solidarity is equivalent to affirming that other persons are at most means to our self-gratification. It may be that what gives me pleasure will give you pleasure, or it may not. If not, I, to the extent that I deny solidarity, will satisfy myself at your expense as much as I am able. Only solidarity, the disposition wherein I affirm that I cannot make myself happy by using you, will overcome such selfishness. The reason that solidarity, so conceived, is opposed to excessive concern with "efficiency" is that efficiency looks only to "getting things done" (cf. #22-23). When my attitude toward others reflects only or primarily such a concern, I will take no account of their good, their flourishing or happiness. When what I want to "get done" is at odds with what they want to "get done," we will be set against one another—precisely the opposite of solidarity.

Remarkably, John Paul describes the culture that arises from these attitudes as "a veritable 'culture of death,'" in which there is "a kind of *conspiracy against life*" (#12). Once it is accepted that I may use others as much as I can, there is no reason in principle why that "use" should regard even the bare lives of others. Hobbes saw this and concluded that "every man has a right to every thing; even to one another's body."[9] I may well have no desire to kill other human beings. I may be so emotionally attached to some others that their deaths would cause me great unhappiness. But if my primary concern is what I want and how to get it, the solicitude that issues from my attachments will be characterized by all the instability that marks the wholly subjective. Any coincidence of the good of others, whether the good of their lives or lesser goods, with my own subjectively-conceived good will be merely accidental and contingent.

Furthermore, we know that many people at least sometimes feel themselves greatly burdened by the presence, condition, or actions of certain others. When those feeling burdened are powerful and the others are vulnerable, the denial of solidarity and excessive concern with efficiency that give rise to the culture of death are therefore likely in fact to endanger some people. It might be objected that a rational view, looking to the long term, would cause me to restrain myself when I have the desire and the opportunity to use others even to the point of killing them. But apart from the likelihood that the emotions of the moment will sometimes overwhelm such considerations, there is the further problem that the decisions about what I will be allowed to get away with will frequently be made at the societal level. Whereas I as an individual might want to take into account the possible repercussions of my own lack of concern for the vulnerable when I am, perhaps, rendered vulnerable by age or sickness or other factors, it is harder to make the case that a relatively powerful group will need to worry about the long term, even if its members, who come and go, will. And it is groups—factions—whose interests tend to dominate on the level of society. What will result, John Paul says, is "a *war of the powerful against the weak*" (#12).

In any case, the notion of freedom that denies solidarity and exalts efficiency will be that of a "freedom of 'the strong'" (#19). Hence, "social life" in the culture of death "ventures on to the shifting sands of complete relativism. At that point, *everything is negotiable, everything is open to bargaining:* even... the right to life" (#20). For as freedom requires strength, "rights" too become either what the strong desire, or what the not-entirely-strong can get in return for something else.[10] The more vulnerable, the weaker, a group is, the more ineffective will be its negotiating position. So society recognizes the "right to choose" an abortion but not the "right to life" of unborn babies (cf. #18).

POWER POLITICS

To construct anything resembling a society, some negotiation will be necessary. Now, reference to "negotiation" brings us back to the level of politics, for it is in the political sphere that negotiations concerning rights take place. But insofar as politics expresses and serves culture, an attempt to solve politically the question of what rights-claims are to be respected or overridden will never rise above the level of raw power in a "culture of death." And classical liberal politics is inextricably linked with the culture of death.

The social contract, and the classical liberal politics of negotiation that write, sign, and enforce it, presuppose that there is in principle a genuine conflict of interest or of "rights" among human beings. The social contract is necessary only if I see your good as at odds with mine. If I see my serving your good as my own good as well, I will not ask you to give anything up in return for my serving it; and vice-versa. But if our goods are incompatible, a "war of the powerful against the weak" over rights-claims will arise. And because no one is all-*powerful*, this war will be inconclusive. A protracted state of war will make life "solitary, poor, nasty, brutish, and short."[11]

The social contract presupposes such a natural state of war. It presupposes that we are naturally each other's enemies, not partners or friends. "Naturally" here means "born or made to be." That is, what is at issue is the relationship of politics and law to human flourishing, to our noble aspirations. For the classical liberal, such aspirations lead to war. The pacifying function of politics is at odds with those aspirations.

Even as classical liberal politics imposes peace, it does not seek to reconcile enemies. Therefore it only institutionalizes the culture of death that manifests the conflict that arises when I see you and your rights as, at best, instrumentally good for me. Insofar as the culture of death is institutionalized, furthermore, it is reinforced. The very practice of a politics that sets as its goal mediating between conflicting rights-claims further encourages one to see such claims, such conflict, as reflecting the structure of reality in principle or by nature. Such politics itself teaches its practitioners to see the other as enemy by nature.

There is then, as if the result of a self-fulfilling prophecy, nothing to the political task but en-*force*-ment. This has particular consequences for the politics of a democracy. We are given to associate democracy with consent rather than with force. In fact, of course, the "majority" consents and then forces the "minority" to do its will. This becomes especially problematic when the majority's consent to legislation is based upon the maximization of its power—when it considers itself free to enforce anything it can get away with and to reject any imposition on itself except as a necessary exchange for something more desirable. That is, democracy becomes problematic when it becomes merely a relatively peaceful channel for the conflict that is really still the war of the powerful against the weak.

It is clear that this is to a great extent what has become of democracy.[12] Politics in general, and democracy in particular, conceived as I have explained cannot even deliver on their promise of peace, let alone bring about justice. The relativism of radical autonomy does not, as John Paul notes, guarantee tolerance; crimes have been committed in its name (#70). Strangely, in fact, liberalism permits totalitarian legislation, because all actions of others colorably affect me without my consent.[13] At the very best, a compromise that is founded upon a principled denial of any common ground other than the desire for enforced peace as a necessary evil will be as unstable as the subjective conviction that such peace is better than principled war, however hellish, against one's natural enemies.

But even to the extent that the search for compromise is sincere, it probably remains incompatible with a successful appeal for legal protection of vulnerable lives, for example, protection of the unborn through restriction of abortion. Once it is accepted in principle—as the liberal politics of negotiated compromise cannot but admit as its foundation—that the other, including the unborn, is an enemy, the logical response to the most conclusive of arguments that the unborn baby is an-*other* person becomes (to paraphrase Stalin), "How many divisions does the unborn baby have?" And so on, *mutatis mutandis*, with respect to all who are vulnerable. Accordingly, we should not be surprised that attempts to argue the pro-life position in the political sphere from the social contract have not been successful. This reflects no inconsistency on the part of our society. It is wholly consistent with the common origin of the social contract and the culture of death. It reflects the very calculation that leads to the social contract.[14]

As a final consideration, someone might propose that our

Declaration of Independence offers a foundation for "rights" that is stronger than that of pure social contract theory. We are endowed by our Creator with rights, first among these the right to life. It is the purpose of politics to secure these rights. Democratic consent is a means whereby the success of politics in this mission can be judged. This understanding of rights and of politics even seems consistent with John Paul's concern for the recognition of certain rights as objective and fundamental (#71). And it is indeed a good beginning.

However, if subjectivistic individualism is to be overcome, this endowment of rights must be seen as something more than what might be called "divine positivism." Otherwise all we have done is shifted the motivation for my respect for your rights from your power to God's. You remain for me but an instrumental good, albeit now to the end of my salvation and not just to the maximization of my earthly life and happiness. This is a more powerful motive—but the question remains open whether a motive *qua* "powerful" can ever really be satisfying, can ever really avail. At some point I may decide that it is "better to reign in hell than to serve in heaven," that divine positivism is an ignoble foundation for justice. God may have more divisions than an unborn baby, but as long as I am used to seeing Him and the baby as my enemies, as obstacles to the happiness of autonomy, I may well continue to fight them in a tragic war.[15]

THE BEAUTY OF LIFE

Evangelium Vitae suggests a way of explaining how my doing what is good for you is good for me; that is, it proposes a vision of justice (and, in view of the Gospel, love) as our common good. A new account of politics will follow from this explanation. John Paul stands in continuity with an ancient tradition that what is "in it for me" when I render justice to others is *beauty*. Human life's value is manifest in beauty; and as beautiful, life invites us to act toward it in a manner commensurate with its beauty (#83). But so to act gives me a share in the beauty of the object of my action. Because beauty is a transcendental quality, it can genuinely be common to you and me. Unlike our sharing of an apple, wherein any part that is yours cannot be mine as well and vice-versa, in our simultaneous sharing in beauty my share does not diminish yours.[16]

In its full and classical sense, "beauty" encompasses the discernible perfection wherein a thing is exactly as it should be. It expresses a comprehensive fittingness. This implies, of course, reference to the kind of being that a thing is. The beautiful will not include the same features for a river as for a tulip, for a tulip as for a dog, for a dog as for a human person. For a human person, the beautiful encompasses dispositions or habits, loves, as well as actions. That is, it includes those mysterious qualities that we attribute to the soul.

As Aristotle explains, human excellence or virtue is made fully real and perfect by beauty—it is attaining beauty that makes virtue, virtue.[17] The disposition to the good that is moral or ethical virtue makes possible, and is in turn expressed in action by, the practical intellectual virtue of prudence, or excellence in deliberation, which being given its right bearings by ethical virtue chooses actions that are beautiful as well as efficient.[18] Thus, when I do what is right (just or loving), what is to the good of other persons (or even things, over which I have dominion, but which, John Paul says [#42], I may not "'use and misuse'"), this is to my good as well because it gives me a share in beauty. And the loss of human beauty that results from evil actions is greater than even the loss of this life. John Paul can therefore affirm that wrongs against persons "do more harm to those who practice them than to those who suffer the injury" (#3, quoting *Gaudium et Spes* #27; cf. also #48).[19]

This implies that being, and dispositions and actions respecting being, have meaning, meaning not given by me. It implies, that is, that there is a real and gratuitous "fittingness" about certain ways of seeing and treating other persons (or things). It implies that our attitude toward reality must be one of reception, prior to any possible manipulation.[20] It implies that we will learn from the meaning of personhood how we ought to treat persons. Some actions (for example, the direct killing of an innocent person) will always be incompatible with the beautiful—they are un-integrable into beautiful life. This establishes the minimal requirements for justice.[21]

John Paul's explanation of the "culture of life" for which he calls includes significant reference to these principles. The members of such a culture are precisely "those who see life in its deeper meaning, who grasp its utter gratuitousness, its beauty and its invitation to freedom and responsibility... who do not presume to take possession of reality but instead accept it as a gift...." In view of such an outlook, and in response to the "invitation" of which it takes note, it will be possible "to *revere and honor every person*" (#83).[22]

It might be asked how we can know that we have this capacity. For Aristotle, any capacity or potentiality of soul is known from its activity. That is, we observe that we recognize beauty, and we conclude that the soul has the capacity so to do. No *a priori* epistemological justification for this or any other kind of knowledge is necessary. Aristotle therefore says that "activities and actions are prior to potentialities according to reason," even though potentialities are existentially prior.[23] Hence, claims concerning the beautiful can be made and judged only by those who have experienced beauty.

John Paul calls the outlook of which he speaks *"a contemplative outlook."* By contemplation, we dispose ourselves to receive and accept rather than to manipulate. We allow the world to affect us rather than insisting, or before we insist, upon changing the world. Another way to describe this is to say that we "celebrate." In fact, John Paul says that to develop a culture of life, it is necessary that the Gospel of life be proclaimed, celebrated, and served; and he places the above remarks at the start of his explanation of "celebrating the Gospel of life."

To celebrate something is precisely to allow oneself to be affected by its beauty. So far has our culture departed from "a contemplative outlook" that we are perhaps not immediately inclined to this understanding of celebration. Even celebration becomes an act of creation on our part, rather than our response to creation that presents itself to us gratuitously. Thus we become almost obsessed with self-expression through novel forms of "celebration," even that celebration of the life of the Reign of God that is the Church's liturgy. But approached with a contemplative outlook, the liturgy is in fact most important for developing our appreciation of the beauty of life (#84).[24]

Pope John Paul's effort in this encyclical can also be characterized as an attempt to show the beauty of human life and respect for life. Inasmuch as proclamation of, celebration of, and service to the Gospel of life are what are necessary to develop a culture of life, and inasmuch as *Evangelium Vitae* is a call for such a culture, it would in fact be surprising if the encyclical did not include those elements of proclamation, celebration, and service. Most relevant for our understanding of how the encyclical seeks to persuade are the elements of proclamation and celebration.

John Paul gives a rational account of the beauty of life in relationship to its Creator and Redeemer, its Beginning and End. But the essence of the proclamation within which the pope gives this account is not syllogistic argument, but rather depiction of life in its fullness so as to put on display its beauty and the beauty of affirmation of life, beginning with and modeled after that living affirmation of life that is God's creative and saving work (cf. #1, 29-51 [ch. 2, "The Christian Message Concerning Life"] especially). This is not John Paul's first use of such an approach.[25] Celebration too, which flows from proclamation as a "setting in which the beauty and grandeur of this Gospel is handed on" (#83), is included in the approach. This is especially evident when in his conclusion the pope looks contemplatively "to the Lord Jesus... 'the Life' which 'was made manifest'" (#102), leading to prayer in union with the Mother of the living.

And concerning the persuasive utility of this approach: Despite the degree of continued resistance of our world to the pope's message, of late he seems to some extent to be disarming, if not yet converting, the world. The press seems, of late, to respect this man and what he says, even while not yet sure why. The coverage of *Evangelium Vitae's* release in particular was positive, at least by comparison to some of the coverage given related stories during the past decades, and in a way that cannot be fully explained by the press's edification at some of the more "progressive" conclusions such as those concerning capital punishment or respect for the environment. I modestly propose that souls are not yet so altogether damaged as to be wholly unable to recognize beauty when they see it. By an act of will, radical rebellion may (and certainly does) persist, but even the confirmed rebels occasionally fall silent in awe.[26]

A POLITICS OF THE BEAUTIFUL

The politics that expresses this view of the world is related to classical liberal politics as the contemplative or receptive attitude is related to the merely manipulative. That is, it is a politics that responds to the invitation of reality and of the human person in particular to beauty, rather than a forceful, if calculated, expression of untutored desire. It seeks to instantiate the common good that beauty in human action represents.[27] It is a politics of friends, not of enemies. As such it is much more than a system or a set of techniques. No mere cleverness, but the practical wisdom that results from experiences of beauty in action, makes possible understanding of political deliberation.[28] And this conception of politics implies no moral/political distinction. The moral is *ipso facto* the political. While identifying an action as moral or immoral does not sufficiently warrant the political conclusion that the action should be prescribed or proscribed by civil law, prudential delimitation of the sphere of the political does not reflect a difference in kind between the principles of morality and the principles of politics.[29]

Especially important in this connection is the relevance of Christian love, the perfection of justice, for politics. As has been indicated, the ultimate reason that the direct killing of the innocent is evil is that it is contrary to love (#41, 77). John Paul's celebration of the beauty of life and of respect for life takes its bearings from this ultimate principle. And loving affirmation of life requires more than does justice alone. But prudence seems rather narrowly to delimit the degree to which the civil law should compel acts of love beyond justice.

At least one distinction is in order, however: that between what prudence allows by way of legal requirements concerning the actions of individuals, and what may be asked of the political community as such. Just as individuals should regard themselves as required by the moral law to be more virtuous than the civil law may prudently command, it may also be the case that the political community should hold itself in its actions *qua* community to a higher moral standard than that to which it could prudently hold its citizens in their actions *qua* individuals. And a recognition that attention to love beyond justice better corresponds to the common good of human dignity underlies the reservations John Paul has developed concerning capital punishment, as I understand his argument (#56, with its use of the *Catechism* #2267; cf. #9, 27, 40).[30] In this and closely related matters at least, John Paul calls the political community to act with love.

There remains room, in a politics oriented toward beauty, for political appeals pointing to the dangerous consequences, for all people, that result when we fail to protect some human lives. These consequences include not only the famous "slippery slope" but also physical and psychological harm to women and others, and the destruction of human relationships.   Such consequences must, however, be presented as signs and effects of the disruption by violations of human life of the order of justice and love that is the common good.   Appeals of this kind have as a necessary, positive counterpart appeals to the beauty of a society in which the integrity of persons and relationships is safeguarded.   Women, uniquely able to know the beauty of motherhood (as well as the wounds inflicted by abortion), are irreplaceable as teachers in these matters (#99).

The characterization of a politics that seeks beauty as a "politics of friends" should not be taken to suggest that spirited argument concerning what is good and the resolve prudently to enact and enforce just laws are inappropriate.   "Divisiveness" is dangerous to the imposed peace of the classical liberal social contract, but true political friendship will not put "getting along" before honest confrontation of even potentially "divisive" issues like social issues in general or life-issues in particular.   The root of friendship is not so much warm feelings as it is partnership in pursuit of true goodness. One does not ignore, but rather tries to supplement and remedy, one's friends' shortcomings in that pursuit.   Good feelings are a response to such help, not a substitute for it.[31]

John Paul gives the political "system" of democracy special treatment.   He says, "If today we see an almost universal consensus with regard to the value of democracy, this is to be considered a positive 'sign of the times,' as the Church's Magisterium has frequently noted." But consistent with what has been elaborated concerning politics, he goes on to add that "the value of democracy stands or falls with the values which it embodies and promotes.   Of course, values such as the dignity of every human person, respect for inviolable and inalienable human rights, and the adoption of the 'common good' as the end and criterion regulating political life are certainly fundamental and not to be ignored" (#70).   Democracy, then, must consist in common deliberation about what laws will respond to the invitation of beauty.[32] But democracy is to be especially valued among possible means to the end of instantiating the values that constitute a society that serves the common good—such that one can speak of a putative movement toward democracies as "positive." That is, if attention to beauty is a criterion for right means to an end, democracy is an especially fitting "means."

Now, the presuppositions of classical liberalism make it difficult to explain the value of democracy. If politics is enforcement of peace, it is unclear that democracy will necessarily be the most efficient means to this end. Presumably, consent being the criterion whereby peace is chosen over war and whereby the details of the peace are justified, any form of government to which consent is given will be equally to be valued. There is nothing in principle better about a form that legislates by popular consent than a form wherein, say, a monarch, to whose office consent has been given, legislates.[33] If, on the other hand, politics is the establishment of the right order or beauty in relations among citizens that is the common good, as well as (and ontologically prior to being) an instrument for pacification, then one can argue that where democracy is possible, it is most fitting. My participation in the search for the beauty in which my life in society is to be a participation is especially congruent. My life of ordered freedom will then express the potentialities of the human person under God.

PRO-LIFE POLITICS AND EVANGELICAL RENEWAL

Pope John Paul writes, "Like the yeast which leavens the whole measure of dough (cf. *Mt* 13:33), the Gospel is meant to permeate all cultures and give them life from within, so that they may express the full truth about the human person and about human life" (#95). Insofar as a culture "expresses" truth or falsehood through politics, this implies the necessity of a politics itself grounded in the truth about the human person. This truth includes our natural communion with one another. Nobility or beauty is not attained at the expense of others but in solidarity, including respect for innocent life that refuses directly to take such life and that seeks to nurture it. This same truth therefore implies a politics that is a common search for the beauty of solidarity.

The pro-life movement must take account of this and teach this. We must not fall into the trap of arguing for respect for the right to life as an instrumental good, which is false, and by which we undermine ourselves. "To be actively pro-life," John Paul teaches, "is to contribute to the *renewal of society* through the promotion of the common good" (#101). Political action, while "taking into account what is realistically attainable" (#90), must never obscure the common good of the right to life by encouraging members of society to continue to view one another, especially the vulnerable, as enemies. Renewal of society and its political dimension is, finally, inseparable from the *"evangelization"* whereby the love of mother for unborn child, man and woman for aged parent, family and friend for the sick and disabled, and each for each at each stage of life, comes to be celebrated as "Good News."

NOTES

1. The relationship between the encyclicals becomes especially clear in *Evangelium Vitae's* ch. 3 on "God's Holy Law." John Paul begins this chapter with reference to the story of Jesus' encounter with the rich young man, the same story upon which ch. 1 of *Veritatis Splendor* is an extensive meditation. The story is used to explain the relationship between the gift of law and the gift of life. Concluding *EV* ch. 3 (#75), John Paul explicitly cites *VS* #81-82 on the meaning of exceptionless negative precepts.

2. In this respect too *Evangelium Vitae* takes up *Veritatis Splendor*; cf. *VS* #97 and 99, which are cited in *EV* #70. Treatment of such other magisterial documents on socio-economic issues as those of John Paul, the Second Vatican Council, and earlier popes, which reflect the same principles, is beyond my scope.

3. Concerning this approach, cf. the *Catechism of the Catholic Church* #1901: "Regimes whose nature is contrary... to the fundamental rights of persons *cannot* achieve the common good..." (emphasis added).

4. Cf. St. Thomas Aquinas, *Summa Theologiae*, I-II, q.96, a.2.

5. For the social contract, see especially Hobbes' *Leviathan*, part 2, ch. 18. More precisely, Hobbes speaks of a "covenant," but this is a species of "contract" (part 1, ch. 14). Cf. John Locke's *Second Treatise of Government*, ch. 8, #97, 99. The liberalism that influenced the American founders was mediated by Locke.

David L. Schindler ("Christological aesthetics and *Evangelium Vitae*: Toward a definition of liberalism" in *Communio* 22 [1995] 193-224) argues that the liberal political culture to which John Paul is responding has as its point of departure from a Christian perspective "the loss of contact with God's wise design" of which the pope speaks (*EV* #22). This gives rise to a rupture between "form and love," which are in reality united as beauty. Schindler criticizes even the principles of the American founding on this basis.

My exegesis and conclusions overlap greatly with Schindler's. I shall add two main things. First, I shall give attention to the roots of contractarian liberalism to identify with greater specificity how liberalism's technological approach to the world, discussed by Schindler, departs from John Paul's principles in the political sphere. Second, I shall show that those principles are not peculiarly Christian. Justice already gives beauty to form. Liberalism loses contact not only with the Persons of the Triune God, but, as the pope precisely says, even with that God's "wise design." John Paul affirms that the Gospel of life *"can ... be known in its essential traits by human reason"* (#29, emphasis in the original; other references to reason's ability to discern good and evil regarding human life are found in ch. 3 and summarized in #77). Therefore, liberalism is anti-Christian for the reason that it opposes a vision that is presupposed by authentic Christianity.

At the same time, Christians know that God's "wise design" includes the economy of salvation, including revelation. Central to John Paul's message is that justice is but the beginning of love. One of his favorite texts from the Second Vatican Council's Pastoral Constitution on the Church in the Modern World *(Gaudium et Spes* #24), teaches that persons find themselves only by making gifts of themselves. *Evangelium Vitae* is informed by this principle (#96 cites *Gaudium et Spes* explicitly, but other allusions abound throughout). And this love is known only in Christ (#29, 51).

Beauty therefore finds its full explanation and perfection in Christianity. Herein lies the importance of evangelization and of "Christological aesthetics." John Paul has gone so far as to speak of the inadequacy of justice apart from love in the form of mercy *(Dives in Misericordia* ["Rich in Mercy," 1980] #12). One might consider this a special case of our inability to attain knowledge of saving truth apart from revelation, except "after a long time, and with the admixture of many errors" (Aquinas, *Summa Theologiae,* I, q.1, a.1).

6. To cite but one example from a classic text of the movement, one finds this as a strand of the argument in Dr. and Mrs. J. C. Willke's *Abortion: Questions and Answers* (Cincinnati: Hayes, 1985) 3-4, 7-9, 175-76; cf. 225-26ff. To note that there is a certain appeal to self-interest in the Willkes' (or anyone else's) argument for restriction of the practice of abortion is in no way to suggest that their opposition to that practice is selfishly motivated.

7. Cf. the *Catechism* #1869: "Sins give rise to social situations and institutions that are contrary to the divine goodness. 'Structures of sin' are the expression and effect of personal sins. They lead their victims to do evil in their turn."

8. In his first encyclical, *Redemptor Hominis* ("The Redeemer of Man," 1979), John Paul emphasizes the need for solidarity in Christ if the modern world is not to threaten humanity with subjection (#16). Here too the Christological focus upon which Schindler ("Christological Aesthetics") concentrates is elaborated. At the same time, working from another of his favorite texts from *Gaudium et Spes* (#22, referring to the revelation of the human person in the revelation of God's love), John Paul shows that the solidarity Christ brings about is a response to the aspirations of the human spirit (#7-12).

9. Hobbes, *Leviathan,* part 1, ch. 14.

10. Hobbes, *Leviathan,* part 1, ch. 14.

11. Hobbes, *Leviathan,* part 1, ch. 13.

12. Russell Hittenger has observed that, seemingly in view of this, *Evangelium Vitae* evinces a return to a cautious approach to democracy like that taken by 19th and earlier 20th century popes ("The Gospel of Life: A Symposium" in *First Things* 56 [Oct. 1995] 33-35). As we shall see, "caution" is not incompatible with a recognition of value.

The American founding presupposes the problematic conception of democracy herein described. According to the defense of the Constitution in *The Federalist Papers,* "The diversity in the faculties of men, from which the rights of property originate, is... an insuperable obstacle to a uniformity of interests. The protection of these faculties is the first object of government" (#10). The authors' talk of "rights" must be understood in the context of the Lockean goal of mediating between competitors for property. Rights are the maximum feasible expressions of autonomy, and in fact are given up as necessary to the government (#2). The authors also speak of "the public good." This is primarily the peace without which property is intolerably insecure. It is because the peace of a stable democracy is rendered precarious by the power of factions that the founders turned to the contrivance of an extended republic. They could not envisage transcending a "science of politics" looking only to "efficacy" (#9).

13. Cf. Hobbes, *Leviathan,* part 2, ch. 18: Those who will not obey the sovereign place themselves back in the "state of war" and may "justly be destroyed." Locke's *Second Treatise* presents the appearance of comparatively moderate traditionalism. Most specifically, Locke says that one's property may not be taken (ch. 11, #138-39). But this does not exclude taxes, the sole criterion for the acceptability of which is the majority's consent (#140). Underlying this is the principle that one who joins the social contract thereby "submits to the community those possessions, which he has, or shall acquire" (ch. 8, #120). More broadly, in the community one has "only so much [power over others] as the law of nature gave him" (ch. 11, #135); yet this is much power indeed, for the same "law of nature" that proscribes violations of others entitles anyone to decide and undertake to punish anyone else to the extent one feels necessary for one's own self-preservation (ch. 2, #6-8). In the end, whatever one thinks of Straussian exegeses in general, Leo Strauss is probably right that Locke is more polite, but more revolutionary, than Hobbes. (The judgment that Locke is *more* revolutionary owes to the centrality of labor or striving in Locke's conception of the good life.) See *Natural Right and History* (Chicago: Univ. of Chicago Press, 1953) 220-51.

14. This analysis replicates—and the formation of my own thoughts is much indebted to—the analysis presented by James M. Rhodes in "Variations on a Theme by Hobbes," a response to a panel on political obligation at the Midwest regional meeting of the American Political Science Association (Chicago, 1988). The problem of the calculation to which I have referred as

essential to classical liberal politics, and which is likely to rule the unborn out of the law's protective sphere, is a special case of the problem Rhodes discussed, wherein utility calculation simply cannot give rise to political obligation.

15. This is the "postliberal" approach of which Schindler ("Christological Aesthetics," 208) speaks. The consequence of liberal politics that is postliberalism's point of departure is explicated clearly by Jean-Jacques Rousseau: "The one who dares to undertake to establish a people ought to feel that he is, so to speak, in a position to change human nature; to transform each individual, who by himself is a perfect and solitary whole, into part of a larger whole, from which this individual receives in some way his life and his being... to substitute a partial and moral existence for the physical and independent existence which we have all received from nature" (*On the Social Contract*, book 2, ch. 7; my translation).

The status of this "partial and moral existence" would seem to be ambiguous at best. Friedrich Nietzsche therefore contended that "we need a critique of moral values.... What if, in the 'good,' there even lay a symptom of retrogression, indeed a danger, a temptation, a poison, a narcotic, through which, perhaps, the present lived at the expense of the future?" (*Genealogy of Morals*, preface #6, my translation). Nietzsche was concerned that willed self-destruction (*Genealogy*, esp. essay 1, #13; essay 2, #16-17) was replacing willed self-transcendence such as that attained by his ersatz "savior" Zarathustra (cf. *Genealogy*, essay 2, #24-25 and *Thus Spoke Zarathustra*, esp. part 1, "Zarathustra's Prologue" #2-4; "On the Three Metamorphoses"). This is *inter alia* a rejection of (Judeo-)Christianity (*Genealogy*, essay 1, #7-8, 14-16; essat 2, #20-22) along with all "trans-earthly hopes" (*Zarathustra*, part 1, "Prologue," #3).

16. The species of the beautiful (*kalon*), Aristotle explains, are "order and due proportion and boundedness" (*taxis kai symmetria kai to hōrizmenon*, *Metaphysics* 1078a36-b1; all references to Aristotle are to the Oxford texts; translations are mine). These seem to suggest, respectively, right relation of parts to whole, of parts to each other, and of whole to larger whole. Hence the *kalon* encompasses at the same time both a being's internal order and its relationship to other beings. Both stand or fall together. To the extent that my relations to you in disposition and action are not beautifully constituted, neither am I of myself beautifully constituted.

17. Aristotle says that a courageous person will endure pains "for the sake of the beautiful (*tou kalou*); for this is the perfection of excellence (*telos tēs aretēs*)" (*Nicomachean Ethics* 1115b12-13). St. Thomas Aquinas does not speak of beauty in this context. However, his understanding of the realities involved can be shown to be the same as Aristotle's. In summary, virtue denotes a perfection and therefore goodness, which requires conformity to the rule of (practical) reason, which apprehends goodness. But goodness as form, that is, as cognitively apprehended, is beauty. See *Summa Theologiae*, I, q.5, a.4; I-II, q.55, aa.1,3; q.64, a.1; q.94, aa.2,3.

18. Deliberation, Aristotle says, involves consideration of "the most efficient and most beautiful (*kallista*)" of means to an end (*Nicomachean Ethics* 1112b17; I am grateful to Darrell Dobbs for bringing the importance of this passage to my attention). And prudence is the excellence of the intellectual faculty of deliberation. But in order for prudent deliberation to make right our movement toward an end, it is necessary that our aim or sight be made right by ethical excellence: *hē men gar aretē ton skopon poiei orthon, hē de phronēsis ta pros touton* (1144a7-9; cf. 1144a29-b1).

19. These contentions imply that just actions toward a person who does evil will be different from just actions toward a comparatively innocent person. This underlies what has come to be known as "retributive justice." The pope makes implicit reference to this principle in his discussion of capital punishment (#56). He affirms that the "primary purpose" of punishment is "to redress the disorder caused by the offense" (quoting the *Catechism*), or, apparently equivalently, to "redress the violation of personal and social rights" entailed in a crime (John Paul's own words). Relative to this purpose of punishment, its utility for public order and safety and its rehabilitative value are secondary. An account of punishment not acknowledging the reality and primacy of retributive justice would make punishment merely an act of use—an expression of the culture of death.

20. For a fuller treatment of this, see Josef Pieper, *Leisure: The Basis of Culture* (New York: Random House, 1963) 24-37.

21. Hadley Arkes ("The Splendor of Truth: A Symposium" in *First Things* 39 [Jan. 1994] 27) writes, "Many students of Leo Strauss, and a flock of Aristotelians, may suffer trauma over the references in [*Veritatis Splendor*] to truths that are categorical—unyielding and uncompromising." The same teaching grounds *Evangelium Vitae,* and a further comment is in order. Strauss (*Natural Right and History,* 157-64) interpreted Aristotle's statement about the mutability of natural right (*Nicomachean Ethics* 1134b29-30) to exclude such truths. As I hope to have made clear, Aristotle's own understanding of the foundation of virtue or excellence makes possible exceptionless prohibitions. For an interpretation of the mutability of natural right that clarifies its compatibility with such prohibitions, see James M. Rhodes, "Right by Nature" in *Journal of Politics* 53 (1991) 317-38.

22. A debate about the meaning of natural law has been taking place. A helpful account of the issues that explains and defends the contentions of the "new" theory of Germain Grisez et al. is that of Robert P. George, "Recent Criticism of Natural Law Theory" in *The University of Chicago Law Review* 55 (1988) 1371-1429. The claims in *Evangelium Vitae* are, implicitly, claims concerning natural law, and might profitably be tentatively located with reference to this debate. The view that "our (practical) knowledge of human good(s) is methodologically prior to our (speculative) knowledge of human nature" (George, "Recent Criticism," 1416) may be compatible with John Paul's, though perhaps one should say "coeval with" instead of "prior to." More problematic, however, is the new theory's isolation and identification

as pre-moral of those goods, and what strikes me as its deontological accent on rationality as a criterion for moral action (George, "Recent Criticism," 1396ff). Human perfection is something that, for John Paul, can be approached, and that can be intellectually discerned insofar as it is beautiful. This perfection and its advancement is the standard for moral goodness. Hence, perfected human nature as bringing together being (form, to use Schindler's term) and goodness (justice and love) is a moral category, and arguing from nature is not arguing from a bare "is" to an "ought."

23. *Proterai gar eisi tōn dynameōn hai energeiai kai hai praxeis kata ton logon* (*De Anima* 415a18-20). Consistently, Aristotle does not call the study of the soul a deductive science (*epistēmē*) that proceeds from *a priori* principles, but rather an "inquiry" (*historian*, 402a4) into what potentialities of soul would explain the activities we observe.

24. Cf. Pieper, *Leisure*, 56-64; and Joseph Cardinal Ratzinger, *The Feast of Faith: Approaches to a Theology of Liturgy* (San Francisco: Ignatius Press, 1986) 61-75.

25. Cf. Joseph F. Chorpenning, "The Holy Family as Icon and Model of the Civilization of Love" in *Communio* 22 (1995) 77-98.

26. This is the worst-case scenario, and in fact there are signs of conversion as well. The phenomenon has also been noted elsewhere; John Mallon reports ("Catholic Essentials" in *Crisis* 14 [April 1996] 8) that the pope and *Evangelium Vitae* have brought about "[a] resurgence of interest in human life" in Italy.

27. The existence of justice as such a common good, and our ability to discern what is just, in fact underlie Aristotle's argument that "man is by nature a political animal" (*Politics* 1252b27-53a39). Moreover it, not consent, is what makes just laws binding in conscience (cf. Aquinas, *Summa Theologiae*, I-II, q.96, a.4; also q.93, a.3 and q.95, a.2; and the *Catechism* #1902-03).

28. Aristotle says that "a young man is not a proper listener to the political, for he is inexperienced in actions of life, but reasonings (*hoi logoi*) [about laws for human action] *proceed from these* and concern these" (*Nicomachean Ethics* 1095a2-4). Remarkably, Aristotle speaks of listening (*a fortiori*, political speaking is presumably excluded as well). The one who has not become aware, through experience, of the beauty that is the principle of political discourse literally will not know the first thing about politics. And even listening to political discourse will be dangerous, not merely unproductive, for such a person. Not knowing what he does not know, he will come fundamentally to misconceive what he is hearing and therefore the nature of politics.

29. Cf. Aristotle, *Nicomachean Ethics* 1141b23-24ff.

30. For more on this, see William L. Portier, "Are We Really Serious When We Ask God to Deliver Us From War? The Catechism and the Challenge of Pope John Paul II" in *Communio* 23 (1996) 47-63.

31. Aristotle speaks of friendship appearing in proportion to the justice of the constitution of a political community (*Nicomachean Ethics* 1161a10-11ff; cf. 1158b13-14). The possibility of friendship between ruler and ruled is consistent with the more general principle that the good do not let their friends err (1159b6-7).

32. Alain Woodrow's criticisms of *Evangelium Vitae* ("The Pope's Challenge to Western Democracy" in *The Tablet* 249 [1995] 448, 450) fail to take any account of these conclusions.

33. Thus, according to Hobbes (*Leviathan,* part 2, ch. 19), monarchy is most efficient. Locke suggests a preference for democracy (*Second Treatise,* ch. 2, #13; ch. 7, #94; ch. 8, #97-99), but accepts any form of government to which consent is given (ch. 10, #132). The Declaration of Independence seems to make consent necessary only at the stage at which a government is "instituted," wherefore it was necessary to establish "a long train of abuses" to condemn the British monarchy, as Martin Diamond has pointed out (*The Founding of the Democratic Republic* [Itasca: F. E. Peacock, 1981] 3-6).

EDITH STEIN: CONTRIBUTION
TO A CULTURE OF LIFE

Sr. M. Stanislaus, O.P.

I. BACKGROUND

Biographical

1891	Born in Breslau, youngest child of an orthodox Jewish family
1916-18	Doctorate in philosophy at University of Freiburg-im-Breisgau and assistant to Husserl
1922	Baptized into the Catholic Church
1923-32	Instructor at the Teachers' College of the Dominican Sisters at St. Magdalena, Speyer. Lecturer in pedagogy
1932-33	Docent at the German Institute for Scientific Pedagogy
1933	Entered the Carmelite Order at Cologne with the religious name Sr. Teresa Benedicta of the Cross
1934-38	Life in the Carmelite convent at Cologne
1938	Fled to Carmelite convent in Holland
1939-42	Life in Carmelite convent in Holland
1942	Arrest and deportation to the East (August). Gassed at Auschwitz, August 9, 1942
1987	Beatified by John Paul II

Significant Dates in the Nazi Regime

1933 (Jan.)	Hitler becomes German Chancellor
1933 (April)	"Law for the Restoration of the Professional Civil Service" (aimed at excluding Jews from the public sector)
1933 (July)	Sterilization law ("Law for the Prevention of Offspring with Hereditary Diseases"), compulsory.
1935 (Oct.)	"Marriage Health Law" (couples needed a Marriage Fitness Certificate)
1936 (June)	Abortion permitted, with the woman's consent, to prevent the birth of a handicapped child
1939 (Aug.)	"Requirement to Report Deformed, etc., Newborn"
1939 (Sept. 1)	World War II began
1939 (Sept.)	Registration of hospitals and nursing homes (also involved

	listing persons with various handicaps and those "not of Germanic blood")[1]
1939 (Oct.)	Hitler authorized physicians, as specified, to kill handicapped children.[2] (He pre-dated this to Sept. 1, 1939). The killing of handicapped children began. This was later expanded to include the aged, the insane, and the incurable, in hospitals and nursing homes.
1940 (spring)	Decision to kill handicapped Jewish patients as a group
1940 (July)	Announcement of the creation of the Reich Committee's first "children's ward" (killing center)
1941 (June)	Killing expanded to include all Jews
1942	Killing of Gypsies

II. CULTURAL CONDITIONS OF HER TIME

A. VIEWS OF WOMAN

Since the 19th century a great cultural change had been taking place in Germany regarding the roles of man and woman. The question of feminism was a burning one in Edith Stein's day. The pioneering struggles in the 19th and early 20th centuries to open up educational and professional opportunities to women had achieved much. The distinctiveness of woman was accepted and there was growing awareness of the value of this difference. The emphasis of the early days on the opportunity for the development of the *individual* woman's potential was giving way to a social attitude that the distinctive value of woman would also benefit society. At the same time other currents of thought were operating. The "Romanticist" view held that woman's place was only in the home. Another position considered woman only from the biological point of view.

B. UNREST, DISUNITY, LOSS OF VALUES

Speaking in 1928, Stein called attention to certain sicknesses of society: dehumanization, disunity, a lack of principles. Some sought escape through pleasure, some through one-sided activity. Others were being drawn to revolutionary groups, e.g., the National Socialists and the Communists. Many held a material view of the human being. There was no comprehension of the spiritual dimension of the human person. In this view woman was understood only in biological terms, an attitude which Stein terms "brutal."[3] The Nazi party, with its racist ideology, saw Aryan women as useful for continuing the superior race (CW 2: 145). Stein also notes the breakdown of marriage and family life, the increase of promiscuity, and the influence of false theories about marriage.

C. EUGENICS, RACISM

There was a growing influence of the outlook which viewed human beings in terms of race and blood. This had been preceded by several decades of seemingly scientific writings claiming to show that certain races were superior and others inferior. Jews, blacks, and gypsies were labeled inferior. In the U.S. also such racist and eugenic ideas were published.[4] Some scientists maintained that there was a link between certain undesirable social traits and "inferior" races. They believed that social problems had biological roots and therefore could be solved in biological ways. "Feeble-mindedness" was a favorite target of eugenicists both in Germany and America. In turn, low intelligence was believed to be related to criminal behavior and immorality.[5] Human beings were classified on a scale of human worth, and this was joined to a type of Social Darwinism or "survival of the fittest." By a logical progression the ideology of National Socialism moved from a policy of exclusion to one of extermination. The goal was a "pure gene pool" which would ensure the development and rule of the superior races.

The work by Binding and Hoche, "Permitting the Destruction of Unworthy Life," published in Germany in 1920, was very influential. Binding was a professor of law and philosophy; Hoche was a medical doctor. They argued for the legalization of euthanasia. One of the primary targets was mental patients. De-humanizing terms such as "idiots" and "dead weight existences" were applied to them.[6] The lives of certain human beings were rated as "absolutely worthless." Contrasting the scene of dead soldiers on a battlefield with the care given to patients in mental hospitals, Binding writes:

One will be deeply shaken by the strident clash between the sacrifice of the finest flower of humanity in its full measure on the one side, and by the meticulous care shown to existences which are not just absolutely worthless but even of negative value, on the other.[7]

By 1932 conditions had worsened. Edith Stein speaks about the fundamental moral and spiritual upheaval taking place in her *Essays on Woman.* The persecution of Jews became more and more open. Jews were being forced out of professional positions. In a letter of May 7, 1933, she writes: "I am not permitted to give any lectures this semester (because of my Jewish descent).... I do not believe... in any return to the Institute [for Scientific Pedagogy, Münster] nor... in any possibility of a teaching career in Germany" (CW 5: 141).

D. EUTHANASIA KILLINGS

Theories about the "worthlessness" of certain races and groups of peoples progressively led to the crucial step of taking *action* against them. The violence against the handicapped in state hospitals and nursing homes began "in 1933 with sterilization and a reduced standard of care."[8] A plan for killing handicapped children was worked out in the spring of 1939; in August 1939 there was a requirement to report the birth of handicapped babies; the first killings of children took place around October 1939.[9]

III. EDITH STEIN'S RESPONSE

Edith Stein lived at a time when society was permeated by a "culture of death." Millions of human beings were marked for death; others were subjected to forced labor. Death-dealing objects were invented and produced by the human mind and hand: lethal gas, gas vans, crematoria, concentration camps, and war munitions. At the same time Edith Stein's life and work can be seen as a contribution to the culture of life.

A. HER POSITION ON THE NATURE OF THE HUMAN BEING

1. *A somatic-psychic-spiritual unity.* Trained in the school of Phenomenology, Stein endeavored to look at things freshly. Regarding the human being, her studies are serious and expressed in an original way. Contrary to the biological view, she points to the somatic, psychic, and spiritual dimensions of the human being. Moreover, the human being is not just spirit; the body belongs essentially to the unity of the human person. For that reason all the operations and activities of the human being are taken up into the unity of the person and have a personal value.[10]

2. *The human being: marked by potentiality and actuality.* Every

human being, from the very beginning, is a person in the unity of body and spirit. The spirit, because it is spirit, does not evolve from potency to act. It is drawn from nothingness into existence (ESW 2: 162). The existence of the human person begins "all at once," but it begins in time, for the spirit is united to a particular body. Moreover the powers of the human being are not perfected in the beginning. Thus our being is marked by both potentiality and actuality, and time is needed to reach perfection.

A person's powers may not unfold, but he/she is still a human being. Based on our own experience, we realize that we are never wholly conscious nor wholly free. My life endures, but I am not conscious all through its duration. Nor am I completely free to shape myself. My freedom is limited, yet I am still a human being. Therefore, conscious life and free action are not synonymous with my being (ESW 337, 342).

Edith Stein often used the analogy of the growth of a seed in order to speak about the development of a human being. There are influences which come from without as well as from within. In addition, there is the primary formative power, the causal agency of the person, who because of the free will has the power to form him/herself.

3. *Spiritual dimension.* The powers of intellect and will give evidence of a spiritual dimension. The person can transcend the sensory level through free acts. In contrast to the animal, the human being has its life in its own hand. In a free action the person in a sense "brings forth its own life" (ESW 2: 343). This does not mean that the human being is its own creator, nor absolutely free. A person's freedom "is *given* to it, and the 'livingness' which it develops in a chosen direction is given to it..." (*ibid.*). Moreover, human freedom is not the freedom of a pure spirit. It is united to the bodily and sensory levels (ESW 344).

4. *Uniqueness of each human being.* Edith Stein gave much attention to the question of the uniqueness of each person, maintaining that it was grounded not just on the body, but more fundamentally on the uniqueness of each human soul. Her reasoning is that human life comprises two aspects. It is not only matter-shaping, as in the case of plant and animal life, but it is also "spiritual-personal" (ESW 2: 458). This, she concludes, must have consequences for individuation. The innermost of the human soul,

what is deepest and most personal, constitutes the essential uniqueness of the human being. In each human soul there is "an unchangeable kernel, the personal structure" (CW 3: 110). This feature, which is most its own, constitutes the essential difference between one human being and another (ESW 2: 458-60). Stein was concerned that those who form and educate others respect this uniqueness and foster its development. This would be particularly important for parents and for teachers. She fiercely opposed the idea that human beings are only atoms in a mechanized society or nameless parts of a collective (CW 2: 197).

5. *Response to Heidegger's view of the human being.* Stein maintains that Heidegger's definition of the human being as a being-toward-death appears circular: first, the meaning of human existence is taken from death, and yet death is taken as the end of human existence. Secondly, to treat the ontological essence of death fully, one must ask what comes after death. Is death "the end of existence" or is it a "path from one mode of being to another" (ESW 4: 101-02)?

Heidegger puts much emphasis on *Angst* or solicitude as characterizing the human being. Stein says that neither this nor temporality are the ultimate meaning of human existence. Rather, these are "precisely what as far as possible must be overcome if" human existence is to attain its end (*ibid.* 111). What really concerns the human being is attaining eternal happiness: endless joy, love, and life. Heidegger views human existence as a course from nothing to nothing. His work seems to leave out "joy, happiness, love," and yet these are what "give the human being fullness" (*ibid.* 110).

6. *Basic equality and dignity of every human being.* Stein affirms the special value of the human being, who, because of the spiritual nature of the human soul, transcends the material world: "In the area of our common experience, the human being is the highest among creation since his personality is created in the image of God" (CW 2: 249).

Whereas the ideology of the National Socialist party wanted to create a "super-race," excluding those deemed inferior, Edith Stein viewed the whole of humanity as an organism of which each human being is a member with a unique calling and a unique role. Her view of the human person was inclusive, not exclusive. A person's powers may not develop, their personality may not completely unfold, as in the case of mental or physical impairment. But each is still a human person" (CW 3: 111-12).

7. *Perfected Humanity*. In contrast to the goal of a "super-race" based on race and blood, Edith Stein sees the goal as the perfection or completion of the human race. In each person there is a longing for the perfection of their being. This involves the harmony of powers and the transcendence of the limitations of the sensory level by choosing what is truly good. At the highest level, the person is united with God. This is *truly* "superhumanity" (CW 2: 262). The highest development of the person consists in acting for love of God and neighbor. God is love, and the person filled with God's life imitates His love, "ready to serve, compassionate, awaken, and foster life..." (CW 2: 52). The goal of a perfected humanity also involves a social dimension. Humanity can be viewed as an organism, built up through the contributions of the members across the ages. In addition, those who are incorporated into Christ form a Mystical Body" (CW 2: 186). One of the errors of the National Socialist party was to believe that the human race could be perfected by physical and mental development, without moral or religious development.

B. INSIGHTS REGARDING EMPATHY

Edith Stein always had an interest in the question of our knowledge of other persons. Her doctoral dissertation in 1917 was "On the Problem of Empathy." She held that the specific uniqueness of a human person, "the uniqueness of the innermost of every human soul" (ESW 2: 460) is, in a certain sense, graspable from the outside: "We can feel ourselves touched by it as by something kindred" (ESW 2: 459). At the same time, the specific difference of an individual is not, strictly speaking, comprehensible.

In a world of growing dehumanization and impersonal relations, Stein grasped the importance of trying to understand others, of sympathizing with them, of perceiving them "with the heart." She noted the importance of this for an individual's growth and held that women had a particular gift for grasping the uniqueness of persons and understanding their specific needs.

C. THE NATURE AND ROLE OF WOMAN

1. *Woman's nature*. Edith Stein was convinced of the distinctiveness of woman's nature and of its intrinsic value. It was

not inferior, but complementary to man's nature. Thus woman as woman had her specific calling. Stein was interested in authentic feminism and made original contributions to this field. Moreover, she tried to go back to the very roots of things in order to have a solid basis for conclusions and practical applications. She noted the following distinctive traits of woman:

* Because of woman's vocation to motherhood, the unity of the physical and the spiritual is more intimate in the case of woman than of man:

Woman's soul is present and lives more intensely in all parts of the body, and it is inwardly affected by that which happens to the body; whereas, with men, the body has more pronouncedly the character of an instrument which serves them in their work and which is accompanied by a certain detachment. This is closely related to the vocation of motherhood. The task of assimilating in oneself a living being which is evolving and growing, of containing and nourishing it, signifies a definite end in itself. Moreover, the mysterious process of the formation of a new creature in the maternal organism represents such an intimate unity of the physical and spiritual that one is well able to understand that this unity imposes itself on the entire nature of woman. (CW 2: 95)

* Woman has an interest in what is living, personal, and whole, rather than what is impersonal and objective (CW 2: 101).
* The emotions play a central role in the life of a woman (CW 2:96).
* Woman is particularly gifted with the powers of empathy, intuition, and feeling (CW 2:81). She grasps the uniqueness of a being and desires to help it toward completion.
* "By nature woman is attracted to moral and spiritual values" (CW 2:81). "She is sensitive to beauty and goodness" (CW 2: 122).
* Woman desires to remedy human need.
* Woman has a desire to reach wholeness, to become what she should be (CW 2: 178).
* Finally, woman has a longing to give herself completely in love (CW 2: 52). She desires "to achieve a loving union which, in its development, validates this maturation [of her humanity] and simultaneously stimulates and furthers the desire for perfection in others..." (CW 2: 93).

2. *Woman's calling.* The characteristics above correspond to *the particular calling of woman* which is to be *spouse and mother.* In speaking of the call of woman to motherhood, Edith Stein notes that motherhood "must be interpreted as supernatural as well as natural" if it is to reach full development (CW 2: 241). Moreover, spiritual or supernatural motherhood is possible without physical motherhood (*ibid.*). Likewise, to be *spouse* is not restricted to married women. Eve was called to be a helpmate for Adam. In addition to the companionship of husband and wife, there is also a spiritual companionship, whereby a woman is a support and help to all she comes in contact with (CW 2: 119). Revelation also teaches of the calling to be "spouse of Christ," either in the restricted sense of the woman consecrated to Christ in a life-long companionship, or in the general sense that every Christian soul is wedded to Christ the Bridegroom (CW 2: 194). *From her primary call to be spouse and mother* woman is thus called to:

* care for and protect human life, to nourish it and lead it to perfection (CW 2: 249). "The care and development of human life and humanity" is "woman's specific duty" (CW 2: 111).
* serve others and provide for them. This is the service of love (CW 2: 149).
* keep the family together; be the heart of the family (CW 2: 141).
* fight against evil. Because of her duty to protect life, and this can be taken to mean natural as well as supernatural life, woman is called to fight against what threatens that life. Stein sees in the Biblical passage, "I will put enmity between you and the woman," a reference to woman's vocation to fight evil (CW 2: 63).

Edith Stein sums up the specific value of woman in one word, motherliness. "Everywhere the need exists for maternal sympathy and help, and thus we are able to recapitulate in the *one* word *motherliness* that which we have developed as the characteristic value of woman" (CW 2: 258).

3. *Contributions woman can make to a culture of life.* In order to fulfill their calling, women must first be "whole persons" themselves. This means an inward order whereby the sensory powers are governed by intellect and will, and the will is directed by the intellect. This guards against a one-sided development of the

emotions which, without the light of the intellect, would present a distorted view of reality. Stein speaks of developing one's authentic humanity. By this she means a human being "in whom God's image is developed most purely," whose gifts and talents have blossomed, and whose inner powers are in harmony (CW 2: 249). Stein gives certain qualities of the ideal woman's soul. The seed of these qualities is present in all women but needs to be cultivated (CW 2: 119). She describes this ideal as follows:

The soul of woman must... be *expansive* and open to all human beings; it must be *quiet*, so that no small weak flame will be extinguished by stormy winds; *warm*, so as not to benumb fragile buds; *clear*, so that no vermin will settle in dark corners...; *self-contained*, so that no invasions from without can peril the inner life; *empty of itself*, in order that extraneous life may have room in it; finally, *mistress of itself*, and also of its body, so that the entire person is readily at the disposal of every call. (CW 2: 119)

Women can bring their specific gifts to every sphere. (a) *In the home* she makes the concerns of her husband her own, stands by him and supports him. She strives to make the home a place where he can find relaxation and renewal when he returns to it. She can counteract the tendency in the masculine nature to become totally absorbed in work. She tries to ensure that "he does not permit his humanity to become stunted, and that he does not neglect his family duties as father" (CW 2: 110).

Her particular sensitivity to the individual and to growth enables her to care for and to foster the development of her children:

This demands, on the one hand, an even more refined gift of sympathy because it is necessary to comprehend the dispositions and faculties of which the young people themselves are as yet unaware; she has to feel her way towards that which wishes to become, but which as yet does not exist. On the other hand, the possibility of influence is greater. The youthful soul is still in the formative stage and declares itself more easily and openly because it does not offer resistance to extraneous influences. However, all this increases the mother's responsibility. (CW 2: 110)

To help her husband and children toward true humanity requires selflessness. She must not become possessive nor use them simply as means for her own ends (CW 2: 110). Rather, she should see them "as gifts entrusted to her" by God, and for whom she has a responsibility (CW 2: 111).

Speaking of the spiritual ills present in her day, Stein said that perhaps the most important thing for the renewal of the country was good mothers: mothers who are firm in their convictions, who know the meaning of marriage and the purpose of life, who are open to the potentials of their children, but also know the necessity of curtailing dangerous tendencies; mothers who realize that they cannot "do everything themselves, but, on the contrary, are able to let go of their children and place them in God's hand when the time comes, when the children have outgrown them. *Such mothers are probably the most important agents for the recovery of the nation*" (CW 2: 254, emphasis added).

If a married woman also works, still she must see her primary responsibility in being "the heart of the family and the soul of the home" (CW 2: 110). If social conditions are such that a woman is forced to work and cannot take care of the home, Stein labels this situation as "unhealthy" (CW 2: 80).

(b) *At work*: Stein believed that any work in which woman's specific nature is able to develop and which can be formed by woman's nature is suitable for a woman. The presence of women in these areas could be a blessing. By their sympathy and concern for the concrete person, they could counteract some of the impersonality and mechanization of the work-place. Even if the work is monotonous or demands abstract thought, one is usually working with other people. With that there is the opportunity for the woman to develop her feminine gifts (CW 2: 48-49).

Stein notes certain professions especially in accord with woman's nature: teaching, the medical profession, and the social services. Such professions call particularly for sympathy, concern for the individual, and interest in the development of the whole person. As to the medical profession, she says that in a time of increasing specialization it is important not to lose sight of the whole person. Woman has a particular gift for being interested in the whole person and for sensing individual's needs, including spiritual needs (CW 2: 256).

The social services also call for persons with sympathy, a desire to help, concern for growth and development. "Everywhere, the problem is to save, to heal endangered or demoralized humanity, to steer it into healthy ways" (CW 2: 257).

Teaching is in harmony with feminine nature since it involves the formation of persons. Stein notes that with the breakdown of the home the responsibility of the school is greater than ever. To have any lasting influence the teacher must win the love and trust of the students. Her heart must be open to all, even the most difficult: "this love and trust must be won by means of a nature which loves consistently. And truly supernatural forces are needed to offer such equal, motherly love to *all*, even to the unlovable, the difficult, the intolerable children—and especially to them because, indeed, they are in most need of it" (CW 2: 255-56). In order truly to foster the growth of the students, the teacher must have firmness. "She herself must be firm in her principles and convictions and know what provides solid nourishment for the young" (CW 2: 255). With respect to conditions in her day Stein says: "Millions of children today are homeless and orphaned, even though they do have a home and a mother. They hunger for love and eagerly await a guiding hand to draw them out of dirt and misery into purity and light" (CW 2: 245).

(c) *In the political sphere* women now hold responsible positions at all levels of government. Here, too, woman's specific gifts can be a contribution. For example, if there is, on the part of the men, an exaggerated, one-sided devotion to party involved in a piece of legislation, it may be counteracted by women who can discern the meaning of the legislation as a whole and its effect on concrete human beings (CW 2: 258). Even if not serving in political office, women have a responsibility to be informed of political affairs, for they are members of the nation and co-responsible for it:

Those who are not interested in political affairs today must remind themselves that the whole political situation depends on how they use their political rights; and it depends on the political situation whether their husband and children will have work and bread, whether they will find opportunities to develop and utilize their intellectual gifts, whether they will be allowed to practice their faith and live. (CW 2: 141)

Elsewhere she notes that in her day "the State was interfering with the right of the family to educate its children" (CW 2: 200).

D. THE ROLE OF SCHOLARS AND EDUCATORS

A great part of Edith Stein's life was spent in the academic world. A deep love of truth led her to pursue the study of philosophy under Husserl, and she continued her research in this field up until her last days. Her writings also included religious and educational topics. A scholar herself, she appreciated the importance of intellectual work for the progress of humanity. Whether dealing with deeply metaphysical subjects or with practical questions of the day, she looked on her activity as helping to bring truth to others:

That it is possible to worship God by doing scholarly research is something I learned, actually, only when I was busy with [the translation of] St. Thomas [Aquinas's *Quaestiones de veritate* from Latin into German].... Only thereafter could I decide to resume serious scholarly research.... Even in the contemplative life, one may not sever the connection with the world. I even believe that the deeper one is drawn into God, the more one must "go out of oneself"; that is, one must go into the world in order to carry the divine life into it. (CW 5: 54, letter of Feb. 12, 1928).

She spoke strongly about the need for those in the academic world to be concerned about the social problems of the day. In an address to Catholic academic women in Switzerland in 1932, she said:

Do we grasp social problems, the burning problems of today? Do they concern us also? Or are we waiting until others find some solution or until we are submerged by the billows of chaos? Is such an attitude worthy of an *academic woman*? Must we not try to help in deed as well as in thought? (CW 2: 266)

Edith Stein also taught for nine years at a teachers' training college run by Dominican Sisters. So she had practical experience from which to draw her ideas about the questions connected with women's education. She called attention to the need to be aware that the material shaped by educators was not inert matter but living human beings, who themselves were the primary agents of their formation. Regarding the education of women, she held that there were three dimensions to be cultivated: their human nature, their nature as women, and their individual nature. She believed that one of the ways whereby the human race progresses is through the creative contributions of individuals. For this reason she sought to encourage an educational method which would promote creativity. She also emphasized the importance for those in the academic profession to understand the youth of their day if they wanted to help them CW 2: 265).

Despite the great difficulties presented by the conditions of her time, she never lost hope. In the same lecture of 1932 to Swiss Catholic women, her closing words were:

In hoc signo vinces runs youth's slogan. Could this not also be our slogan? We will not overcome this mountain of difficulties by our own power, but we will do it well through *that sign*! We will be *victorious* in the sign of the cross; that is, we will live our lives fully as Catholic academics—successfully or unsuccessfully—as a blessing of our society, our nation, and our Church. (CW 2: 268).

IV. CONCLUSION

What contribution did Edith Stein make to a culture of life? Surely her love of truth and her intellectual efforts in its service are a contribution, for life and truth are inherently related. The lives of human beings and the life of a nation are safeguarded and promoted only to the degree that they are guided by truth. A culture flourishes according as it advances in the truth. At a time when many were blinded or confused by false ideologies, Edith Stein continued to fulfill her responsibilities as a member of the academic profession, investigating the truth and communicating it to others. her intellectual work has shed new light on the nature of the human person. Her efforts to foster dialogue between medieval and contemporary thought, and in particular between the philosophy of St. Thomas and Phenomenology, has helped to give a new impulse to Catholic philosophy. As a teacher she sought to encourage the development of the whole person, to respect the uniqueness of each, and to prepare the young for life.

She has brought a deeper understanding of the nature of woman. In this way she has promoted greater recognition of the dignity of women and of their role. The more opportunity there is for the specific gifts and talents of women to develop and to be put at the service of society, the more hope there is for authentic cultural progress.

A culture of life has room for every human being. It does not try to eliminate sickness, abnormality, and poverty by eliminating the sick, the abnormal, and the poor. Rather, it recognizes that imperfection marks the human race and, while seeking to solve these problems, tries to help those in need live as fully as possible. Edith Stein, with maternal love, sought to restore, as far as possible, those who were wounded and impaired.

A *culture of life* must be a culture *from the heart*. One of her important contributions is her recognition of the importance of the "heart" in building up a culture worthy of the human being. In her person she combines the light of truth, which she loved so much, with the warmth of love. One of the last pictures we have of her, as told by someone who saw her in the Dutch concentration camp before deportation, shows her caring for the children and calming their fears, since many mothers, in despair, had ceased to do this:

Sister Benedicta at once took care of the poor little ones, washed and combed them, and saw to it that they got food and attention. As long as she was in the camp she made washing and cleaning one of her principal charitable activities....[11]

Her death in Auschwitz appears, from the human point of view, to be the victory of death over life. In reality her death was a birth to the fullness of life. In the same lecture to the Swiss Catholic women in 1932, speaking of how a person's individuality reaches its highest development (CW 2: 261), she quoted Nietzsche: "You must desire to be consumed in your own flame: how did you intend to become new if you were not ashes first?" Then she quoted Christ's words: "The grain of wheat must die, only then does it bring forth fruit. Whoever wants to save his soul must lose it" (CW 2: 261).

NOTES

1. Henry Friedlander, *The Origins of Nazi Genocide: From Euthanasia to the Final Solution* (Chapel Hill: Univ. of North Carolina Press, 1995) 76.

2. *Ibid.* 67.

3. Edith Stein, *Essays on Woman*, tr. Freda Mary Oben, vol. 2 of *The Collected Works of Edith Stein*, ed. L. Gelber and R. Leuven (Washington: ICS Publ., 1987) 144-45. [Hereafter citations from the English edition will be identified in the text as CW, followed by volume and page.] Vol. 3 (1989) is entitled *On the Problem of Empathy*; vol. 5 (1993) is entitled *Self-Portrait in Letters*.

4. Friedlander 5ff.

5. *Ibid.* 6-7.

6. Alfred Hoche and Karl Binding, "Permitting the Destruction of Unworthy Life" (Leipzig: Verlag von Felix Meiner, 1920), tr. in *Issues in Law and Medicine* 8/2 (1992) 248, 262.

7. *Ibid.* 246.

8. Friedlander 39.

9. *Ibid.* 44.

10. Edith Stein, *Endliches und Ewiges Sein*, vol. 2 of *Edith Steins Werke*, ed. L.. Gelber and R. Leuven (Freiburg: Herder, 1962) 242. [Hereafter citations from the German edition will be identified in the text as ESW, followed by volume and page.] Vol. 4 (1962) is entitled *Welt und Person*.

11. Hilda Graef, *The Scholar and the Cross* (Westminster: The Newman press, 1955) 15.

THE ANTI-LIFE FAMILY CONFERENCES OF THE UNITED NATIONS

Mercedes Arzu Wilson

AS THE SUN ROSE over Communist China on a September morning in 1995, the Western forces marched on to the conference-center determined to start a sexual revolution in the developing world. The pro-family forces from the developing countries, encouraged by a determined group of volunteers, also streamed toward the conference-venue. Though severely outnumbered, these courageous pro-family veterans of two previous United Nations conferences (Cairo and Copenhagen) felt wiser and braver.

THE REVOLUTION

This was clearly an undeclared war. At issue was a document under consideration by conference-delegates representing virtually every country of the world. It calls for worldwide population-control on a colossal scale, which would be achieved through abortion, pills and other man-made technologies. It includes the universal recognition of not two genders but possibly five. It is hostile to the two-parent family and to motherhood in particular. It is also antagonistic toward religion and religious people. It promotes sexual experimentation and homosexuality—anything that does not result in childbirth. In short, the UN document is riddled with every possible attack on the family. It would effectively make Planned Parenthood's mission-statement international law through compulsory treaty. Parents would have to take a back seat in this new tyrannical system.

This battle, pitting the world's most powerful Western countries against its most weak and impoverished, entails changing cultural values and religious traditions worldwide. The most vocal countries in the Western coalition were the European Union (comprised of 15 European countries and most Scandinavian countries, Canada, Australia, New Zealand, and the U.S.). Under the auspices of the UN, they seek to make universal population-control and an attack on the traditional family the cornerstone of a new world.

CONTROLLING MARRIAGE AND MOTHERHOOD

The UN Universal Declaration on Human Rights provides for the "recognition of the inherent dignity" of each human being. It also calls equal rights of all human beings the "foundation of freedom, justice and peace." Despite these earlier statements made by the UN's member-states, the Western coalition vigorously insisted upon the removal of all references to human dignity from the document considered in Beijing in September 1995.

The Universal Declaration makes marriage a fundamental right. It also provides that, "The family is the natural and fundamental group unit of society and is entitled to protection by society and the state." In contrast, the Beijing document portrays marriage and the family as obstacles to a woman's self-realization. Marriage and family are associated with violence against women within a family.

The Western negotiators did not stop there. They insisted on changing the term *family* to the ambiguous word *families*. This is an ominous change, for it implies that any group of unrelated people could call themselves a family. While pro-family delegates were successful in preventing this change, other provisions of the document extended the actual meaning of the term *family*.

The Universal Declaration of Human Rights provides that "motherhood and childhood are entitled to special care and protection." The Western countries repeatedly requested the deletion of any references to the word *mother* except when it appeared in a negative light. In effect they argued that the role of women is to be an executive, a politician, a producer—anything but a mother.

"IMAGINE THERE'S... NO RELIGION, TOO"

The UN Universal Declaration on Human Rights provides that, "Everyone has the right to freedom of thought, conscience and religion... freedom, either alone or in community with others, and in public or private, to manifest his religion or belief in teaching, practice, worship and observance." Yet in Beijing the anti-family coalition aggressively sought to remove all reference to religion, spirituality, morals or ethics—except where they were portrayed negatively, such as when associated with intolerance or extremism. To these delegates, there is nothing good about religion, especially the Catholic Church. After all, it is argued, it is the Church that has kept women down and, therefore, has been responsible for overpopulating the earth.

According to this document, every country in the world must recognize that "human rights and fundamental freedoms," as defined by the feminist-controlled Western countries, are more important than cultural or religious traditions and beliefs. Imagine the actual impact on your life, if you hold your religious views to be more important than this UN decree.

MY PARENT, THE STATE

The Universal Declaration on Human Rights and the Convention of the Rights of the Child made special provision for parents' rights and responsibilities regarding the education and upbringing of their children. The Western delegations worked to eliminate recognition of parental rights and responsibilities from key sections of the draft—even rejecting direct quotations from the Convention of the Rights of the Child. One pivotal paragraph was changed to give first mention to "rights of the child to access to information, privacy, confidentiality...." The implication here is that these supersede the parents' rights.

In Beijing special committees (called "contact-groups") were set up to allow for discussion and consideration of recommended action on various topics. In the contact-group on parental rights, the Guatemalan delegation suggested two possible additions to the Beijing document. Under the proposals, one of the following would be added: (1) "with the support and guidance from the parents and in conformity with the Convention on the Rights of the Child" or (2) "recognizing the rights and responsibilities of parents and persons legally responsible for adolescents to provide in a matter consistent with the Convention on the Rights of the Child, appropriate support and guidance in matters of sexual and reproductive matters." The end result would be recognition of basic parental rights. Number two was approved by a majority of delegates attending the meeting of the contact-group.

Two days later the Canadian chairman suddenly produced copies of a totally different option with a significant change in the language. The new version read: "Taking into account the rights of the child to access information, privacy, confidentiality, respect and informed consent, as well as the rights and duties of the parents and legal guardians to provide in a manner consistent with the capacities of the child, appropriate direction and guidance in accordance with the Convention of the Rights of the Child, and in conformity with non-discrimination against women, in all actions concerning children, the interest of the child should be a primary consideration." This was an unacceptable paragraph, but was nevertheless adopted.

If the Western delegates were to have their way, children were effectively to be property of the state—which would decide not only how they are raised, but if they should live or die.

NOT TWO GENDERS, BUT FIVE

From the very beginning in Beijing, the main strategy of conference-leaders was to bring up the most controversial points first. This would give the minority-coalition of Western nations an advantage before the various delegations from the poor countries got used to the dubious strategies of the opposing forces. They did not want the poor countries to align with each other in the closed-door meetings. This was a very clever move. On the first day, September 4, the chairman brought forth to the delegations the most controversial of all the points in the draft document—the lack of a precise definition of the word *gender*.

This controversy erupted in the preparatory committee-meeting at the UN in New York in the spring of 1995. Originally only three countries (Argentina, Guatemala and Honduras) questioned the meaning of the term. They requested that the word *gender*, which appears over 200 times in the 145-page document, be adequately and clearly defined. This caused a tremendous uproar from the developed countries which wanted to leave the word without a definition.

On September 4 the chairman reported at the main committee the ambiguous language that had been approved in New York by about 40 countries—with the exception of Guatemala, which offered a clear definition and dissented from leaving it undefined. When this point was brought up in Beijing, Guatemala requested the floor and offered this definition: "The term gender in this document refers to male and female as the two sexes of the human being." Unfortunately, no support was given to the Guatemalan delegation—even from those expected to support the amendment.

This was a very sad and tragic day. No support was given to oppose what is going to become a very dangerously ambiguous definition of a word that has now been given official acceptance by

182 countries around the world. It was decided that *gender* would be "interpreted and understood as it is in ordinary and generally accepted usage." The extremists—anti-womanhood and anti-motherhood feminists— claim that gender-roles are socially constructed. In other words, one is not born male or female, but society imposes such constructs. Paragraph 28 says "Socially constructed gender roles" and "socially ascribed gender roles" also appear in paragraph 50 of the draft. Consequently, recognition of five genders could emerge: male, female, homosexual, bisexual, and transsexual.

This not an unimportant point. Acceptance of the definition of *gender* as "socially constructed, socially determined or socially ascribed roles" imposes an alien and radical ideology on the women of the world. Such an ambiguous definition of *gender* carries with it the implication that motherhood and heterosexuality are not natural, but artificially created social constructs. It is a denial of the natural differences between men and women—which must be respected if women are to be truly equal as women and not as "imitation-men" as indicated in these documents. The language accepted at the conference is actually promoting the masculinization of women. It would be equally destructive and wrong to promote the femenization of men.

"AN OFFER YOU CAN'T REFUSE"

Marilyn McAfee, the American ambassador to Guatemala, was so incensed by my challenge to the Beijing document that she wrote to the Guatemalan Minister of Foreign Relations about my statements to the press. The following are excerpts from her letter, a copy of which was sent to my brother while he was still a candidate to the presidency.

Through this letter I wish to express to you my preoccupation on the comments to the press by a member of the Guatemalan delegation, Mrs. Mercedes Arzú Wilson, during the Fourth Woman's Conference....

The government of the United States has maintained a very active program of foreign aid for more than 30 years in this country [Guatemala].... The U.S. Congress is currently in the process of defining the budget of foreign aid for the 1996 Fiscal year and will substantially reduce the levels of aid for this year.... In light of the current deliberations by the U.S. Congress, the comments made by Mrs. Wilson arrive at an especially inopportune moment and we hope it will not have a negative effect on the U.S. aid to Guatemala.

It would be unfortunate if it was thought that certain public comments, lacking prudence, ...reflect the reaction of Guatemala toward our aid.

Was the American ambassador concerned that I was speaking, or was she really seeking to censor the content of my speech?

After receiving Ambassador McAfee's threatening letter, I sent a copy to Congressman Bob Livingston (R-LA), chairman of the House Appropriations Committee, and Rep. Christopher H. Smith (R-NJ), chairman of the House Subcommittee on International Operations and Human Rights. Rep. Livingston soon responded:

I feel distressed and deeply concerned that our American Ambassador to Guatemala would write a letter accusing you of criticizing U.S. foreign aid because of your strong stand in defending life, motherhood, parental rights, and high moral grounds....

As Chairman of the Appropriations Committee..., I can assure you that there is no political bias in Congress against Guatemala for your courageous stand as a delegate from Guatemala in Beijing. On the contrary, there is much admiration and esteem for your work.

Rep. Smith was even more blunt:

I am deeply disappointed that our ambassador to your country has seen fit to disparage your participation in the [UN] Conference. In particular, her expression of "hope" that your comments "will not have a negative effect on the U.S. aid to Guatemala" implies a threat that is entirely inappropriate.

Often countries are singled out as dissenters for standing up for the family, motherhood and parental rights. Many countries are sacrificing their moral values and ethical principles in the hope of economic concessions that may never come. Why do we always have to be beggars? How can we eradicate poverty, hunger and misery when the so-called humanitarian aid is really used as a bribe?

POPULATION-CONTROL AND SEX-EDUCATION TO ADOLESCENTS: THE ROOT OF ALL PROBLEMS

The time has come for the truth to unfold with regard to the so-called "humanitarian" family-planning programs that are nothing more than chemical warfare against women and families. As a Guatemalan, I can tell you that government officials and the people of my country have long been pressured to accept such pernicious programs. I can assure you there is nothing humane about them.

The Western world, led by the U.S., has financed the most shameful and repressive population-control drama in history. In India, for example, millions of men were hauled away in trucks and forcibly sterilized. Women are often offered financial incentives—which are difficult to refuse when you are among the poorest of the poor—in an effort to lure them into destroying their delicate reproductive organs. The West is also responsible for inspiring the notorious one-child population-control policy that enforces compulsory sterilization and abortion in China—all while claiming to oppose such abhorrent practices.

The contraceptive mentality has degenerated to such a degree that doctors generally fail to inform their patients of all the dangers to their health and the abortifacient effect of the many methods of artificial birth-control. These include the most commonly used methods, such as the Pill, Norplant, Depo-Provera and the Intra-uterine device. (All of them were first experimented with using the poor in Third World countries.) Their proponents ignore studies which show a link between the hormones in such chemical devices and a significant increase in cancer among women, as well as numerous other serious consequences.

Writers from around the world detail violations of women's rights by population-programs when they are coerced to have fewer children than they desire in order to meet governmental goals. [1] Frequently, women in the Third World are not told of the side-effects of the various contraceptive methods. These adverse reactions may be more severe for poor women than for women in the West given widespread malnourishment and their generally poor health.

Implants like Norplant and injectables like Depo-Provera promise protection against conception for months and even years. However, if a woman changes her mind and wants a child, she may be forced to continue the use of these methods. If the government has set population-reduction goals, she may be unable to find medical personnel willing to assist her by removing implants.

As shown in "The Human Laboratory," [2] a video documentary filmed by the British Broadcasting Company:

[T]hrough [BBC's] moving filmed testimony, HORIZON uncovers a catalogue of claims that Norplant is destroying women's lives. Serious side effects have been reported.... The film follows the diminutive Farida Akhter on her mission of mercy through the slums of Dhaka to uncover what she believes is the truth of the [Norplant] trials: side-effects often not reported; women pleading for removal of Norplant, but being turned away or asked to pay large sums of money; claims that they did not even know it was an experimental drug. And harrowing tales of bad science and coercion come from the poorest slums in the Western hemisphere, in Cité Soleil, Haiti, which health workers believe has become America's offshore human laboratory. Farida Akhter says: "It's cheaper for them to use Third World women than to use an animal in a laboratory in the West."

Narrator: Norplant is at least an officially approved contraceptive. But there are other, less regulated methods already in use... there are... a whole range of private foundations that are funding the building of a population-control movement. One private organisation is run by two doctors [Dr. Elton Kessel and Dr. Stephen Mumford] from America's southern states who believe they've found the answer for Third World Women in a drug called Quinacrine.

Dr. Elton Kessel: We have trials of the Quinacrine method going in some 17 countries like India, China, Bangladesh, and the trials are going very well. 10,000 women have had this method without a single fatality being reported.

Narrator: Dr. Elton Kessel was the founding director of Family Health International. He now researches Quinacrine in a worldwide operation, masterminded from Dr. Mumford's basement in Chapel Hill, North Carolina. Quinacrine is inserted into the top of the womb where it causes inflammation and scarring in the Fallopian tube, in theory blocking the tube with scar-tissue and preventing the sperm from reaching the egg.

Stephen Mumford: It's a very simple procedure, takes only a few minutes. It can be done in very primitive settings by people who do not necessarily have a lot of clinical skills....

Narrator: But some scientists believe the drug could put women's lives at risk—from cancer and ectopic pregnancy. And they question this entire approach to sterilisation.

Professor Shree Mulay: This method of producing scar-tissue is extremely barbaric. To try to damage the tissue so that you produce inflammation and block the tubes that way I think is extremely crude. It is imprecise for sure because one does not know where exactly that is going to take place and it causes a tremendous amount of pain because of the inflammation. There has been a long history of chemical-sterilisation research and this history is really an ugly one and its quite a shocking one because all kinds of agents have been used—sulphuric acid, formaldehyde—all of these agents which actually burn the tissue and cause production of scar-tissue. Chemical sterilisation was first tried out by the Nazis in their very first experiments in the death camps. That it has been picked up in the 60ˢ, 70ˢ and the 80ˢ and been promoted as rescue for the women of the Third World I think is quite extraordinary.

In a field-trial prior to marketing it for general use, a fertility-regulating vaccine (FRV) is being injected with tetanus-toxoid into young women in India. According to a World Health Organization document, the vaccine, anti-human chorionic gonadotrophin (hCG), is being injected without the strict controls imposed on such experiments by most developed countries where governments regulate the introduction of new vaccines to ensure that there are no serious, unwanted side-effects.

The motives behind such attacks on individuals and families—after all, real human beings are targets when "population" is criticized—often include unfounded opinions about economic reality. Yet as many astute observers have pointed out, they also include the puzzling and sinister notion that other people are bad—that human beings are the problem, rather than social injustice, faulty distribution of goods and services, and lack of economic opportunity and freedom. The population-controllers never seem to see themselves as part of an "overpopulation-problem," only the defenseless poor, whom they belittle, coerce and seek to reduce in number.

Time and time again I demanded that women should be properly informed of such abuses, reminding them that the Beijing Conference was supposed to be for the benefit of women. Nevertheless, my petitions were repeatedly denied, my factual information from US government sources was ignored, and my requests that programs of abstinence and the promotion of "self-control" instead of "birth-control" be implemented, were continually ridiculed.

The medical profession has lost credibility and respect for treating fertility—one of the greatest gifts God has given to us—as a disease that must be controlled, destroyed, regulated, altered, or manipulated at will. Most doctors do not encourage couples to practice natural family planning, preferring to hold to the pharmaceutical and abortion-industry hysteria of a poor effectiveness-rate. In reality, independent studies worldwide have proven that the latest and most scientific Ovulation Method, for example, has a 98-99% effectiveness.

Governments, schools and universities in the United states apparently hold to this same fallacious ideology. They throw condoms, pills and other technologies to boys and girls who, they presume, are incapable of living chaste lives. Isn't it time we challenge our younger generation to practice self-control instead of birth-control? Not only will it bring back respect and appreciation for the natural laws and their gift of fertility, but it will also serve as a remarkable teaching-tool that will have positive impact on young people in many other areas of life. Only through this approach can we begin to reverse the shameful statistic that one in every five Americans has a sexually transmitted disease. Of course, this is largely because of the irresponsible promotion of birth-control products by medical, academic and government institutions.

It is high time to recognize that, historically, every country that has embraced the contraceptive mentality has invariably succumbed to the legalization of abortion. Furthermore, national and international population-control programs—which ignore cultural and religious traditions of peoples throughout the world—are not only very expensive for the taxpayers, but very lucrative for the industries involved. To the poor countries of the developing world it becomes a financial nightmare, for the following reason. While the West can absorb the enormous medical costs associated with artificial birth-control, lesser developed countries who can barely treat common diseases, are unable to cope with the expenses for treating such serious side effects. The international programs have been dismal failures, heartbreaking and destructive to the people of the Third World. As the influence of such programs spreads, so do divorce rates and other socially troubling behavior.

The only beneficiaries of these programs are entities such as Planned Parenthood, whose strong influence was felt throughout all UN conferences, the pharmaceutical industry, and the irresponsible physicians who continue to prescribe the harmful chemicals and mechanical devices. They seem insensitive as they go about destroying both human life and the health of uninformed men and women.

Abortion, which was unthinkable a mere 30 years ago, has become the most commonly performed surgical procedure in the United States. The medical profession should be up in arms rather than embracing and promoting what they have pledged to oppose: "first do no harm."

Nowhere in the Constitution of the United States or that of any country of the Western World do we find a statement requiring or even encouraging these governments to impose population-control programs all over the world, violating their sovereignty. While most poor nations naturally appreciate true humanitarian aid, it is time to stop the abuses in the name of "humanitarianism."

According to the Beijing document, which would have the force of international law by treaty, unlimited access to birth-control and other population-control measures would be considered the norm. In fact, poor countries would be expected to advocate population-control programs and policies strongly. It is ironic that this policy was being pushed in Communist China where the Ovulation Method of Natural Family Planning was tested and found to have a 98.7% effectiveness-rate. But that would not fit into the overall, ideologically-based agenda. Whenever we advocated the use of natural family planning, the Norwegian delegate, backed by the U.S. delegate, would reply that "it is not natural for couples to have to abstain", or "we will have to check and see if natural family planning is an acceptable method of birth-control." In other words, the laws of nature, created by God, are being questioned by men.

When the Western delegates promote sex-education, they mean from kindergarten on. By the time children get to the fourth grade, they are to be instructed on condoms as the most effective barrier against AIDS and other sexually transmitted diseases. But the Family Research Council raises this fact: "In 1984, 7% of San Francisco's homosexuals were HIV positive; seven years of safe-sex later, the figure is 50%."[3] Further, C. M. Roland, editor of *Rubber Chemistry and Technology* for the National Research Laboratory, wrote:

[T]here exists direct evidence of voids in condom rubber. Electron-micrographs reveal voids 5 microns in size (50 times larger than the virus), while fracture-mechanics analyses, sensitive to the largest flaws present, suggest inherent flaws as large as 50 microns (500 times the size of the virus).[4]

This means that over the course of a year, the average woman whose partner uses condoms has one in six chances of becoming pregnant.

The chance of contracting AIDS is even higher because HIV is 500 times smaller than a human sperm and one-tenth to one-third the size of the smallest detectable hole in a condom. Moreover, while a woman can become pregnant only one hundred hours each month, given the nature of her ovulatory cycle, HIV can be transmitted at *any* time.

Whether among heterosexuals or homosexuals, AIDS is clearly linked to promiscuous and/or unnatural sexual activity, such as sodomy (anal intercourse), as well as intravenous drug use.[5] Consider the following breakdown:

male homosexual/bisexual contact	61%
intravenous (IV) drug-use (female and heterosexual male)	21%
male homosexual/bisexual contact and IV drug-use	7%
heterosexual contact	5%
receipt of contaminated blood-transfusion or tissue	2%
other/undetermined	3%

A recent UN program of several million dollars suggested for Guatemalan kindergarten and primary-school children was recently drafted. The goal was to implant in their innocent minds the notion that human beings are destructive, and therefore there should be less of them. They also presented these children (kindergarten to second grade) with explicit pictures of their anatomy, asking them to give the "correct" names, plus the appropriate function of each organ of the body.

The UN wants documents demanding that children have complete confidentiality (meaning, of course, that we parents cannot find out what our children are doing) in matters of sexuality. They can get pills, condoms, IUDs, Norplant, abortions, and so on—all without parental knowledge. After all, it is argued, it is best that parents do not know about such things. Once again, government-officials, bureaucrats, and radical anti-family movements are telling parents how to raise their own children.

HOMOSEXUALITY: STOPPING PREGNANCY

The most controversial discussion, which contained the topic of "sexual orientation," was left for the last day of the conference. The anti-family coalition knew that the developing nations would not accept any language in the document that promoted or condoned homosexuality.

Once it was brought to the floor, Benin, Egypt, Sudan, Jordan, Iran, Ecuador, Syria, Uganda, Belize, Senegal, Ghana, Guatemala, Bangladesh, Algeria, Ivory Coast, and Yemen strongly objected. There were another 25 or 30 countries seeking to be recognized as well, all of which wanted "sexual orientation" deleted from the document. It was an overwhelming response. They said it offended them, irrespective of religious beliefs, or their ethical and aesthetic sense. They said, "We came here to discuss the problems of hunger and poverty, not the things some women—with very few worries or things to do—want to do by imposing abnormal practices on the rest of the world. Such delegations want to legalize illegality."

There was a dramatic response from the poor nations of the world. The countries wanting to retain the language of "sexual orientation" included Canada, the United States, the European Union, New Zealand, Switzerland, South Africa, Slovenia, Cuba, Barbados, Chile, Latvia, Brazil, Colombia, and Cook Island. The chairman stopped the deliberations because it was apparent that there was an overwhelming number of countries requesting the floor to speak against it and there was no point in continuing the debate. The chairman removed the topic from discussion and deleted "sexual orientation" from the paragraphs. Canada, which had brought the issue to the floor for approval, was angry about the defeat of this provision, as was the United States. Both twice requested that the language be reinserted.

"SHOW ME A WINDOW OF YOUR PARADISE"

A Sudanese delegate was engaged in an interesting conversation with a French delegate at the UN Fourth World Conference on Women in Beijing:

"Why are you so angry?" the Sudanese delegate asked. "You have all those rights you want us to accept—artificial birth-control, sterilization, abortion, fetal experimentation."

"Because we want the whole world to have them," the French delegate responded.

Then the Sudanese delegate replied: "But please show me a little window of your paradise, because you have all of these things and you are still not happy. All I see in your world is increased promiscuity among young people, increased divorce, increased abortion, homosexuality, venereal diseases in epidemic proportions. I don't see your paradise."

The French delegate turned away in anger.

In another tragic incident, the Western delegates were trying to pass a dubious proposal entitled "Sexual Rights."

"Sexual rights!" the Moroccan delegate exclaimed in exasperation at the insistence of the West to push programs and so-called rights that would not be even in the imagination of the poor of the world. "I have no idea what level of affluence you people are coming from, but our people need food, clean water, clothing, housing and you are fighting for 'sexual rights.' Can you imagine what my people would think if I go back to my country and I tell them, I did not get you food, I did not get you water, I did not get you clothing or housing, but........I got you SEXUAL RIGHTS!!! They would think I had gone mad!"

Delegates opposed to any section of the Beijing document had the right to make a "reservation" at the end of the conference. "If you don't like what we are doing," we would be told over and over again, "make a reservation." Needless to say, those reservations can be deleted by a new administration that receives more pressure from the West to accept the whole document.

It is a matter of basic principle that family, motherhood, parental rights and moral values do not belong in a "reservation." The words *God, marriage, husband,* and *father* are nowhere to be found.

We pleaded repeatedly with Western delegates to renounce such impositions on our poor nations. Our countries are poorly equipped and would be unable to handle the accompanying consequences of a promiscuous lifestyle, as is happening in the West—sexually transmitted infections in epidemic proportions resulting from the increase in promiscuity among young people, increase of cancer resulting from hormonal therapy and artificial birth-control, increase in prostitution, infections from massive sterilization, artificial birth-control programs and abortion. Why does the West insist on exporting failure? So a few organizations and corporations can make billions of dollars? So a narrow ideology can be imposed on the entire world?

The truly sad reality is that the programs being imposed through the Beijing document are already being practiced in the countries of the West, much to the detriment of their own people. We are talking about abortion, fetal experimentation, sterilization, sex-education programs without morals and values, the usurpation of parental rights, marketing of human organs, the expansion of homosexual practices, and so on. What the Western delegates now want is to expand these evil and degrading programs to the poor nations of the world. After all, poor people are defenseless and they know their only hope is that someone will stand up for them. The poor countries are courageously trying to defend themselves from such calamities, but often they give in so that the Western nations will not single them out and deny them future international loans and assistance.

WHAT CAN ALL OF US DO?

Words are most inadequate to express to the world the drama taking place behind closed doors. Most people on the street ignore the strategies plotted against humanity taking place at the United Nations. The principal questions for us as teachers and educators are "Why?" and "Who is behind it?" Such clever manipulations orchestrated with such precision, particularly over the last thirty years, are no coincidence.

How is it possible that Supreme Court Judges, as well as the President of the most powerful nation on earth, who received, supposedly, the best education from the most prestigious institutions of learning, apparently learned nothing about the difference between good and evil? Surely, they must have been taught that the violation of the natural law, the killing of an innocent human life, born or unborn, is murder. In their pride and arrogance, such heads of state and legislators are questioning the wisdom of the Creator of Nature and the natural law as though they were superior to them. Their blindness is leading us ever deeper into the culture of death, that which the Holy Father has been warning us to change.

THE CULTURE OF DEATH

We are living in a world where a minority of powerful groups and individuals are imposing a secular humanist doctrine on the rest of the world. The sophistical ways in which these powerful adversaries disguise their programs as benevolent protectors of the family are repugnant. The majority of the citizens of the West are not aware that this culture of death, funded with their own taxes, is contributing to their own destruction. In addition, Western populations have been depleted below replacement-levels. According to the UN, the population of the world will begin its decline at the beginning of the next century, at which time, it is predicted that their retirement systems will tumble.[6] The countries of the West already do not have enough tax-paying young people to finance the retirement of each retiree. Hence, the next step of the advocates of the culture of death will be to eliminate the elderly and handicapped by officially legalizing euthanasia by using the subtle arguments of "death with dignity" and "living wills." Already we are witnessing the brainwashing of these populations, preparing people to accept less health-care and to be "considerate" by not becoming a financial burden to future generations. The linguistic "warfare" against the powerless is already taking place. Just as they legalized the killing of the unborn child, they are rushing to pass the legalization of the elimination of the disabled and infirmed.

A few decades ago, an abortionist would be put in jail for his crime. Today those who protest the massive murder of innocent life are the ones being punished and incarcerated. The inborn modesty and natural innocence of the young are being destroyed under the disguise of "sex-education" without morals and values, totally excluding the rights of their parents. Sodomic practices once considered an abomination are now being protected by law. The statistical failure of such programs is ignored and the epidemic of deadly venereal diseases keeps expanding all over the world while special-interest groups continue to profit from the consequences of promiscuous behavior.

THE CULTURE OF LIFE

The future of humanity is in our hands. We must rescue the family from the jaws of darkness. As we enter the third millenium, we must unite with those who are sincerely concerned about the future of mankind. As Pope John Paul II said in his Sunday Angelus address of February 13, 1996, "Authentic love is not a vague sentiment or a blind passion. It is an inner attitude that involves the whole human being. It is looking at others, not to use them but to serve them. It is the ability to rejoice with those who are rejoicing and to suffer with those who are suffering. It is sharing what one possesses so that no one may continue to be deprived of what he needs. Love, in a word, is *the gift of self*.... The family, the great *workshop of love* is the *first school*, indeed, a lasting school where people are not taught to love with barren ideas, but with incisive power of experience. May every family truly rediscover *its own vocation to love!* Love that absolutely respects God's plan, love that *is the choice and reciprocal gift of self* within the family unit."

Our influence as parents and educators can defeat the forces of darkness. We must not underestimate the power of self-control that young people naturally possess and should be challenged to put into practice. "True love waits for marriage" is the answer to their future happiness.

Married couples do not have to remain slaves to the lucrative market of artificial birth-control, sterilization or abortion. By respecting the natural functions of the human body, and being able to space children through the natural regulation of conception (Natural Family Planning), the couple can also increase communication and respect for each other, resulting in dramatically low divorce rates (between 2% to 5%).

In his October 1995 speech to the UN General Assembly, His Holiness Pope John Paul II said:

We must not be afraid of the future. We must not be afraid of man. It is no accident that we are here. Each and every human person has been created in the "image and likeness" of the One Who is the origin of all that is. We have within us the capacities for wisdom and virtue. With these gifts and with the help of God's grace, we can build in the next century and the next millennium a civilization worthy if the human person, a true culture of freedom. We can and must do so! And in so doing, we shall see that the tears of this century have prepared the ground for a new springtime of the human spirit.

NOTES

1. Doctors from around the world include Drs. Evelyn and John Billings from Australia, Kevin Hume from Australia, Sr. Dr. Brigitta Schnell from Tanzania, Dr. Andrew Kjura from Kenya, Dr. Maria Lorena de Casco from Honduras, Dr. Maria Ines Girault from Mexico, Dr. Christine Vollmer from

Venezuela, and Dr. Julian Simon from the United States.

2. "The Human Laboratory" in *Horizon* (Nov. 6, 1995).

3. *Washington Watch*, October 1991.

4. Letter to the Editor, published in *The Washington Post* on July 3, 1992.

5. Robert A. Hatcher, Felicia Stewart, James Trussell, Deborah Kowal, Felicia Guest, Gary K. Stewart, and Willard Cates, *Contraceptive Technology: 1990-1992*, 15th rev. ed. (New York: Irvington Publ., 1990) 70-71.

6. See the graph of this decline in *World Tables*, 3rd ed., Vol. II, World Bank, Recent Demographic Developments in the Member States of the Council of Europe (1986).

CONFRONTING THE LANGUAGE OF THE CULTURE OF DEATH

William Brennan

IN *THE GOSPEL OF LIFE* Pope John Paul II makes an eloquent plea for the creation of a culture of life to displace the encroaching culture of death.[1] This paper focuses primarily on one of the major forces powering the culture of death: the degrading language directed against society's weakest individuals both before and after birth. The terminology underpinning the culture of death consists of an extensive vocabulary of dehumanization that engulfs the most defenseless victims of today as well as throughout history. The paper also explores the significance of positive, life-affirming definitions of the vulnerable for replacing the demeaning rhetoric that has been in use from antiquity to modern times.

SEMANTIC WARFARE AGAINST THE VULNERABLE

The following set of semantic classifications provides a comprehensive framework for detecting and analyzing a host of pejorative expressions invoked to devalue individuals and groups now and in times past: *deficient human, subhuman/nonhuman, lower animal, parasitic creature, infectious disease, inanimate object, waste product*, and *nonperson*. These demeaning designations have been and continue to be so extensively resorted to that they constitute a veritable *war of words*.

The culture of death, then, consists of two wars: a verbal war and a physical war. Sequentially, the verbal war often precedes and leads to the physical war. When applied to abortion, the war of words against the unborn took place in the minds of the perpetrators long before it was implemented in hospitals and clinics. As so aptly stated by Pulitzer Prize winning editor Paul Greenberg of the *Arkansas Democratic-Gazette*: "Those we want out of the way must first be dehumanized.... The least of these must be aborted in words before it becomes permissible to abort them in deed."[2]

Any war, semantic or otherwise, requires an identifiable enemy upon whom to impose the derogatory classifications. At one time or another almost every imaginable racial, ethnic, religious, age, and social group has suffered the consequences of linguistic abuse, ranging from discrimination to outright annihilation. The victimized groups selected for analysis in this study include some of the most oppressed on record: *the unborn* (unwanted human lives before birth in contemporary society), *the dependent and disabled* (mainly young children, people with disabilities, debilitated patients, and the elderly), *women* (past and present), *those exterminated in the Nazi Holocaust* (primarily Jews, but also Gypsies, "asocials," the handicapped, Poles, and others), *the victims of Soviet tyranny* (peasants, religious groups, "deviationists," and others), *African Americans* (especially enslaved blacks before and during the Civil War), and *Native Americans* (North American Indians on the frontier).

Deficient Human. Although those placed under this category are officially acknowledged as members of the human species, it is an ambiguous and questionable status fraught with constant scrutiny and endless qualifications. The imposition of such words as "stupid," "defective," "inferior," "unfit," "potential life," and "lives not worth living" are intended to consign those so labeled to the margins of the human race. The image persistently projected is that of hopelessly flawed human beings whose lives are considered so devoid of value that they can be placed in serious jeopardy and exploited at will.

Today unborn humans are viewed as at best "only potential life,"[3] and severely disabled people are seen as "lives not worth living."[4] Down through the ages, women were frequently characterized as a "defective" and "inferior sex,"[5] Jews and others in the Third Reich as "inferior" life unworthy of life,[6] and peasants in the Soviet Union as a "stupid, turgid people."[7] Black people in the pre-Civil War American South were regarded as a "subordinate and inferior class of beings" incapable of independent existence,[8] and Indians on the frontier as an "inferior" breed destined to disappear with the coming of white civilization.[9]

Subhuman/Nonhuman. For some perpetrators the *deficient human* classification is not demeaning enough because those relegated to this status are still granted recognition, at least implicitly, as members of the human race. In the world of massive oppression, acknowledgement of even a semblance of humanity is often considered too risky. Extensive victimization therefore requires stripping away all vestiges of humanity from the victims and reducing them to totally "subhuman" or "nonhuman" creatures existing entirely outside the most remote borders of the human community.

Contemporary abortion and euthanasia proponents often call their respective victims "not human," "subhuman," "only human forms," and "nothing." Sociologist Amitai Etzioni, for example, once called the so-called "previable" unborn "subhuman and relatively close to a piece of tissue,"[10] while situation-ethics founder Joseph Fletcher referred to the child with Down's syndrome as "a sadly non- or un- or subhuman creature."[11] The expressions "not human" and "nothing" comprise mainstays in the longstanding war of words against women.[12] Images of Jews as "not human," "subhuman," and "nothing" furnished a semantic foundation for racial genocide in Nazi Germany.[13] The designation "not human" was imposed on farmers who resisted the Soviet collectivization of agriculture.[14] Acceptance of slavery was helped along by perceptions of African Americans as "not human" and "subhuman."[15] Portrayals of Native Americans as "not human" and just human "shapes" supplied a rationalization for their extermination on the frontier.[16]

Lower Animal. A commonly employed method of removing undesired individuals completely from membership in the human race is to re-classify them as a species of "lower animals." Animal analogies are meant to denigrate the victims in two basic ways: the victims are reduced to the insignificant level of primitive animals whose fate is of no consequence, or they are portrayed as dangerous, wild beasts that need to be subdued, hunted down, or destroyed.

Today's abortion and euthanasia defenders compare the expendable preborn and born to "lower animals." Neurologist Hart Peterson likens fetal movement to "that of a primitive animal that's poked with a stick"[17] and animal-liberation philosopher Peter Singer reduces severely handicapped infants to a status below that of some animals.[18] For millennia women have been referred to as "domestic animals."[19] The Nazis relegated disabled people to entities "far down in the animal kingdom" and Jews to "experimental animals."[20] Marxists labeled Russian peasants "beasts of burden."[21] Slaveholders viewed African Americans as "work animals" ordained to serve white civilization.[22] Native Americans were frequently maligned as "wild animals" doomed to extinction.[23]

Parasitic Creature. Another degrading metaphor involves relegating the unwanted to the despicable level of "parasites," "vermin," and "lice." The two most common parasitic qualities attributed to undesired human beings are their total dependence on the host and the threat they pose to the survival of the host. The fact that the parasite is an alien organism differing markedly from the host serves as a convenient pretext for depicting vulnerable human beings as a repugnant species with no rightful claim to membership in the human family.

Currently unborn humans are depicted as "parasites" in the woman's body[24] and debilitated patients as "parasites" on the health-care system.[25] Women have been persistently portrayed as "parasites" on men,[26] Jews as "parasites in the body of other peoples,"[27] Kulaks as "parasites" on the Soviet economy,[28] African Americans as "parasites" in need of bondage for survival,[29] and Native Americans as "vermin" necessitating eradication.[30]

Infectious Disease. Likening human beings to "infectious diseases" ranks among the most degrading uses of metaphor. In many instances people suffering from real illnesses have borne an enormous brunt of the disease-infested rhetoric. For the most part, however, the malignant metaphors have nothing to do with real diseases; they are aimed at perfectly healthy human beings whose main deficiency is being unwanted. When combined with the expressions "infection," "contagion," "epidemic," "plague," and "pestilence," disease-analogies are intended to project an ominous image of undesired, vulnerable humans as dangerous epidemics that threaten the health and life of those who count—the wanted segments of society.

Today unwanted pregnancy is defined as an "infection," a "venereal disease" and an "epidemic,"[31] while troublesome patients are viewed as "diseases" and forms of "pathology."[32] Down through the years women have been equated with "plagues" and "contaminations."[33] The Nazi nomenclature is replete with images of Jews as a "pestilence," "plague," and "syphilis."[34] Soviet propagandists reduced their victims to "diseases," "epidemics," and "contagions."[35] Images of black people as a "contagion" and "pestilence" were widely circulated in the American South before and after the Civil War.[36] North American Indians were linked with the spread of "syphilis," "contagions," and "pestilences."[37]

Inanimate Object. The semantic transformation of undesired humans into inanimate objects—mere things with no semblance of personality, humanity, consciousness, or vitality—comprises one of the most radical and pervasive forms of denigration. In this process of extreme objectification, the perpetrators view themselves as owners of others who are reduced to the level of simply "matter" and "material" or as mere "property," "possessions," "merchandise," and "commodities" to be used, exploited, and disposed of at the owner's whim.

Contemporary portrayals feature the unborn as "property" of the woman and "material" for fetal research,[38] and nursing-home patients as discardable "objects."[39] For centuries rape was defined in law, not as violence against the woman, but as "trespass against" another man's "property."[40] The targets of Nazi genocide were processed as "merchandise" for shipment to the death-camps where they were exploited as "experimental material" in terminal research projects and "raw material" in the I.G. Farben factories at Auschwitz.[41] Prisoners in the Soviet Gulag became "raw material" for death-inducing work projects.[42] Slaveowners viewed African Americans as "a species of property" for slave labor and "articles of merchandise" for public auction.[43] Native Americans have been frequently exiled to the status of "anthropological specimens" and "museum pieces."[44]

Waste Product. Equating human beings with noxious "waste matter" places them at the lowermost depths of the subhuman scrap pile. Such terms as "garbage," "trash," "rubbish," "debris," and "refuse" have been invoked against victims at all phases of the human life cycle. The oppressors consider garbage-designations as especially apt characterizations because many victims share the same ultimate fate as real waste-matter: disintegration through incineration.

The epithets "garbage," "refuse," "debris," and "rubbish" are regularly imposed on today's unwanted before and after birth.[45] Women's bodies have been commonly referred to as "sewers" for the emptying of "refuse."[46] Nazi word distorters labeled Jews "garbage," "rubbish," and "trash" for disposal in crematory ovens.[47] People, groups, and ideas viewed with disfavor by the Soviet regime were consigned to "garbage," "debris," "rubbish," and "refuse" on history's "garbage heap."[48] African American culture was once maligned as "a heritage of organic and psychic debris" and slaves as "refuse."[49] Native Americans on the frontier were equated with "garbage" and accused of reducing the environment to a vast "red wasteland."[50]

Nonperson. Among the expressions constructed to devalue human lives, the term "nonperson" is the most devastating epithet of all because it alone has been enshrined into law and a legal nonperson is an entity devoid of basic rights, including, in many instances, the most fundamental right, life itself. "Nonperson" is fast becoming the designation of choice for devaluing human beings before and after birth. It has inaugurated a new litmus test for survival: no longer is one's humanity a sufficient basis for meriting the right to life. One must also be a person, and the definition of personhood required for existence is an increasingly elitist one whereby expanding numbers of individuals are declared expendable and consigned to the rightless category of "legal nonpersons."

In 1973 the U.S. Supreme Court in its *Roe v. Wade* decision ushered in the modern era of legal nonpersonhood by maintaining that "the unborn have never been recognized in the law as persons in the whole sense" and by ruling that "the word 'person,' as used in the Fourteenth Amendment, does not include the unborn."[51] Today the word "nonperson" is increasingly invoked to devalue debilitated patients after birth.[52] Through much of history women as a class have been treated as "less than persons" before the law.[53] A 1936 German high court decision "refused to recognize Jews living in Germany as 'persons' in the legal sense."[54] The designation "unperson" served as a weapon for erasing from public records people purged by the Soviet regime.[55] According to the *Dred Scott* and other court decisions, slaves were defined as "non-citizens" and "nonpersons" under the law.[56] The longstanding assaults on Native American territories and lives by federal agencies and state-governments were based on a perception of the Indian as "not a person within the meaning of the Constitution."[57]

The above examples of defamatory terminology scratch only the surface. Many others can and should be cited along with the extensive documentation that backs them up. A table, "The Semantics of Oppression," containing some of these disparaging classifications and accompanying documentation can be found in *Dehumanizing the Vulnerable: When Word Games Take Lives.* This highly condensed tabular version reveals at a glance the startling similarities among the demeaning expressions and their pervasive scope. *Dehumanizing the Vulnerable* also includes an extensive analysis of these and other degrading designations as well as insights on how to counteract them.[58]

COMBATTING THE SEMANTIC WAR AGAINST THE VULNERABLE

This research points to an urgent need for a major transformation in language, perception, and thought. Such a transformation will involve challenging the degrading designations and replacing them with positive, life-affirming words and phrases. The following comprise six steps that can be taken to counter the escalating war of words:

1. Bring to greater awareness the pervasive scope of the dehumanizing terminology. The degrading words have become a prominent part of the politically correct discourse dominating contemporary society. Many people, however, remain oblivious to how extensively such terminology has taken hold. The public, therefore, needs to be informed each time the expressions *deficient human, non-human/subhuman, lower animal, parasitic creature, infectious disease, inanimate object, waste matter,* and *nonperson* are invoked against the unwanted unborn and born.

A prime illustration of the deeply rooted nature of the name-calling is Supreme Court Justice John Paul Stevens' ringing defense of the nonperson construct in *Planned Parenthood v. Casey* (1992), almost two decades after *Roe v. Wade* first defined human beings before birth as legal nonpersons:

> The Court [in *Roe*] concluded that... 'the unborn have never been recognized in the law as persons in the whole sense.' Accordingly, an abortion is not 'the termination of life entitled to Fourteenth Amendment protection.'
> From this holding, there was no dissent, indeed, no member of the Court has ever questioned this fundamental proposition.[59]

Similar kinds of fully entrenched and deeply degrading portrayals led Supreme Court Chief Justice Roger Brooke Taney to put forth in the *Dred Scott* decision of 1857 the rationale for declaring that Negroes "have never been regarded as a part of the people or citizens of the State":

They had for more than a century before been regarded as beings of an inferior order... and treated as an ordinary article of merchandise. This opinion was at that time fixed and universal in the civilized portion of the white race. It was regarded as an axiom in morals, as well as in politics, which no one thought of disputing or supposed to be open to dispute.[60]

Thus the *Dred Scott, Roe v. Wade,* and *Planned Parenthood v. Casey* decisions—so completely bogged down by the oppressive weight of prejudicial precedents and pejorative stereotypes—have proven to be totally devoid of the expansive vision needed for recognizing black people and unborn children as legitimate human lives entitled to the same rights and protections enjoyed by other members of the human community.

2. *Expose the draconian ideology underpinning the language of the culture of death.* The dehumanizing designations, it should be emphasized, do not suddenly appear out of the blue in a random, chaotic fashion. Instead, behind almost every widespread proliferation of name-calling is some kind of deliberate, systematically-constructed ideology; that is, a philosophy, a social theory, or a set of interrelated ideas, concepts, and myths that generate and sustain the dissemination of pejorative rhetoric.

A prophetic editorial, "A New Ethic for Medicine and Society," which appeared in the September 1970 issue of *California Medicine*, proposes the ideology needed to bring about the public acceptance of abortion and euthanasia—a quality-of-life ethic intended to "violate and ultimately destroy" the Judeo-Christian ethic of "intrinsic and equal value for every human life regardless of its stage, condition, or status," and replace it with an ethic in which "relative rather than absolute values" are placed "on such things as human lives."[61] It is this elitist ideology which is powering today's culture of death. In the practical order it too often translates to mean the quality of life for some at the expense of life for others.

Few have probed the significance of malevolent ideology with keener insight than Aleksandr Solzhenitsyn. He writes:

To do evil a human being must first of all believe that what he's doing is good, or else that it's a well-considered act in conformity with natural law.... Shakespeare's evildoers stopped short at a dozen corpses. Because they had no *ideology*.

Ideology—that is what gives evildoing its long-sought justification and gives the evildoer the necessary steadfastness and determination. That is the social theory which helps to make his acts seem good instead of bad in his own and others' eyes, so that he won't hear reproaches and curses but will receive praise and honors....

Thanks to *ideology*, the twentieth century was fated to experience evildoing on a scale calculated in the millions.[62]

Throughout history a host of ideologies have furnished the theoretical sparks for igniting scores of inflammatory designations accompanied by aggression on a monumental scale. "The Great Chain of Being," an imposing theory which ranked the world's races according to a hierarchy of worth, was invoked to justify atrocities against Indians and Blacks during the 1800s. The myth of Aryan Supremacy generated an extensive nomenclature of defamation that had its most disastrous impact in the Third Reich. The dogma of reproductive freedom is deployed to justify the tyranny of killing human lives inside the womb.

These and other ideologies, whatever their benevolent guise, share one essential ingredient—they are based on a constricted, elitist definition of the human race. And it is this deplorable notion that has fueled and continues to fuel the unrelenting litany of pejorative expressions directed against vulnerable individuals today and in times past.

3. *Uncover the blatant falsity of the disparaging expressions.* These designations, it needs to be reiterated, are pernicious, outlandish stereotypes completely out-of-line with reality and common sense. Phillip Knightley, a close observer of wartime propaganda, once concluded that when war comes, the first casualty is the truth.[63] Consequently, a feature common to any war of words, whomever the victims, is the patent falsehood of the designations concocted. The words fabricated not only degrade the victims but also totally falsify their human nature. Some in the pro-abortion movement have actually made startling admissions about the necessity of bold-faced lying in the service of killing. Such acknowledgements must be brought to public attention. Biology professor Garrett Hardin's rhetoric furnishes a prime example of how recklessly abortion

proponents manipulate language in order to devalue preborn life:

Whether the fetus is or is not a human being is a matter of definition, not fact; and we can define in any way we wish.... It would be unwise to define the fetus as human..., unwise ever to refer to the fetus as an "unborn child."[64]

The sheer arrogance and arbitrariness in Hardin's admonition to make words mean anything one chooses is comparable to Humpty Dumpty's oration on linguistic abuse delivered to Alice in Wonderland. When Alice challenged Humpty Dumpty's definition of glory as "a nice knock-down argument," he replied:

"When I use a word... it means just what I choose it to mean—neither more nor less."
"The question is," said Alice, "whether you can make words mean so many different things."
"The question is," said Humpty Dumpty, "which is to be master—that's all."[65]

Therefore, in abortionland as in wonderland, he who controls words controls thoughts. And eventually language corrupts thought itself.

In addition to identifying the quality-of-life ideology as a means of obtaining public acceptance of abortion and euthanasia, the 1970 *California Medicine* editorial also proposed a flagrant form of lying about the nature of prenatal life: "avoidance of the scientific fact, which everyone really knows, that human life begins at conception." The editorial places this avoidance of the scientific fact about the intrinsic humanity of the unborn under the heading "semantic gymnastics," an apt classification indeed since it connotes the twisting and manipulation of language. The editorial then likens "the very considerable semantic gymnastics which are required to rationalize abortion as anything but taking a human life" to "a schizophrenic sort of subterfuge" and asserts that "this schizophrenic sort of subterfuge is necessary because while a new ethic [the quality-of-life ethic] is being accepted the old one [the sanctity-of-life ethic] has not yet been rejected."[66] The form of duplicity advocated here involves not just a fib, but lying so extreme that it qualifies as a major mental disorder, schizophrenia.

More recently, leading feminist author Naomi Wolf disclosed that the Second Wave feminists of the early 1970s "reacted to the dehumanization of women by dehumanizing the creatures within them": "The fetus-is-nothing paradigm of the pro-choice movement," she admits, is based on deliberate deception. "Clinging to a rhetoric about abortion in which there is no life and no death, we entangle our beliefs in a series of self-delusions, fibs, and evasions." Wolf is especially alarmed that "too often our rhetoric leads us to tell untruths" and to "a hardness of heart," resulting in "callous, selfish and casually destructive men and women who share a cheapened view of life." Her remedy is to take what she considers the high moral ground: "a new abortion rights language" devoid of lying which squares "a recognition of the humanity of the fetus, and the moral gravity of destroying it, with a pro-choice position," a moral framework of "sin and redemption" in which abortion is defined as "a necessary evil" and "the mother must be able to decide that the fetus, in its full humanity, must die."[67]

Wolf's revelations are nothing short of revolutionary. They violate two sacrosanct principles of semantic gymnastics—denial of the humanity of the preborn and the portrayal of abortion as something other than killing. Her call for abandoning the deceitful rhetoric bolstering the killing while continuing to justify the killing, however, is seriously flawed. She fails to comprehend that once the destruction-inducing terminology is exposed for what it is, it would be difficult, if not impossible, to keep on rationalizing the destruction accompanying this terminology. Abortion proponents depend upon the oppressive language to continue justifying their defense of the indefensible.

Whether this atypical foray into the alien world of truth-in-telling constitutes the beginning of the unraveling of the "pro-choice" rhetoric, only time will tell. But it is, nevertheless, a pertinent example to cite in demonstrating the blatant duplicity powering this rhetoric.

4. Reveal the awesome power of semantic gymnastics under socially impeccable auspices. One need only quote again from the *California Medicine* editorial of 1970 to demonstrate the indispensable role played by prestigious individuals in transforming the big lie about abortion and prenatal life into the new truth: "The very considerable semantic gymnastics required to rationalize abortion as anything but taking a human life would be ludicrous if they were not often put forth under *socially impeccable auspices.*"[68]

Not too long ago anyone who went around calling human beings, either before or after birth, "deficient humans," "nonhumans," "animals," "parasites," "diseases," "inanimate objects," "waste products," or "nonpersons" would have been deemed deranged. Today, however, when these ludicrous expressions of semantic gymnastics are put forth under the socially impeccable auspices of organized medicine, academia, the law, or the media elite, they are embraced as gospel. What had once been the undisputed "scientific fact, which everyone really knows, that human life begins at conception" has been reduced to the suspect status of an outmoded, sectarian bias. Thanks to the awesome power of semantic gymnastics in the hands of prestigious purveyors, no longer does everyone really know that human life begins at conception.

It should also be emphasized that throughout history highly respected personages rank among the most steadfast purveyors of degrading terminology. George Washington, a prominent slaveowner, called slaves "a very troublesome species of property."[69] One of America's greatest historians, Francis Parkman, equated Indians with "leeches" and "contagions."[70] Nobel Prize-winning scientist Francis H. Crick once stated that "no newborn infant should be declared human until it has passed certain tests regarding its genetic endowments and that if it fails these tests it forfeits the right to live."[71]

Such revelations are not intended to detract from the monumental achievements of these individuals, but to demonstrate that even they became agents of the prevailing rhetoric. The weakest and most defenseless victims have much more to fear from the relentless outpouring of name-calling constructed by society's so-called "best and brightest" than from the occasional outbursts of invective from mobs in the streets.

Furthermore, it needs to be underscored that the widespread resort to semantic gymnastics in the service of oppression by so many professors, physicians, scientists, jurists, and other impeccable sources constitutes a deplorable assault on some of the core elements intrinsic to any academic discipline or profession—the pursuit of truth, knowledge, and understanding.

5.   *Document   the   extraordinarily   close   kinship   between   the
dehumanizing   designations   of   the   present   and   the   past.*   Today's
perpetrators must be continually confronted with the alarming reality
that the words they are using against the unwanted unborn and born
are, in many instances, the exact same words invoked against some
of history's most reviled peoples.

Whenever, for example, individuals such as astronomer Carl Sagan
call the preborn human "a kind of parasite" that "sucks blood from
capillaries,"[72] they should be made aware that Hitler, Lenin, and
Stalin resorted to identical terminology against their respective
victims: Hitler referred to Jews as "a parasite" that repeatedly
"squeezed and sucked... blood" from "the masses,"[73] Lenin branded
farmers "parasites" that "sucked the blood of the working people,"[74]
and in 1934, after millions of peasants had been eradicated, Stalin
announced "the elimination of the parasitic... kulak-exploiters, the
bloodsucking usurer."[75]

When the radical feminists Lori Andrews and Rachel Conrad
Wahlberg reduce the unborn child to "personal property" and the
woman's "possession,"[76] they need to be reminded that throughout
history some men often defined women as the man's "property"[77]
and the *Dred Scott* decision of 1857 consigned slaves to being "articles
of property."[78]

When doctors such as Martti Kekomaki label aborted babies "just
garbage... just refuse"[79] and emergency room physicians refer to
troublesome patients as "a lot of rubbish,"[80] they should be told that
pornographers portray women's bodies as "sewers" for the emptying
of "refuse,"[81] Nazi extermination specialist Christian Wierth equated
Holocaust victims with "garbage,"[82] 1938 Purge Trial prosecutor
Andrei Vyshinsky maligned former Communist officials as a "heap
of human garbage,"[83] Virginia plantation-owner William Fitzhugh
relegated black slaves to the status of "refuse,"[84] and poet Christopher
Brooke characterized Native Americans on the frontier as "garbage...
of Earth."[85]

When the wording in *Roe v. Wade* is cited to justify reducing the
unborn to the status of legal nonpersons, it should be compared with
the wording in court decisions of the past defining other groups as
nonpersons before the law:

"The word 'person,' as used in the Fourteenth Amendment, does not
    include the unborn." (*Roe v. Wade*, 1973)[86]
"The word 'person' as used in the act could not rightly be interpreted to
    include women in those entitled to sit in the House of Lords."
    (*Viscountess Rhonda's Claim*, 1922)[87]
"The unborn have never been recognized in the law as persons." (*Roe v.
    Wade*, 1973)[88]
"In the eyes of the law... the slave is not a person." (*Bailey et al. v.
    Poindexter's Ex'or*, 1858)[89]
"The unborn have never been recognized in the law as persons." (*Roe v.
    Wade*, 1973)[90]
"Standing Bear was not... a person under the law." (District Attorney,
    Standing Bear v. Crook, 1879)[91]

Thus a compelling way of discrediting today's dehumanizing
rhetoric is to document how it ranks with the most extreme forms
of name-calling in the annals of inhumanity.

6. *Replace the language of dehumanization with a life-affirming lexicon
of humanization.* It is not enough to curse the darkness by revealing
the pervasiveness, shortcomings, perniciousness, falsity, and absurdity
of the demeaning terminology. Positive, life-affirming
characterizations of vulnerable individuals at risk possess an
enormous potential in their own right for challenging and
supplanting the derogatory rhetoric. Even during historical periods
when the most defamatory definitions of the oppressed dominated
the public consciousness, countervailing voices could be heard
referring to those being victimized as "human beings," "brothers,"
"sisters," "men," "women," "brethren," and "children." Today right-
to-life proponents, disability-rights activists, and like-minded
defenders of society's most defenseless groups are employing the same
life-sustaining words to counter the demeaning designations
prevailing against undesired human beings inside and outside the
womb. Forging links between the humanizing images of the present
and the past places the contemporary pro-life movement where it
rightfully belongs: on common ground with the great human rights
movements throughout history.

In today's world where the global slaughter of the unborn is
dismissed as the mere removal of "fetal material" and "waste
products," Pope John Paul II emphasizes the urgent need "*to call*

things by their proper names." Words celebrating the humanity and sacredness of all human lives, especially the most defenseless individuals, comprise a cornerstone of his compelling, evangelical call for building a new and enduring culture of love and life.[92]

Against the contemporary view of severely disabled persons as parasitic, vegetative lives not worth living, nursing-administrator Jeryl Turco opposed the removal of a feeding-tube from Nancy Ellen Jobes by insisting that Jobes "is not a vegetable but a human being who is as deserving of food and water as you and I."[93]

When characterizations of women as inferior beings, plagues, and domestic animals dominated the historical scene, the Bible served as an authoritative source for calling attention to the equality, humanity, nobility, and spirituality of women.[94]

Aleksandr Solzhenitsyn countered the Soviet regime's definitions of prisoners as raw material for slave labor in the Arctic death-camps of the Gulag with portrayals of them as "human beings," "wise spiritual beings," "our own people," "the innocent," "my own Brothers."[95] On August 3, 1941 in response to the thousands of mentally ill and handicapped patients being exterminated in German hospitals and institutions, Bishop August von Galen gave a powerful anti-euthanasia sermon in which he declared: "We are speaking here of human beings, of our neighbors, our brothers and sisters."[96] While African American slaves were being sold as "articles of merchandise," Angelina Grimke asserted, "Man cannot rightfully hold his fellow man as property."[97] When the war of words against Native Americans was at its zenith during the 19th century, Lydia Maria Child in her *An Appeal for the Indians* maintained that North America's original inhabitants were "human beings," "members of the human family," and "red brethren."[98]

CONCLUSION

Exposing the pernicious nature of denigrating language and substituting positive, personalized terminology will not alone put an end to massive oppression, but they constitute long overdue steps toward achieving such an essential goal. The war against the vulnerable will never end until the war of words against them also ceases and is replaced by a vocabulary of life-supporting designations. The purpose of historical inquiry is not merely to learn about the past, but also to learn about the present from the past. The comprehensive set of degrading classifications and their life-affirming replacements furnish indispensable frameworks for a better understanding of what happened then and how it relates to what is happening now. Heightened awareness of these past and present linguistic parallels provides an essential perspective for recognizing and challenging modern-day threats to human life before and after birth as constituting an unconscionable repetition of some of history's most horrendous atrocities. Only when we draw lessons from the past, and apply them to the present, can there be hope for the future.

NOTES

1. Pope John Paul II, *The Gospel of Life [Evangelium Vitae]* (Boston: Daughters of St. Paul, 1995).

2. Paul Greenberg, "The Power of a Cartoon" in *National Right to Life News* (13 Dec. 1994) 18.

3. *Roe v. Wade*, 410 U.S. 159 (1973).

4. "Care for Retarded in Dispute on Coast" in *The New York Times* (26 Nov. 1978) 38.

5. Arthur Schopenhauer, *Essays: From the Parerga and Paralipomena: Studies in Pessimism*, trans. T. Bailey Saunders (London: George Allen and Unwin, 1951) 65, 68.

6. Robert Proctor, *Racial Hygiene: Medicine Under the Nazis* (Cambridge: Harvard Univ. Press, 1988) 175, 215.

7. Robert Conquest, *The Harvest of Sorrow: Soviet Collectivization and the Terror-Famine* (New York: Oxford Univ. Press, 1986) 20.

8. *Dred Scott v. Sanford*, 19 Howard 404 (1857).

9. Richard Drinnon, *Facing West: The Metaphysics of Indian-Hating and Empire Building* (Minneapolis: Univ. of Minnesota Press, 1980) 140.

10. Amitai Etzioni, "A Review of the Ethics of Fetal Research" in *Society* (March-April 1976) 72.

11. Joseph F. Fletcher, "The Right to Die: A Theologian Comments" in *Atlantic Monthly* (April 1968) 62.

12. Lloyd Vogelman, *The Sexual Face of Violence: Rapists on Rape* (Johannesburg: Ravan Press, 1990) 68-69; Otto Weininger, *Sex and Character* (New York: AMS Press, 1975) 286, 297.

13. C. C. Aronsfeld, "The Nazi Design Was Extermination, Not Emigration" in *Patterns of Prejudice* 9 (May-June 1975) 22; Clarissa Henry and Marc Hillel, *Of Pure Blood*, trans. Eric Mossbacher (New York: McGraw-Hill, 1976) 32.

14. Vasily Grossman, *Forever Flowing*, trans. Thomas P. Whitney (New York: Harper & Row, 1972) 144.

15. Ariel [Buckner H. Payne], *The Negro: What Is His Ethnological Status?* (Cincinnati, 1867) 21; William T. English, "The Negro Problem from the Physician's Point of View" in *Atlanta Journal-Record of Medicine* 5 (October 1903) 466, 468.

16. Daniel Marder, ed., *A Hugh Henry Brackenridge Reader, 1770-1815* (Pittsburgh: Univ. of Pittsburgh Press, 1970) 100.

17. "Abortion Controversy—The Silent Scream" in *Nightline*, transcript #972 (12 February 1985) 3.

18. Peter Singer, "Sanctity of Life or Quality of Life?" in *Pediatrics* 129 (July 1983) 72.

19. H. R. Hays, *The Dangerous Sex: The Myth of Feminine Evil* (New York: G. P. Putnam's Sons, 1964) 201.

20. Karl Binding and Alfred Hoche, *Permitting the Destruction of Unworthy Life: Its Extent and Forms*, trans. Walter E. Wright (1920), reprinted in *Issues in Law and Medicine* 18 (Fall 1992) 262; Philippe Aziz, *Doctors of Death*, trans. Edouard Bizub and Philip Haentzler, 4 vols. (Geneva, Switzerland: Ferni, 1976) 1:232.

21. Esther Kingston-Mann, "Marxism and Russian Rural Development: Problems of Evidence, Experience, and Culture" in *American Historical Review* 4 (Oct. 1981) 742.

22. *American Slavery As It Is: Testimony of a Thousand Witnesses* (1839; reprint: New York: Arno Press and The New York Times, 1968) 110.

23. Dr. Josiah C. Nott, "Statistics of Southern Slave Population" in *De Bow's Review* 4 (Nov. 1847) 280.

24. L. W. Sumner, *Abortion and Moral Theory* (Princeton: Princeton Univ. Press, 1981) 52, 67, 71.

25. Interview with Janine Thomas (pseudonym), intensive care nurse (27 May 1989).

26. Rene Guyon, *Sexual Freedom*, 2nd ed., trans. Eden and Cedar Paul (New York: Knopf, 1958) 207.

27. Adolph Hitler, *Mein Kampf*, trans. Ralph Manheim (Boston: Houghton Mifflin, 1943) 304.

28. V. I. Lenin, *Collected Works*, trans. Joe Fineburg and George Hanna, 45 vols. (Moscow: Foreign Languages Publishing House, 1960-70) 27:396.

29. Daniel Drake, *Letters on Slavery to Dr. John C. Warren, April 3, 5, and 6, 1851* (New York: Schuman's, 1940) 31.

30. Francis Parkman, *The Conspiracy of Pontiac and the Indian War After the Conquest of Canada*, 2 vols. (Boston: Little, Brown, 1897-98) 2:42.

31. Willard Cates, David A. Grimes, and Jack C. Smith, "Abortion as a Treatment for Unwanted Pregnancy: The Number Two Sexually-Transmitted Condition" in *Advances in Planned Parenthood* 12/3 (1978) 115-21.

32. Terry Mizrahi, *Getting Rid of Patients: Contradictions in the Socialization of Physicians* (New Brunswick: Rutgers Univ. Press, 1986) 101.

33. Hugh Lloyd-Jones, *Females of the Species: Semonides on Women* (Park Ridge: Noyes Press, 1975) 54; Simone de Beauvoir, *The Second Sex*, trans. H. M. Parshley (New York: Vintage Books, 1974) 168.

34. Hitler, *Mein Kampf* 58, 78, 249-53.

35. Lenin, *Collected Works* 18:432, 24:54; Conquest, *Harvest of Sorrow* 199.

36. William Lloyd Garrison, *Thoughts on African Colonization* (1832; reprint: New York: Arno Press and The New York Times, 1968) 125; Sterling A. Brown, "American Race Problem Reflected in American Literature" in *Journal of Negro Education* 8 (July 1939) 281.

37. Parkman, *Conspiracy of Pontiac* 2:123; Francis Parkman, *The Jesuits in North America in the Seventeenth Century*, 2 vols. (Boston: Little, Brown, 1902) 2:224; Sherburne F. Cook, *The Conflict Between the California Indians and White Civilization* (Berkeley and Los Angeles: Univ. of California Press, 1976) 26-27, 270.

38. Lori Andrews, "My Body, My Property" in *The Hastings Center Report* 16 (Oct. 1986) 37; Ake Seiger, "Collection and Use of Aborted Central Nervous System Material" in *Fetal Therapy* 3 (1988) 8-13.

39. Andrea Fontana, *The Last Frontier: The Social Meaning of Growing Old* (Beverly Hills: Sage Publications, 1977) 144, 155-56.

40. Susan Brownmiller, *Against Our Will: Men, Women, and Rape* (New York: Simon and Schuster, 1975) 17-18, 163.

41. Claude Lanzmann, *Shoah: An Oral History of the Holocaust, The Complete Text of the Film* (New York: Pantheon Books, 1975) 103-04; Nürnberg Military Tribunals, *Trials of War Criminals*, 15 vols. (Washington, D.C.: U.S. Government Printing Office, 1945-47) 1:142; Joseph Borkin, *The Crime and Punishment of I.G. Farben* (New York: The Free Press, 1978) 126.

42. Aleksandr Solzhenitsyn, *The Gulag Archipelago, 1918-1956: An Experiment in Literary Investigation*, 3 vols. (New York: Harper & Row, 1973-74) 2:104.

43. Kenneth M. Stampp, *That Peculiar Institution: Slavery in the Ante-Bellum South* (New York: Alfred A. Knopf, 1968) 204; *Dred Scott v. Sanford*, 19 Howard 393 (1857).

44. Frederick E. Hoxie, "Red Man's Burden" in *Antioch Review* 37 (Summer 1979) 336-38; Donald A. Kaufmann, "The Indian as Media Hand-Me-Down" in *Colorado Quarterly* 23 (Spring 1975) 503.

45. Naomi Wade, "Aborted Babies Kept Alive for Bizarre Experiments" in *National Examiner* (19 August 1980) 20-21; Dorothea Kersale and Donn Casey, "Abortion Induced by Means of the Uterine Aspirator" in *Obstetrics & Gynecology* 30 (July 1967) 37, 43; Roger Jeffrey, "Normal Rubbish: Deviant Patients in Casualty Departments" in *Sociology of Health and Illness* 1 (June 1979) 92, 94.

46. Henry Miller, *Quiet Days in Clichy and The World of Sex: Two Books* (New York: Grove Press, 1978) 110.

47. Gitta Sereny, *Into That Darkness: From Mercy Killing to Mass Murder* (London: Andre Deutsch, 1974) 201; David S. Wyman, *The Abandonment of the Jews: America and the Holocaust, 1941-1945* (New York: Pantheon Books, 1984) 4; Leon Poliakov, *Harvest of Hate: The Nazi Program for the Destruction of the Jews of Europe*, revised and expanded edition (New York: Schocken Books, Holocaust Library, 1979) 115, 128.

48. Robert C. Tucker and Stephen F. Cohen, eds., *The Great Purge Trial* (New York: Grosset & Dunlap, 1965) 520; Lenin, *Collected Works* 1:353; 26:480; 14:313.

49. English, "Negro Problem" 469; Willie Lee Rose, ed., *A Documentary History of Slavery in North America* (New York: Oxford Univ. Press, 1976) 40.

50. Richard F. Berkhofer, *The White Man's Indian: Images of the American Indian from Columbus to the Present* (New York: Alfred A. Knopf, 1978) 20; Theodore Roosevelt, *The Strenuous Life: Essays and Addresses* (New York: Century Company, 1902) 38.

51. *Roe v. Wade*, 410 U.S. 162 (1973).

52. Michael Tooley, *Abortion and Infanticide* (Oxford: Oxford Univ. Press, 1983) 411-12.

53. *Commonwealth v. Welosky*, 177 *North Eastern Reporter* 660 (1931).

54. Ernst Fraenkel, *The Dual State: A Contribution to the Theory of Dictatorship*, trans. E.A. Shils with Edith Lowenstein and Klaus Knorr (New York: Oxford Univ. Press, 1941) 95.

55. "1984 Revisited," a CBS television special, narrated by Walter Cronkite (7 June 1983).

56. *Dred Scott v. Sanford*, 19 Howard 404 (1857); *Bailey v. Poindexter's Ex'or*, 14 Grattan 432 (1858).

57. George F. Canfield, "The Legal Position of the Indian" in *American Law Review* 15 (January 1881) 28, 33.

58. William Brennan, *Dehumanizing the Vulnerable: When Word Games Take Lives* (Chicago: Loyola Univ. Press, 1995).

59. "Excerpts from the Justices' Decision in the Pennsylvania Case" in *The New York Times* (30 June 1992) A8.

60. *Dred Scott v. Sanford*, 19 Howard 411-12 (1857).

61. "A New Ethic for Medicine and Society" in *California Medicine* 113 (Sept. 1970) 67-68.

62. Solzhenitsyn, *Gulag Archipelago* 1:173-74.

63. Phillip Knightley, *The First Casualty: From the Crimea to Vietnam: The War Correspondent as Hero, Propagandist, and Myth Maker* (New York and London: Harcourt, Brace, Jovanovich, A Harvest Book, 1975).

64. Garrett Hardin, "Abortion—Or Compulsory Pregnancy?" in *Journal of Marriage and the Family* 30 (May 1968) 250-51.

65. Lewis Carroll, *Through the Looking Glass and What Alice Found There* (London: Macmillan, 1872) 124.

66. "A New Ethic for Medicine and Society" 67-68.

67. Naomi Wolf, "Our Bodies, Our Souls" in *New Republic* (16 Oct. 1995) 26-35.

68. "A New Ethic for Medicine and Society" 68.

69. David Brion Davis, *The Problem of Slavery in the Age of Revolution, 1770-1823* (Ithaca and London: Cornell Univ. Press, 1975) 171.

70. Francis Parkman, *The Oregon Trail: Sketches of Prairie and Rocky Mountain Life* (Boston: Little, Brown, 1925) 173; Parkman, *Conspiracy of Pontiac* 1:243, 2:123.

71. Francis A. Schaeffer and C. Everett Koop, *What Happened to the Human Race?* (Old Tappan: Fleming H. Revell, 1979) 73.

72. Carl Sagan and Ann Druyan, "Is It Possible to Be Pro-Life and Pro-Choice?" in *Parade Magazine* (22 April 1990) 6.

73. Hitler, *Mein Kampf* 313.

74. Lenin, *Collected Works* 27:396; 28:56-58.

75. Josef V. Stalin, *Works*, 13 vols. (Moscow: Foreign Languages Publishing House, 1953-55) 13:340, 342.

76. Andrews, "My Body, My Property" 37; Rachel Conrad Wahlberg, "The Woman and the Fetus: One Flesh?" in *New Women/New Church* (September-October, 1987) 5.

77. Francis Power Cobbe, "Wife-Torture in England" in *The Contemporary Review* (April 1878) 62.

78. *Dred Scott v. Sanford*, 19 Howard 393 (1857).

79. Naomi Wade, "Aborted Babies Kept Alive for Bizarre Experiments" in *National Examiner* (19 August 1980) 20-21.

80. Jeffrey, "Normal Rubbish: Deviant Patients in Casualty Departments" 92, 94.

81. Henry Miller, *Black Spring* (New York: Grove Press, An Evergreen Black Cat Book, 1963) 144.

82. Gitta Sereny, *Into That Darkness: From Mercy Killing to Mass Murder* (London: Andre Deutsch), 1974) 201.

83. Tucker and Cohen, *The Great Purge Trial* 520.

84. William Lee Rose, ed., *A Documentary History of Slavery in North America* (New York: Oxford Univ. Press, 1976) 40.

85. Berkhofer, *The White Man's Indian* 20.

86. *Roe v. Wade*, 410 U.S. 162 (1973).

87. Cited in *Commonwealth v. Welosky*, 177 *North Eastern Reporter* 660 (1931).

88. *Roe v. Wade*, 410 U.S. 162 (1973).

89. *Bailey et al. v. Poindexter's Ex'or*, 14 Grattan 432 (1858).

90. *Roe v. Wade*, 410 U.S. 162 (1973).

91. Kay Graber, ed., *The Ponca Chiefs: An Account of the Trial of Standing Bear* (Lincoln: Univ. of Nebraska Press, 1972) 92.

92. Pope John Paul II, *Gospel of Life*, #58, pp. 94-95.

93. Jeryl Turco, "A Message to the Community and Staff of Morristown Memorial Hospital," advertisement in *Daily Record* (Northwest New Jersey, 2 August 1987).

94. Katherine Usher Henderson and Barbara F. McManus, eds., *Half Humankind: Contexts and Texts of the Controversy about Women in England, 1540-1640* (Urbana and Chicago: Univ. of Illinois Press, 1985) 49.

95. Solzhenitsyn, *Gulag Archipelago* 1:549, 184, 614, 76, 549.

96. August Clemens von Galen, *The Bishop of Munster and the Nazis: The Documents in the Case*, trans. and ed. Patrick Smith (London: Burns Oates, 1943) 43-45.

97. Hugh Hawkins, ed., *The Abolitionists: Means, Ends, and Motivations* (Lexington: D. C. Heath, 1972) 59.

98. Lydia Maria Child, *An Appeal for the Indians* (New York: William P. Tomlinson, 1868) 8, 10, 14-15.

ABORTION AND NAZISM:
IS THERE REALLY A CONNECTION?

John Hunt

SHE USED THE WORDS "shallow" and "disgraceful," or words like these, as I recall, in describing William Brennan's work, *The Abortion Holocaust*, in which he connects many of the actions and attitudes of those who believe in legalized abortion with many of the actions and attitudes of the Nazis.[1] She was the commentator on a panel devoted to reproductive policies at the Fall 1994 meeting of the New England Historical Association.[2]

Right To Life groups certainly do make the connection between abortion and the Nazi Holocaust. Brennan's work is the best known when it comes to making this connection. In the beginning of his book he compares abortion in the United States today to the killing of "postnatal discards" by the Nazis, that this linkage involves the "universality of the victimization process."[3]

Brennan's work came on the heels of many others who drew the same parallel. Let us observe just a few examples:

- *The National Catholic Register* stated on May 13, 1979: "Six million is the number generally assigned not only to Jews who died under Hitler but to babies who have died under the Supreme Court."[4]
- A sign at a 1979 RTL convention read: "Auschwitz, Dachau, and Margaret Sanger, Three of a Kind."[5]
- *The Abolitionist*, an anti-abortion newsletter published in Pittsburgh, stated: "We are not headed for a Holocaust. We are living in the very midst of one."[6]
- *The Wanderer*, a Roman Catholic periodical, has stated that there is no difference between the U. S. Supreme Court that legalized abortion and the Nazi civil service that carried out the final solution."[7]
- Terence Cooke, former Cardinal of New York, has stated: "Buchenwald, Dachau, Auschwitz—they say it would never happen here. But it has already happened. It is happening all around right

now." The Cardinal was referring to legalized abortion.[8]

■ C. Everett Koop, distinguished physician and former Surgeon General of the United States, in 1977 came up with the slippery slope idea when he wrote: "...I see the progression from abortion to infanticide, to euthanasia, to the problems that developed in Nazi Germany.... I guess I favor the title: 'The Subtle, Slippery Slope to Auschwitz'."[9]

It is still William Brennan's work, *The Abortion Holocaust*, however, which makes the most thorough attempt to establish the connection between abortion and the Nazis. This paper has neither the time nor the space to analyze all of Brennan's arguments. What this paper will do, is to address itself to the specific criticisms made by those who say that there are no parallels between abortion and the Nazi Holocaust. It will then analyze these criticisms.

CRITICISM OF THE ABORTION-NAZI CONNECTION

We will analyze here the statements of five prominent organizations and three prominent individuals. These organizations and individuals have had an important influence in this country concerning the subjects of Nazism and/or abortion.

The National Organization of Women (NOW) has been in favor of legalized abortion since its founding in 1966. Perhaps because of its interest in many issues relating to women other than abortion, it is not interested in the very specific issue of abortion and a Nazi connection. NOW has no official position on the subject.[10]

The Holocaust affected Jews more than anyone. Due to the percentage killed and the deliberate singling out of Jews by the Nazis, the Jews suffered more than anyone.[11] Yet, the Anti-Defamation League has told me concerning Nazism and abortion: "We have nothing on this."[12]

An organization that has pushed for legalized abortion since the death of its founder, Margaret Sanger, in the mid-1960s is Planned Parenthood. When queried about a position concerning abortion and Nazis, an official of Planned Parenthood told me that they usually "do not dignify" with a statement, right-to-life charges of a connection.[13] I took this answer to be like the positions of NOW and the Anti-Defamation League, i.e., no position. Later, the representative informed me that she was unable to locate anything written or specific about Planned Parenthood's position on abortion and the Holocaust.[14]

I then turned to the American Civil Liberties Union (ACLU). This organization, along with NOW and Planned Parenthood, had pushed hard since the mid-1960ˢ (especially in court) for legalized abortion. Yet, when it came to a refutation of any connection between legalized abortion and Nazism, the ACLU had no official position. A speaker for the group did inform me orally that the Nazis performed abortions for eugenic reasons, while the ACLU did not have this motive in pushing for legalized abortion.[15] The only other response to the subject was an article written by the former head of the ACLU, Aryeh Neier, in the *Civil Liberties Newsletter*, a publication by the ACLU in the 1960ˢ and 1970ˢ. Neier, a Jewish refugee from Nazism, claimed that anti-abortionists, not pro-abortionists, were closer to the Nazi position,[16] a charge this paper will analyze.

These pro-legalization-of-abortion sources had no official position on the subject, although their unofficial positions are clear. Let us analyze four other pro-legalization forces that do take an official position on the subject.

We will begin with the National Abortion and Reproductive Rights Action League. This is the third name of this organization, but it has always used the acronym NARAL. Founded in 1969 by Betty Friedan, Lawrence Lader, Bernard Nathanson and others, the purpose of the organization was to make abortion legal and keep it legal. Unlike NOW, whose interests in women go far beyond the issue of abortion, NARAL has concentrated solely on this issue and, as a result, has had much influence. It is perhaps only natural that they would have a position on our question under discussion. The NARAL position is this:

Hitler used racial grounds to exterminate Jews and other "undesirables." The reproductive rights movement has no genocide component—no one is out to kill all embryos. It is an insult to the memory of the alive and conscious human beings murdered by the Nazis to equate them with embryos for anti-abortion propaganda.[17]

A careful reading here can discern two points: (1) legalized abortion is not genocide; and (2) the unborn are not (it is implied) human.

NARAL also maintains that Nazism was anti-abortion, and thus implies that those who are anti-abortion today are the ones closer to Nazism.[18] So they also make a third argument, that of anti-choice.

Gloria Steinem, a leading feminist, founder of *Ms* magazine, and author, makes the same three arguments in an essay written in 1980, but not published until 1983; the same year as the NARAL position was adopted. The essay is entitled: "If Hitler Were Alive, Whose Side Would He Be On?," and became an unnumbered chapter in her 1983 book *Outrageous Acts and Everyday Rebellions.*[19]

Specifically, Steinem here points out that Afro-Americans have a higher abortion rate than whites because of lack of access to good health care and contraception.[20] Legalized abortion is not genocide as is often charged.

She makes much of Hitler's demanding the subordination of the individual to the Nazi state and how this hurt the feminists in Germany. Her emphasis here is on born females, and she does not address herself to the unborn.[21] The implication here, as in the NARAL position, is that the unborn are not worth counting.

Finally, Steinem mentions the sterilizations and forced abortions carried out by the Nazis, but condemns them only because they were involuntary. Here we have that third argument, i.e., the Nazis were against choice.[22]

Whereas NARAL mentioned Nazi anti-abortion policies as being against choice, Steinem emphasizes forced abortions as being against choice. This is a critical distinction and will be explained more later; *it involves a discussion of the nature of abortion itself, that is, why the Nazis forbade it to one group but forced it on others.* Steinem uses phrases such as "anti-equality groups," "authoritarianism," and "right-wing" throughout the chapter to describe groups that are anti-individualistic, racist, sexist, and afraid of change. To her, pro-life people fit here and are thus closer to Nazis than are pro-choice people.[23]

We turn now to Ellen Goodman, author and influential syndicated newspaper columnist. In one of her columns she echoes two of the three arguments put forth by NARAL and Steinem. Agreeing with Argument #2 of NARAL and Steinem—the implication that the unborn are something less than human—she states: "Anti-abortion groups talk about the abortion-holocaust—comparing fetuses to Jews and the doctors [who do the abortions] to Joseph Mengele."[24]

Again, like NARAL and Steinem, but particularly like NARAL, she invokes Argument #3, that of choice: "As far as pinning the Nazi label on the supporters of abortion rights, the propagandists surely know that Hitler was a hard-line opponent of abortion. (Did that make him pro-life?). Tell the ditto-heads [right-to-lifers] that feminists were a prime target of the Nazis."[25]

Finally, we must explore the work of Professor Robert Weisbord. Professor Weisbord is not as well known as the groups and people mentioned so far. Weisbord, however, who is a history professor at the University of Rhode Island, teaches a course on the Holocaust, and has written four books and thirty articles on Jewish and Black history. He represents, therefore, a good bit of pro-choice thought in academia, especially our topic under discussion.

Weisbord's arguments are contained in an article entitled: "Legalized Abortion and the Holocaust: An Insulting Parallel," which he wrote for a Jewish publication. His arguments concern questions of the unborn's humanity (#2), and the argument about choice (#3). Here he is like Ellen Goodman. Let us deal here with his choice argument first. Like NARAL, Steinem, and Goodman, Weisbord stresses the anti-choice elements in Nazi abortion thinking. NARAL and Goodman, you might recall, stressed Nazi anti-abortion policies as being against choice, while Steinem emphasized forced abortions as being against choice. In this matter, Weisbord stresses both when he says: "Thus the Nazis followed a coercive pro-natalist policy for fellow Germans and a coercive anti-natalist policy for vanquished peoples. Denial of reproductive freedom, the absence of truly free choice, and disregard for women's rights were the common elements."[26]

Weisbord, more than anyone else, focuses attention on the nature of abortion itself, by focusing on the question of why the Nazis forbade it to healthy Germans but forced it on unhealthy Germans and non-Germans. This is the second time we raise this question in this paper. Weisbord condemns both (those who forbid and those who force abortion). He implies that if a woman wants an abortion she should be allowed to have one, and that if she does not want one, she should not have it imposed on her. The whole focus is on the born woman and her choice, and not the unborn life involved.

This brings us to his statements about unborn life (#2). NARAL, Steinem, and Goodman only imply that a fetus is not fully human; Weisbord comes right out and says that it definitely is not:

We must never forget who the principal targets of the Nazis were... men, women and children, each possessing his or her own name, identity and personality. They were living, human beings. How can any reasonable person liken them to the fetuses destroyed when unwanted pregnancies are terminated? The fetuses in question do not exist independently of their mothers in whose wombs they are nourished and nurtured.... The destruction of a fertilized egg, we are told, is the moral equivalent of gassing or shooting a human being because he is a Jew. Surely, to equate the two is to trivialize the tragedy of the Holocaust.... The equation of legalized abortion and the Holocaust... is more than deceitful. It is insulting to the memory of the six million who perished in the nightmare of Nazism.[27]

Weisbord's article contains a picture of a Jew just before being shot by a Nazi, and this is juxtaposed against a picture of a six week old fetus. There is a caption stating that the two can hardly be equated.[28]

Hence, to Weisbord, the unborn are not human (#2), and thus the choice (#3) of whether or not to terminate a pregnancy should be left to the born woman. In the beginning of his article, which I will use here to summarize, he states: "In their zeal to buttress their case, anti-abortionists often show symptoms of that age-old malady, selective historical amnesia."[29]

AN ANALYSIS OF THE CRITICISMS

To repeat, the criticisms of those who say there is no connection between Nazism and abortion can be boiled down to three points:

(1) Legalized abortion is *not genocide*—this is the view of NARAL and the unofficial view of the ACLU.
(2) The unborn are *not human*—this is implied by NARAL, Steinem, Goodman, but stated openly by Weisbord.
(3) The Nazis, like pro-lifers, were *against choice*—all four of those with officially stated positions (NARAL, Steinem, Goodman, Weisbord) make this point, while at least three other organizations (NOW, Planned Parenthood, ACLU) would no doubt agree, even though they have not made official statements.

Let us analyze each of these three points.

(1) Legalized abortion is *not genocide*—the dictionary defines "genocide" this way: "the deliberate and systematic extermination of national, racial, political, or cultural group."[30] Another definition comes from Raphael Lemkin in his book, *Axis Rule in Europe*, published in 1944. Lemkin is the one who actually coined the term "genocide." He states that genocide is "the coordinated and planned annihilation of a national, religious, or racial group by a variety of actions aimed at undermining the foundations essential to the survival of the group as a group."[31]

These two definitions would seem to back the NARAL and ACLU criticisms. According to the two, genocide must be "systematic" or "planned," in other words, deliberate. In addition, the deliberate killing must be aimed at a specific racial, religious, national, political, or cultural group. Since legalized abortion cuts across racial, religious, national, political, and cultural (even gender and class) lines, no one group is deliberately singled out, hence no genocide is involved.

I would like to fine-tune this definition. On December 11, 1946, the United Nations General Assembly passed this resolution concerning genocide: "Genocide is the denial of the right of existence to *entire human groups* [emphasis mine].... Many instances of such crimes of genocide have occurred, when racial, religious, political and *other groups* [emphasis mine] have been destroyed, entirely or in part."[32] "Entire human groups... destroyed... in part" can mean the unborn: those killed for reasons of age, size, stage of development, and temporary place of residence. A law legalizing abortion victimizes an identifiable group of human beings who are just at the start of life's continuum. Even though most unborn are not aborted, the abortion laws in the United States and most western countries *deliberately classify the unborn, as a group*, as being vulnerable to abortion. These laws fit, I believe, into the United Nation's definition of genocide. We must remember that those guilty of genocide do not necessarily kill all members of a given group.

In 1948, the United Nations elaborated on this 1946 resolution with its Convention on the Prevention and Punishment of the Crime of Genocide. Article II condemns as genocide the "imposing of measures intended to prevent births within the [targeted] group."[33]

For many of the born, laws legalizing abortion seem to allow choice; for the unborn, however, those laws certainly are impositions.

Finally, with regard to the matter of genocide and its connection specifically to Nazism, *is it not strange that, with all of the things associated with the Nazis, and condemned by the Nuremberg Trials after World War II, abortion was one of them?* In the RuSHA, or Greifelt Case, the Tribunals condemned Nazi activity in the eastern part of Europe, activities that included murder, deportations, expropriation, enslavement, torture, the kidnapping of children, forced Germaniza-tion of enemy nationals, special persecution of the Jews, and abortion.[34] The prosecutor, in his summation at the RuSHA Trial, stated that abortion, voluntary or forced, was "an act of extermina-tion," and "ill-treatment of a civilian population."[35] *Thus, abortions were used as one of the means of the Nazi genocide.* There is a connection between abortion, in general, and the Nazi Holocaust, in particular, in the matter of genocide.

(3) The Nazis, like pro-lifers, were *against choice*—let us consider this argument before #2. If the unborn are not human, then what the Nazis did was wrong because it was forced or pressured, and because they systematically applied it just to certain groups. The Nazis, in other words, would have violated the born in the matter of abortion. We can deal with this briefly by asking: *Is it not strange, that what many today see as a woman's liberty, Nazis saw as a very useful and efficient means of killing?* Who is right? The question brings us back to the second (and final) argument.

(2) The unborn are not *human*—it is a biological fact that human life is a continuum. It is true that the unborn, as distinct from the born, are very small, young, out of sight, and very dependent on the born. However, to dehumanize the unborn on the basis of size, age, temporary place of residence, and need—all relative things —is to open up a Pandora's Box that could redound badly on the born.

Consider a child in an incubator. He or she is very small, very young, almost out of sight, and highly dependent on others. To kill that child on the basis of its size, age, temporary place of residence, or need would be a great evil. Is their that much difference between the child in the incubator and the child in the incubator of his mother's womb?

There are some who would confuse *"being"* with *"functioning."* If an individual cannot function because he or she is in a coma (a disorder), that individual is still a person. If an individual cannot function because he or she has not fully developed (a child, in or out of the womb), that individual is also a person. *Both are human beings* with the potential to function as a person. In other words, the being in the coma once did function, but does not now, while the born or unborn child does not now function, but in time will. There is not that much difference. The being of each, a continuum, takes precedence over the functioning of each. If we declare as persons (and thus grant to the declaree the protection of the law) only those who can function, we open, to repeat, a Pandora's Box of possibilities. There would be great conflict as to what constituted adequate function, and even greater conflict as to who would set the standards.[36]

History is replete with examples of legal dehumanization and depersonalization: the enslavement of Afro-Americans to help the American economy, the almost-annihilation of Native Americans in the push westward (Manifest Destiny), the low status of women and children throughout most of history because of patriarchy, the victims of the Holocaust due to visions of racial superiority, and abortion of the unborn because of convenience, to name just a few. In all of these cases dehumanizers offered no scientific evidence whatsoever to justify what they were doing. These dehumanized and depersonalized groups, at one time or place or another, were either treated as objects and used, or seen as obstacles and annihilated. Yet today, Western society recognizes the humanity and personhood of all but the last, having withdrawn legal protection during the 1960[s] and 1970[s], after roughly a century of protection (it is ironic to note that the law protected unborn children before born children).

Don Feder, a Jewish syndicated columnist, has had this to say about our subject under discussion: "Jewish abortion advocates cringe at the equation of slaughter of the unborn and the Holocaust. Yet Rabbi Jakobovits [the outgoing Chief Rabbi of the United Kingdom in 1991], himself a refugee from Nazi Germany, declares: 'Jews may be particularly sensitive to any such discrimination (determining which life is worthy of preservation), having witnessed the horror of six million being shoved into the gas chambers because they were deemed inferior [non-human].'"[37]

We must constantly remind ourselves of the Nuremberg Trials, and in the 1947-1948 RuSHA Trial, the prosecutor, in his summation, admitted that Section 218 of the German Empire's Penal Code had been amended by Weimar (1918-1933) and the Nazis (1933-1945), and that these regimes were legal. Nevertheless, the prosecutor still maintained that the Weimar democracy's liberalizing of abortion for women's reproductive liberty, and Hitler's legalizing of abortion for racial reasons, were laws that should not have been passed. He described Nazi use of abortion as "an inhumane act," and ended by saying that even if a woman had an abortion voluntarily, "it constituted a war crime and a crime against *humanity* [emphasis mine]."[38] The Tribunal, in its decision, found that "encouraging," as well as "compelling," abortion constituted war crimes and crimes against humanity.[39] *If the Nuremberg Trials are wrong about this, what else were they wrong about?*

Thirty years after World War II, West Germany legalized abortion on demand for the first trimester of pregnancy. On February 25, 1975, the Federal Constitutional Court of that country (*Bundesverffasungsgericht*) struck the law down as being unconstitutional. In its decision, it said that life was a continuum and that unborn life was to be respected in principle with born life.[40] It stated that "abortion is an act of killing that the law is obligated to condemn," and that the "bitter experience" with Nazism had led the Court to value life highly.[41] The beginning of the decision showed the connection between abortion and Nazism this way:

Article 2 II 1 of the Constitution protects life being developed in the mother's womb as an independent legal entity. The express inclusion of the right to life in the Constitution... in contrast, for example, to the Weimar Constitution, is to be explained primarily as a reaction to the "destruction of life that is not worthy of living," to the "final solution" and to 'liquidations' carried out by the National Socialist [Nazi] regime as governmental measures. Article 2 II 1 of the Constitution contains, in addition to the abolition of the death penalty in Article 102, "a profession of commitment to the fundamental value of human life and to a concept of the state that places it in decisive opposition to the views of a political regime to which an individual life meant little and which for this reason engaged in unlimited abuse of the right it had usurped over the life and death of the citizen."[42]

The German High Court repeated this connection at the very end of its decision:

The basic laws that underlie the state's foundation can be explained only by understanding the historical experience and spiritual-moral explanation of the previous system of National Socialism [Nazism]. Against the omnipotence of the totalitarian state, the boundless power over all aspects of social life claimed for themselves, and with the pursuit of its national goal that the basic life of the individual meant nothing, [Nazism] established as the basic law the principal of order, which subordinated the individual and his dignity to its control. There exists, as the court has already declared... the basic case, that humankind possesses a uniquely independent value of which there is absolute concern for the life of *every single individual* [emphasis mine], which also aids irrevocably the *apparently* social *"valueless"* [emphasis mine], and which, for this reason, excludes exterminating *any life* [emphasis mine] without justified reason. This basic clarification by the court determines the making and interpretation of the entire legal code. Likewise, the lawmaker not in agreement is not free; politically correct considerations of expediency, even state political necessities, could not prevail over these constitutional limits.[43]

In other words, the Nazis had no respect for human life, and to insure human life's protection for the future, we have to respect all human life, including life in the womb. Put yet another way, if, as a society, we do not respect pre-natal life, we will not respect post-natal life, and we will be thinking like the Nazis (those against the death penalty always are stating how capital punishment erodes respect for life, even among the decent). If we say that the German High Court is wrong here, cannot someone also say that the U. S. High Court was wrong with *Roe v. Wade* in 1973? The German High Court's decision, however, must be given much weight, given their awareness of what took place under Nazism in that country.[44]

Is there a connection between abortion and Nazism? The answer is yes. Let us summarize by looking, for the last time, at the arguments of those who say no, arguments that maintain: there is *no genocide*, there is *no human* involved, there should be a *choice*.

(1) The Nazis used abortion as one of the means of their *genocide* during World War II, and this was specifically condemned at the Nuremberg Trials in 1948 when the Nuremberg prosecution described abortion, voluntary or forced, as an "act of extermination" and "ill-treatment of a civilian population." Abortion also fits the definition of the United Nations' definition of genocide, formulated between 1946 and 1948, in reaction to the Nazi experience.

(2) The prosecutor at the RuSHA trial of Nazis at Nuremberg made no distinction between voluntary and forced abortion in declaring abortion a war crime and crime against *humanity*, and the Tribunal stated that encouraging as well as compelling abortion were war crimes and crimes against *humanity*. The German Supreme Court's decision in 1975, in striking down a law legalizing abortion, stated very clearly, that if we do not respect unborn life equally with born life, we will be thinking like Nazis.

(3) Since abortion in general is genocide, and was specifically used as a tool of genocide by the Nazis, and since life in the womb is human, there can be no question about *choice*.

Will concerns about class, race, gender, and sexual orientation have to make room (again) for concerns about age and size in order to preserve respect for life in our society? We will end here with the words of Elie Weisel, a Jewish prisoner of Auschwitz (where he lost his whole family), whose novels, plays, and speeches have kept alive the memory of the Holocaust, and which won him the Nobel Prize in 1986. He has said: "I really have not given the issue [of abortion] enough thought."[45]

NOTES

1. William Brennan, *The Abortion Holocaust: Today's Final Solution* (St. Louis: Landmark Press 1983). A more recent work touching on this subject by the author is *Dehumanizing The Vulnerable: When Word Games Take Lives* (Chicago: Loyola University Press 1995).

2. The Fall meeting of The New England Historical Association, University of Hartford, West Hartford, Connecticut, October 22, 1994. I was on the panel and gave a paper entitled: "A Tale of Two Countries: American and German Attitudes to Abortion Since World War II."

3. Brennan (1983) 3-4.

4. Gloria Steinem, *Outrageous Acts and Everyday Rebellions* (New York: Holt, Rinehart, and Winston 1983) 305.

5. Ibid.

6. Steinem 306.

7. Robert G. Weisbord, "Legalized Abortion and the Holocaust: An Insulting Parallel" in *The Jewish Veteran* (Jan.-Mar. 1982) 12.

8. Ibid.

9. C. Everett Koop, "The Slide to Auschwitz" in *The Human Life Review* 3/2 (Spring 1977) 112.

10. Telephone conversation with Connecticut and national offices of the National Organization of Women, May 3, 1995.

11. Stephen T. Katz, "The Distinctiveness of the Holocaust." Talk given before the 14th Annual Conference on the Holocaust, Millersville University, Millersville, Pennsylvania, April 10, 1995. The speaker was an official of the Holocaust Memorial Museum in Washington, D. C.

12. Telephone conversation with the Anti-Defamation League, New Haven, Connecticut, June 23, 1995. The woman who spoke appeared tense and angry with the question.

13. Telephone conversation with Susan Yolan, Director of Public Affairs and Communications for Planned Parenthood of Connecticut, June 14, 1995.

14. Letter from Susan Yolan, Director of Public Affairs and Communications for Planned Parenthood of Connecticut, to the author, June 23, 1995.

15. Telephone conversation with Cheryl Cohen, Reproductive Freedom Project, American Civil Liberties Union, New York City, June 14, 1995. See also: Letter from Dr. Alan Weston to the author, June 29, 1995. The ACLU directed me to write to Dr. Weston, an ACLU member and one most knowledgeable on the subject.

16. I am recalling this from memory. The article was written in the late 1960⁵ or early 1970⁵. The only place in Connecticut where the *Newsletter* was located was at the University of Connecticut at Storrs, Connecticut. Their collection was very spotty and did not contain the article.

17. Letter from Laurel Tiesinga, MSW, Executive Director of Connecticut NARAL, to the author, May 22, 1995. The position stated in this letter is #45 of 54 points in a point/counterpoint (anti-choice/pro-choice) format, prepared by Polly Rothstein and Marian Williams, Westchester [NY] Coalition for Legal Abortion, and printed, with permission, by the NARAL Foundation, Washington, D. C., 1983. Cited hereafter as NARAL Document.

18. NARAL Document, #46.

19. Steinem (cited in n. 4 above) 305-06.

20. Steinem 307.

21. Steinem 309-310.

22. Steinem 311, 313-314.

23. Steinem's ideas in her 1983 book about authoritarianism, patriarchy, and anti-feminism in the United States and Germany are reflected again later, in shorter form, and with an emphasis on born children, in *Revolution from*

Within: A Book of Self-Esteem (Boston: Little, Brown and Company 1992) 74-77.

24. Ellen Goodman, "Reserve Words About Nazis for the Reich" in *The Hartford Courant* (June 6, 1995) A 9.

25. Ibid.

26. Weisbord 13.

27. Ibid. Weisbord concentrates on the Jews, but an equal number of non-Jews perished in the same death camps.

28. Ibid.

29. Weisbord 12.

30. *Webster's College Dictionary* (New York: Random House 1991) 557.

31. David E. Stannard, *American Holocaust: The Conquest of The New World* (New York: Oxford University Press 1992) 279.

32. Stannard 279-80.

33. Stannard 280.

34. *Trials of War Criminals Before the Nuernberg Military Tribunals, October, 1946 - April, 1949,* Vols. IV-V, "The RuSHA Case" (Washington, D. C.: U. S. Government Printing Office 1949) IV, 609-617. Cited hereafter as *TWC.*

35. *TWC* 685-86. Records of the United States Nuernberg War Crimes Trials, *United States of America v. Ulrich Greifelt, et al.* (Case VIII), October 10, 1947- March 10, 1948 in the National Archives, Washington, D. C., Microfilm Publication 894, Roll 31 (Trial Vols. 12 and 13) pp. 13-14. See also pp. 37-42. Cited hereafter as *NWCT.* The RuSHA (Greifelt) Case covers some 5400 pages of testimony of which about 800 pages have been published in Volumes IV and V of *TWC.*

36. These ideas are more fully developed by Stephen Schwarz, *The Moral Question of Abortion* (Chicago: Loyola Univ. Press 1990) 12-19. In Chapter 7, Schwarz argues forcefully for the personhood of the unborn.

37. Don Feder, "Abortion, Judaism, and Jews" in *National Review* 43/12 (July 8, 1991) 37.

38. *NWCT* M 894, R 31, pp. 13-14. See also pp. 37-42.

39. *TWC* V, 153, 160-161, 166. See also IV, 610, 613.

40. Donald D. Kommers, "Abortion and the Constitution: The Cases of the United States and West Germany" in *Abortion: New Directions For Policy Studies,* eds. Edward Manier, William Liv, and David Solomon (Notre Dame: Univ. of Notre Dame Press 1977) 94-95.

41. Kommers 97-98.

42. Translated by Dr. O. J. Brown in *The Human Life Review* 1/3 (Summer, 1975) 77-78.

43. *Neues Juristisches Wochenblatt*, 1975, XIII, 582. Kommers and Brown, cited in notes 40 to 42 above, do not have this translated. This is my own translation.

44. As late as 1993, the German High Court at Karlsruhe reaffirmed this 1975 decision. In two of its seventeen basic principles it stated: (1) The Basic Law [the German Constitution] mandates the state to protect humankind, including unborn children. This protection has its basis in Article 1, Section 1 of the Basic Law; it is more clearly spelled out in Article 2, Section 2 of the Basic Law. The unborn already have human dignity. The proper approach for the law must be to accept the unique right to life during the unborn's development. This right to life is not established simply by its acceptance by the mother. (4) The abortion must be viewed as being basically wrong for the entire length of the pregnancy and accordingly be forbidden (Confirmation, Federal Constitutional Court, 39, 1 [44] = Basic European Laws, 1975, 126 [140]. The right to life of the unborn should not, if only for a limited time, be in the hands of a third party, even if it be of the mother. See *Europaische Grundrechte Zeitschrift* (June 4, 1993) IX-X, 229.

45. Elie Weisel and John Joseph O'Connor, *A Journey of Faith* (New York: Dr. Fine 1990) 78.

About Our Contributors

J. Bottum is Associate Editor of First Things. A graduate of Georgetown University, he received his doctorate from Boston College in Philosophy.

William Brennan, Ph.D., is a professor in the School of Social Service at St. Louis University. His writings have appeared in such professional and popular periodicals as *Social Work, Crime and Delinquency, Journal of Education for Social Work, Journal of Health and Social Behavior, Liguorian, Social Justice Review, Studies in Prolife Feminism, National Right to Life News, New Oxford Review,* and *The Living World.* Dr. Brennan's most recent book is *Dehumanizing the Vulnerable: When Word Games Take Lives* (Loyola Univ. Press, 1995).

James Carey, Ph.D., teaches in the Graduate School of Journalism at Columbia University in New York.

Keith Cassidy, Ph.D., teaches in the History Department at the University of Guelph, Ontario. His field of interest is modern American social and intellectual history. He is at work on a full-length study of the Right-to-Life Movement.

Rev. John J. Conley, *S.J.* (Ph.D., Louivain) is the Chair of the Philosophy Department at Fordham University, Bronx NY. He has published many articles in ethics and aesthetics.

Marie A. Conn received her Ph.D. in Theology (Liturgical History/Ethics) from the University of Notre Dame. He is Chair of the Religious Studies Department at Chestnut Hill College and has published nearly two dozen articles in such journals as *The New Theology Review* and *Aim.*

John F. Crosby (Ph.D., Univ. of Salzburg, 1970) has tuaght at the University of Dallas, the International Academy of Philosophy (Liechtenstein), and is now professor of philosophy at the Franciscan University of Steubenville.

Rev. Joseph W. Koterski, S.J. (Ph.D., St. Louis Univ.) teaches philosophy at Fordham University, where he is Editor-in-Chief of International Philosophy Quarterly and director of the M.A. Program in Philosophical Resources.

Peter Lubin is Associate Professor at the Southern New England School of Law.

Kevin E. Miller has degrees in molecular biology and political science and is currently pursuing his Ph.D. in Religious Studies at Marquette University. His research interests revolve around philosophical and theological anthropology and ethics in the Aristotelian/Thomistic tradition, especially as these relate to church, politics, and marriage and family. He is writing a dissertation on Pope John Paul II's position on capital punishment.

Mary Nicholas is a physician and a candidate for the M.T.S. degree at the John Paul II Institute of Marriage and Family. She has been active in pro-life activities, including the Preparatory Committees for the International Conferences on Population and Development and the Fourth World Conference on Women. She is founder and executive director of the Stein Research Institute, named after Blessed Edith Stein.

Mary Lee O'Connell, M.S., R.N., F.A.A.C.E., resigned her position as an Assistant Professor at Catholic University of America's School of Nursing to become a student in the Women's Health Nurse Practitioner Program at the University of Maryland at Baltimore. She is a graduate of the Education for Parish Service program at Trinity College, a Natural Family Planning Instructor, and a Childbirth Educator.

Julian Simon is Professor of Business Administration at the University of Maryland and author of The Ultimate Resource II (Princeton: Princeton Univ. Press, revised edition, 1996 [1981]).

Sister M. Stanislaus, O. P., is a member of the Dominican Sisters of St. Mary of the Springs, Columbus, Ohio. She received her M.A. and Ph.D. in philosophy from St. Louis University. She is currently